THE VANDERBILT HEARING AID REPORT II

THE VANDERBILT HEARING AID
REPORT II

Edited by
Gerald A. Studebaker, Fred H. Bess, and **Lucille B. Beck**
In cooperation with the Department of Veterans Affairs

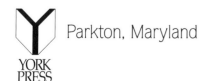 Parkton, Maryland

YORK
PRESS

This book was manufactured in the United States of America. Typography by Brushwood Graphics, Inc., Baltimore, Maryland. Printing and binding by Maple-Vail Book Manufacturing Group, York, Pennsylvania.

Library of Congress Cataloging-in-Publication Data

The Vanderbilt hearing aid report II / edited by Gerald A. Studebaker, Fred H. Bess,
    and Lucille B. Beck, in cooperation with the Department of Veterans Affairs.
        p.   cm.
    Based on a conference held in Nashville, Tenn. 1990.
    Includes bibliographical references and index.
    ISBN 0-912752-26-2
    1. Hearing aids—Fitting—Congresses.   2. Hearing aids—Testing—
Congresses.   3. Signal processing—Congresses.   4. Hearing impaired—
Rehabilitation—Congresses.   I. Studebaker, Gerald A.   II. Bess, Fred H.
III. Beck, Lucille B.   IV. Vanderbilt University.   V. United States. Dept. of
Veterans Affairs.   VI. Title: Vanderbilt hearing aid report 2.
    [DNLM: 1. Acoustics—congresses.   2. Hearing aids—congresses.
3. Hearing Disorders—rehabilitation—congresses.   4. Prescriptions,
Non-Drug—congresses.   5. Signal Processing, Computer-Assisted—
congresses.   WV 274 V228 1990]
RF300.V36   1991
617.8′9—dc20
DNLM/DLC
for Library of Congress   91-4894
                                                                          CIP

Contents

Foreword

The Department of Veterans Affairs (VA) is pleased to have co-sponsored the Vanderbilt/VA Second Conference on Amplification and to participate in bringing you the proceedings of the 1990 conference. Myriad issues continue to surround the clinical and rehabilitative management of hearing-impaired persons. Advances in hearing aid technology have progressed rapidly during the past decade along with major changes in clinical instrumentation techniques, assessment and fitting procedures, and rehabilitative strategies. In reflecting on these activities and their affects on the delivery of services to veterans, the 1982 Vanderbilt/VA Hearing Aid Conference served as a reminder of the significant educational activity needed in this rapidly changing field.

In 1989, Dr. Fred Bess invited VA to join in convening a similar conference to assess our progress and future needs. With our common interests in hearing impairment and a long standing commitment to optimum technology-based services, we were excited with the prospect of convening experts in research and clinical practice to help us chart the course for the 1990s. We were supported with guidance and funds from VA's Rehabilitation Research and Development Service, and the Rehabilitation Education Program of VA's Academic Affairs. Our collaboration was launched with involvement of a planning group comprising scholars and clinicians highly regarded for their expertise with hearing aids.

The conference that emerged was designed to link research and clinical practice, clarifying opportunities for technology transfer that have practical and desirable benefits for users of amplification. Other objectives were to develop recommended hearing aid evaluation procedures for adults and a research agenda for amplification needs in the 1990s. Experts from among the faculty remained after the conference to develop these latter objectives. They are contained in these proceedings for your consideration and use. We are indebted to these individuals for their important contributions.

Appreciation is extended to Vanderbilt University, the planning group, faculty, conference participants, and editors of the proceedings for an initiative that will serve to guide us in years to come.

Allen E. Boysen, Ph.D.

Preface

In 1981, Vanderbilt University and the Bill Wilkerson Center sponsored a major conference, Amplification for the Hearing-Impaired: Research Needs. The conference was supported in part by the Department of Veterans Affairs. The proceedings of this meeting, *The Vanderbilt Hearing Aid Report*, was well-received by professionals throughout this country and abroad and served as a fundamental resource on amplification for almost a decade.

Since 1981, however, considerable change has taken place in both hearing aid technology and the procedures used to select and evaluate amplification systems for the hearing impaired. Alternative approaches to rehabilitation also have occurred. Hence, the Department of Veterans Affairs, Vanderbilt University, and the Bill Wilkerson Center once again pooled their resources to develop a sequel meeting on amplification for the hearing impaired. A special group of recognized authorities on amplification was assembled to develop an innovative and relevant program. The general intent of the conference was to discuss and debate current issues on clinical and research aspects of hearing aids. The format was primarily tutorial with state-of-the-art presentations followed by discussions. In addition, informal workshops were held each evening to foster maximum participant involvement.

Following the meeting, two task forces were assembled to develop consensus statements on the recommended components of a hearing aid selection procedure for adults and the research needs in amplification. The documents developed by these working groups appear in the Appendices to this book.

Similar to the first meeting, the Second Vanderbilt/VA Conference was judged to be an outstanding success. The quality of papers delivered at the conference as well as the discussions were high in content value. It is our sincere hope that this volume will serve to benefit practitioners who are involved with amplification and the hearing impaired, to promote future research, and to highlight the special amplification needs of the hearing-impaired population.

Numerous individuals contributed to the success of the meeting and this book. We are grateful to Vanderbilt and the Bill Wilkerson Center who assisted with various phases of the meeting. Especially helpful were Dorothy Adams, David Chandler, Jeanne Dodd, Kathy Hollis, Susan Logan, and Andrea Williams. We also are grateful to Allen E. Boysen and Manny Suter who recognized the need for an update on amplification for the hearing impaired and utilized their resources to bring the meeting to fruition.

Gerald A. Studebaker, Fred H. Bess,
and Lucille B. Beck, Editors

Contributors

Lucille B. Beck, Ph.D.
Department of Veterans Affairs
Veterans Administration
Medical Center
50 Irving Street
Washington DC 20422

Ruth A. Bentler, Ph.D.
Wendell Johnson Speech and
Hearing Center
University of Iowa
Iowa City IA 52242

Fred H. Bess, Ph.D.
Vanderbilt University School of
Medicine
1114 19th Avenue South
Nashville TN 37212

Carl A. Binnie, Ph.D.
Audiology and Speech Sciences
Purdue University
Heavilon Hall B-13
West Lafayette IN 47907

Allen E. Boysen, Ph.D.
Audiology and Speech
Pathology
Veterans Administration
Medical Center
Washington DC 20422

Gene W. Bratt, Ph.D.
Audiology and Speech
Pathology Services
Veterans Administration
Medical Center
1310 24th Avenue South
Nashville TN 37212

Edwin D. Burnett
National Institute of Standards
and Technology
Room A-149, Building 233
Gaithersburg MD 20899

Denis Byrne
National Acoustic Laboratories
126 Greville Street
Chatswood New South Wales
2067
AUSTRALIA

Cynthia Compton, M.S.
Director, Assistive Devices
Center
Gallaudet University
800 Florida Avenue, NE
Washington DC 20002

Robyn M. Cox, Ph.D.
Memphis State University
Speech and Hearing Center
807 Jefferson Avenue
Memphis TN 38105

David A. Fabry, Ph.D.
L-5 Audiology
Mayo Clinic
Rochester MN 55901

Thomas H. Fay, Ph.D.
Director
Speech and Hearing
Department
Columbia-Presbyterian Medical
Center
622 West 168th Street
New York NY 10032

Sandra Gordon-Salant, Ph.D.
Department of Hearing and
Speech Sciences
University of Maryland
College Park MD 20742

David B. Hawkins, Ph.D.
Department of Communicative
Disorders
University of South Carolina
Columbia SC 29208

Larry E. Humes, Ph.D.
Department of Speech and
Hearing Sciences
Indiana University
Bloomington IN 47405

Jim Kates, Ph.D.
Center for Research in the
Speech and Hearing Sciences
City University of New York
33 West 42nd Street
New York NY 10036

Vernon D. Larson, Ph.D.
Audiology and Speech
Pathology
Veterans Administration
Medical Center
2460 Wrightsboro Road
Augusta GA 30910

Harry Levitt, Ph.D.
City University of New York
Graduate School
Speech and Hearing Sciences
33 West 42nd Street
New York NY 10036

Patricia A. McCarthy, Ph.D.
The University of Georgia
College of Education
Communication Sciences and
Disorders
565 Aderhold Hall
Athens GA 30602

Allen A. Montgomery, Ph.D.
Department of Communicative
Disorders
University of South Carolina
Columbia SC 29208

H. Gustav Mueller, Ph.D.
Division of Audiology
Presidio of San Francisco
Letterman Army Medical Center
San Francisco CA 94129

Wayne Olsen, Ph.D.
Department of Otolaryngology
Mayo Clinic
Rochester MN 55901

David A. Preves, Ph.D.
Vice President of Research and
Development
Argosy Electronics
10300 West 70th Street
Eden Prairie MN 55344

Patricia G. Stelmachowicz, Ph.D.
Audiological Services
Boys Town Institute
555 North 30th Street
Omaha NE 68131

Gerald A. Studebaker, Ph.D.
Memphis State University
807 Jefferson
Memphis TN 38105

Jean Sullivan, M.A.
House Ear Institute
2100 West Third Street
Los Angeles CA 90057

Barbara Weinstein, Ph.D.
10 West 15th Street #9n
New York NY 10011

List of Acronyms

AARP, American Association of Retired Persons
AC, air conduction
ADA, Americans with Disabilities Act
AFR, adaptive frequency response
AGC, automatic gain control
AI, Articulation Index
ALD, assistive listening device
ALDS, assistive listening devices and systems
A/M, acoustic-to-magnetic [adapters]
AMP, amplified auditory only
AMP + VIS, amplified audio plus speechreading
ANOVA, analysis of variance
ANR, automatic noise reduction
ANSI, American National Standards Institute
A/PILL, automatic programmable increases at low levels
ASP, adaptive signal processing *and* automatic signal processing
ASR, automatic speech recognition
ATE, at the ear
AV-AI, auditory-visual articulation index
AVC, automatic volume control
AVI, audiovisual integration
BAHA, bone anchored hearing aid
BC, bone conduction
BILL, bass increases at low levels
BN, background noise
CANS, central auditory nervous system
CAPD, central auditory processing disorder
CCITT, International Telegraph and Telephone Consultive Committee
CCT, California Consonant Test
CPHI, Communication Profile for the Hearing Impaired
CST, Connected Speech Test
CV, consonant-vowel
CVR, consonant-vowel ratio
DAI, direct audio input
DMHA, digital master hearing aid
DSI, Dichotic Sentence Identification test
EM, environmental microphone
FDA, Food and Drug Administration
FFR, fixed frequency response
FG, frequency gain
FM, frequency modulation
FSPHAU, Feasibility Scale for Predicting Hearing Aid Use

HAPI, Hearing Aid Performance Inventory
HCO, high cutoff response
HFA, High-Frequency average
HHIE, Hearing Handicap Inventory for the Elderly
HHIE–S, Hearing Handicap Inventory for the Elderly–Screening Form
HHS, Hearing Handicap Scale
HI, hearing impaired
HPF, high pass filter
HPI, Hearing Performance Inventory
HTL, hearing threshold level
IJ, intelligibility judgment
IM, intermodulation [distortion]
IRIS, Intelligibility Rating Improvement Scale
IROS, ipsilateral routing of signal
ITC, in the canal
ITE, in the ear
KEMAR, Knowles Electronic Manikin for Acoustic Research
LCO, low cutoff response
LDFR, level-dependent changes in frequency response
LDL, loudness discomfort level
MAC, Minimal Auditory Capabilities [test]
MCL, most comfortable level
MCO, mid-cutoff response
MCR, message-to-competition ratio
MLD, masking level difference
MPO, Maximum power output
NAL, National Acoustics Laboratories'
NAS, Nobelpharma Auditory System
NIST, National Institute of Standards and Technology
NST, nonsense syllable test
OUT, Organization for the Use of the Telephone
PAS, personal amplification system
PB, phonetically balanced
PG, prescribed gain
PHAB, Profile of Hearing Aid Benefit
PHAP, Profile of Hearing Aid Performance
PI, performance intensity
PILL, programmable increases at low level
P-MEI, partially implantable middle ear implant
PMR, programmable multifrequency response
POGO, prescription of gain output
PTA, Pure-tone average

PTM, probe-tube microphone measurement
REAR, real ear aided response
REIG, real ear insertion gain
REIR, real ear insertion response
RESR, real ear saturation response
REUR, real ear unaided response
RMS, root mean square
R-SPIN, Revised Speech Perception in Noise Test
RST, repeated sentence task
SBCA (PC), standard bone conduction hearing aid
  (percutaneous)
SBCA (TC), standard bone conduction hearing aid
  (transcutaneous)
SHHH, Self Help for Hard of Hearing People
SIGFR, simulated insertion gain frequency
  response

SL, sensation level
S/N, signal to noise ratio
SPIN, Speech-in-Noise test
SPL, sound pressure level
SRT, speech reception threshold
SSI, synthetic sentence inventory
SSP, speech signal processing
SSPL, saturation sound pressure level
SSW, Staggered Spondaic Word test
TDD, telecommunication device for the deaf
TILL, treble increases at low levels
U/Pill, user-adjustable programmable increases at
  low levels
VA, Department of Veterans Affairs
VLSI, very large integrated [circuits]
WAI, weighted audibility index

Steering Committee

Lucille B. Beck, Ph.D.
Veterans Administration Medical Center
Washington, DC

Fred H. Bess, Ph.D., Chair
Vanderbilt University School of Medicine

Allen E. Boysen, Ph.D.
Department of Veterans Affairs
Washington, DC

Gene W. Bratt, Ph.D.
Veterans Administration Medical Center
Nashville, TN
and Vanderbilt University School of Medicine

David B. Hawkins, Ph.D.
University of South Carolina

Vernon D. Larson, Ph.D.
Veterans Administration Medical Center
Augusta, GA

Harry Levitt, Ph.D.
City University of New York Graduate School

Gerald A. Studebaker, Ph.D.
Memphis State University

Emanuel Suter, M.D.
Department of Veterans Affairs
Washington, DC

CHAPTER 1

Amplification Needs
Where Do We Go From Here?

Lucille B. Beck

During the past decade the profession of audiology has seen a dramatic change in the provision of hearing health care. The communication problems of hearing-impaired persons can now be addressed much more effectively due to the technological advances in personal hearing aids. Improved component parts, such as electret microphones, integrated circuit amplifiers, and broadband receivers along with improved chassis design and better coupling techniques have resulted in hearing aids that are smaller and more versatile, of an improved ergonomic design, and of higher quality than earlier models.

For the audiologist today, hearing aid selection considerations include a wide array of choices for electroacoustic characteristics and special circuit features, all within the context of style, size, cost, and personal preference of the user. A vast array of assistive listening devices (ALDs) have also been developed for communication situations where personal hearing aids are of limited value, such as listening at some distance from the primary source and/or environmental conditions of background noise and reverberation. Alternate technologies to audition, such as speech to text and visual or vibratory alerting systems, offer choices for alleviating communication difficultes, as well. These advances in technology suggest that the future is bright for the hearing-impaired consumer and for the practitioner dedicated to meeting those needs.

The Department of Veterans Affairs (VA), in recognition of the significant limitations imposed by hearing handicap on the quality of life, provides a full complement of clinical and rehabilitative services to hearing-impaired veterans. Mindful of the ever pressing need for improvements in technology and clinical techniques, the VA has made research efforts in hearing a priority. The second Vanderbilt/VA conference provides a special opportunity to focus on the past while planning for the future. The first Vanderbilt conference (Studebaker and Bess 1982) on hearing aids, which was organized as a

state of the art research conference, is the foundation for the second. Nine years later, we come together again to assess our progress in the research effort, highlight research needs, expedite the transfer of the knowledge base to service delivery, and move toward the development of clinical protocols for the acoustic rehabilitative management of hearing loss. It is a time for critical self-appraisal of both the research efforts and the clinical services for hearing aid selection, evaluation, and fitting. It is a time to ask ourselves whether the research effort provides a basis for resolving the dilemmas regarding amplification needs. It is especially a time to ask whether clinical audiology can take a stand regarding methodological issues for hearing aid evaluation. Has the profession of audiology developed a knowledge base that now guides the contemporary art of hearing aid selection? Is there a science of hearing aid selection that skilled clinical practitioners will use with patients in the selection of hearing aids? This question of art versus science is one that all health care professions debate when the research and the clinical communities labor to generalize the results from mean data on groups of subjects to the needs of an individual patient.

It would seem that the proper future direction for determining research needs, clinical requirements, and effective rehabilitation solutions only can be determined through the combined efforts of the research scientist, the clinical practitioner, and the hearing-impaired consumer, each with a distinct role to play. The research scientist seeks the answer to relevant questions through the use of research methodologies. The clinical audiologist practices the contemporary art of hearing aid selection for remediation of the communication difficulties of a particular patient. Both are grounded in science. We have come to understand that an appropriate technique or goal for the research laboratory may not be equally effective for the hearing aid selection process. Strategies for the selection, evaluation, and fitting of hearing aids must be developed through separate endeavors rather than the adaptation of laboratory research techniques and/or diagnostic measurement methods.

Where we go from here will in large part be determined by the degree to which we are able to manage the communicative needs of the hearing-impaired person. Hearing aids, unlike some other sensory devices, most notably eyeglasses, cannot yet fully restore auditory function, and hearing-impaired consumers consistently report that they develop another set of needs when they first wear hearing aids. The ability of the person to use compensatory strategies, a task that the audiologist must include in the rehabilitation package, seems to be the real key to success. Long-term communicative efficiency requires the assistance of a rehabilitative program tailored to individual communicative needs concurrent with, and subsequent to, the fitting of the hearing aid.

In considering the critical issues regarding the research effort and the service delivery need, it is enlightening to view hearing loss from the perspective of consumers—not just hearing-impaired consumers but the general public as well. In 1977, the Food and Drug Administration (FDA), by legislative action, began regulating hearing aid products by requiring a quality control type electroacoustic performance standard and protecting consumers by requiring medical clearance prior to hearing aid use. Clearly, such action identified hearing aids as medical devices related to general health. The profession of audiology, at that time, had come only recently to the issue of service delivery for hearing aids and was not prepared to assume a leadership role in the hearing aid delivery system.

Since that landmark legislation, a number of significant consumer-driven activities have sent a strong message to professionals regarding amplification needs. Self Help for Hard of Hearing People (SHHH) is an eleven-year-old self-help organization dedicated to people with hearing loss who wish to remain a part of the hearing world. The organization has 35,000 members and its founder, Rocky Stone, has made hearing loss an issue of national concern. SHHH has self-help chapters all over the country, its members serve on state committees on the handicapped, and the group has influenced legislation at the federal and state levels. This organization has been critical of hearing aids and the present service delivery system.

In 1982 and again in 1988, Congress passed laws related to telephone use and hearing aid compatibility through induction coupling by means of the telecoil in the hearing aid. Initially, public phones were required to be hearing aid compatible and subsequently all phones were required to have induction-coupling capability. This was quite an accomplishment, considering that the majority of hearing aids sold in this country do not have telecoils. A consumer group known as OUT (Organization for the Use of the Telephone) led that lobbying effort. It should be clear that hearing-impaired consumers view the ability to communicate by telephone to be essential. What should be obvious as well is that consumers can be very effective at achieving federal legislative oversight for communicative purposes.

The passage of the Americans with Disabilities Act (ADA) of 1990, hailed as the most significant civil rights legislation since the 1960s, guarantees Americans with hearing loss, whether that hearing loss is mild or profound, the right to reasonable access in employment, public accommodations, and telecommunications. The implications are far-reaching and the requirements for regulations are already being developed. A prominent hearing-impaired consumer is a member of this preregulatory activity. It should be clear that the effectiveness of personal hearing aids will be carefully scrutinized. Think about the irony of having federal legislation requiring induction-coupling capability for all telephones while few hearing aids have telecoils and, for those that do, useful technical specification on the telecoil performance is limited.

Remediation for hearing loss has emerged as a primary interest of a powerful consumer organization, the American Association of Retired Persons (AARP). Incidence of hearing loss is around 30% for the elderly (Gates et al. 1990), a group that will comprise a large percentage of the population by the year 2000. A consumer report about hearing aids, published in 1989 by the AARP, entitled *How to Buy a Hearing Aid*, addresses all aspects of the hearing aid delivery system including the quality of the device, an appropriate evaluation and fitting procedure, qualifications of the professional, the ensuing adjustment period, and the cost of the device. The complexity of the problem of buying a hearing aid is handled remarkably well, but this brochure points up the chaotic state of affairs in the delivery system. The audiology profession cannot move forward without addressing these issues. Senior citizens are a vital part of our society. At present, unremediated hearing loss is causing many to withdraw socially and to retire early from their employment. Clearly, hearing aid effectiveness is a major issue for consumers.

The VA, in response to the needs of hearing-impaired veterans, established an audiology program for diagnostic hearing services in the 1950s. Shortly thereafter, it became necessary to develop a National Hearing Aid Program for provision of auditory rehabilitative devices including hearing aids, assistive devices, batteries, and repairs. Presently, comprehensive auditory rehabilitative services are concentrated in a network of approximately 80 medical centers located throughout the country.

In 1989 the VA provided 62,000 hearing aids to veterans. Presently, 200,000 veterans are receiving services including hearing aids, batteries, assistive devices, and repairs. Because the vast majority of veterans who receive hearing aids from the VA must have incurred a hearing loss as a result of military service to receive these services, only a small portion of the nation's 26,000,000 veterans are eligible. Nevertheless, the VA is the largest single purchaser of hearing aids in the United States.

The VA hearing aid program and its attendant professional services have been studied by many groups, including congressional committees and consumer advocates, always receiving favorable reviews because the program ensures that high quality hearing aids are provided as part of a comprehensive professional rehabilitative service. To accomplish the goal of selecting high quality hearing aids, the VA developed, under the direction of Edwin Burnett at the National Institute of Standards and Technology (NIST), a comprehensive set of electroacoustic procedures designed to predict performance on the user and determine the effectiveness of hearing-aid circuitry. The NIST has used simulated in situ measures to characterize hearing aid performance since 1976.

Hearing aid models and custom in-the-ear (ITE) hearing aid manufacturers are selected on the basis of these electroacoustic results and other factors such as usage rate, clinical acceptability, and projected needs. The VA's program has a strong electroacoustic foundation to assure selection of hearing aid models with superior technical performance. It is not meant to be an indication of the "best" hearing aid since that decision is based on individual needs including assessment of hearing impairment and resulting communication difficulty, a determination that is made during audiological clinical service delivery to the veteran. This electroacoustic foundation, when combined with professional audiology services, results in good hearing health care. The important feature then becomes the professional services, that is, the selection of electroacoustic characteristics, the evaluation of the hearing aid, the dispensing of the instrument, and the appropriate follow-up care.

Because a consensus of scientific findings and professional opinion regarding the hearing aid evaluation was not available, the VA has subscribed to the philosophy that the veteran receive an evaluation and trial with the actual hearing aid to be dispensed, the nature of that trial to be determined by the audiologist. In short, the VA has had a program of professional audiological dispensing for well over three decades.

Today (1991) the VA has specific research needs in amplification as well as clinical requirements for a set of protocols that will identify the essential elements of a hearing-aid-selection process to ensure that the prospective user will not only receive the most appropriate compensatory technological features in a hearing aid but also will be able to make the best use of a hearing aid for everyday living requirements.

Electroacoustic Measures

At the first Vanderbilt conference, there was discussion regarding the need to develop and refine measurement procedures for hearing aids. Significant progress in electroacoustic specification of technical performance has resulted in techniques that describe the operational performance of circuitry. Directional microphone hearing aid performance can be specified by the use of a directivity index. Compression hearing aids and other adaptive frequency response circuits are measured using a broadband input signal varied in level. The NIST has developed a method for simultaneous presentation of real speech and noise to evaluate noise reduction in hearing aids (Handbook of Hearing Aid Measurement 1989). Work is underway by Kates (1990) to complete development of a sophisticated computer procedure that will evaluate and specify the parameters of even the most complicated hearing aid. Coherence measures as well as other sophisticated approaches to specify distortion characteristics of hearing aids are currently being studied. The continuing development of computer control over dynamic input signals, along with better averaging techniques, suggests that improved methods for operational specification of electroacoustic characteristics will continue.

Significant progress has been made, as well, with regard to coupling techniques. The absolute inappropriateness of the 2-cm³ coupler as a fitting tool that relates to performance on the real ear has been documented. A manikin with attendant ear-like coupler has been developed and a standard for measurement procedure exists to enable simulated real-ear measures. Both linear and nonlinear performance of circuitry can be assessed under simulated real-ear conditions. Perhaps most significant has been the development of clinical instrumentation, probe-tube real-ear systems, that permit direct assessment of these technical characteristics on the user. It is no longer necessary to assume that a particular set of electroacoustic characteristics such as gain, frequency response, and saturation sound pressure level (SSPL), is present in the user's ear. Performance characteristics that had only been available from elaborate research laboratory settings can now be measured reasonably well on users in clinical settings. There has been a consistent evolution of measurement procedures progressing from the 2-cm^3 coupler to the Zwislocki coupler to Knowles Electronic Manikin for Acoustic Reseach (KEMAR) to the hearing aid user directly, resulting in a level of realism that cannot be duplicated by any laboratory coupler measure. The research literature has delineated measurement variables and the specification of methods for reliable and accurate real-ear measures. The dilemma that arises when one uses in situ measures is that the only available technical specifications for hearing aids continue to be provided using the 2-cm^3 coupler. This situation is analogous to speaking in two different languages. As a result, many have developed correction factors to translate from in situ to 2-cm^3 coupler data or vice versa (Killion and Monser 1980; Burnett and Beck 1987). While this correction factor approach is a practical solution to an existing problem, it will always be limited because correction factors can only provide a first-order approximation to real-ear performance. They cannot account for the vent that affects not only the low frequency portion of the response but also the high frequency portion, notably the peaks (Kates 1988). In addition, correction factors use data from a median real-ear unoccluded response and many authors have pointed out that individual characteristics can differ markedly from median data (Shaw 1974; Schum 1986). One of the things badly needed is the routine specification of technical performance in a way that approximates performance as measured on the user. Clinical practitioners should expect to see technical performance specifications under in situ conditions, such that the remaining variable will be the difference between the individual's real-ear data and the median (KEMAR) data. The fact that the

2-cm^3 coupler is an FDA required quality control standard, adopted when stock hearing aid models were widely used, should not preclude implementation of more suitable techniques. Dedicated research efforts have produced superior methods for determining hearing aid performance. Please think about how this explosion of technical information can best be used by practitioners for fitting hearing aids. Are we limited to 2-cm^3 coupler information to which correction factors are applied? Is that the most useful approach? Plans for the future should include delineation of appropriate technical specifications for fitting purposes and a plan to ensure that those data are available to audiologists. Research in this area should focus on ways to relate the measures associated with qualitative factors such as distortion and noise to performance on the user.

New Technology

Technology is an amazing thing and it has come to have special meaning in our society. Our lives are governed by technology and we have come to expect technological solutions to all of our problems. The computer does everything for us and instant access to events around the world is routine. The general public expects a technological solution to hearing loss. An example of a technological breakthrough in the hearing care field is the cochlear implant. That device has significantly benefitted a segment of the hearing-impaired population that was beyond the help of conventional amplification. On the opposite side, many of us have experienced a media blitz about a technological breakthrough regarding a hearing aid that raised the expectation of consumers, only to have their hopes dashed. Many of the consumers that I know are waiting for the "digital" hearing aid because they have been led to believe that this new technology will be the solution for their problems.

Appropriate use of new technology will be expedited if clinical practitioners have answers to some important questions. What does this technology do? Who is a candidate for this technology and how should it be evaluated on the potential user? What is the expectation for communication change in the individual's personal life? Let me suggest that we should expect to see a theoretical basis for the technological approach, followed by performance specifications, including electroacoustic and behavioral data. A set of clinical trials with an established protocol should be conducted that can provide performance data, candidacy, and indications for use. A set of field trials should be undertaken as well, particularly with the final product, to assure that it is reliable and durable.

The general approach to date has been to commercialize the product and let the marketplace decide. If it sells, then it is good. New technology is introduced and the practitioner is in the position of conducting clinical trials to determine the usefulness of the technology. Sometimes a hearing-impaired consumer pays a significant amount to participate unknowingly in a clinical trial, and his or her expectations for performance are not met. In some cases, perfectly good technology is abandoned for the wrong reasons. Think of the havoc that would ensue if drug manufacturers could introduce a new product to the market without efficacy data and professionals were expected to try it as part of their clinical service delivery and thereby find out how well it works. In many cases that is what the audiologist is required to do. Although I am not advocating the same stringent requirements for hearing aids as are necessary for drugs, reasonable documentation of performance should be mandatory.

The advent of digitally controlled, programmable hearing aids and fitting systems has made the need for data and documented technical performance even more apparent. Is the ability to program a circuit for a specific set of electroacoustics a desirable and necessary feature worthy of the additional costs, or have these programmable units simply replaced jeweler's screwdrivers and potentiometers? Until there are assessment and review protocols with attendant data for new technological approaches to hearing loss, benefit will continue to be described by anecdotal reports and marketing/advertising plans that have little staying power or long-term feasibility in hearing health care.

Psychoacoustic Test Battery

An area identified as being an urgent research need in psychoacoustics at the first Vanderbilt conference was the development of a psychoacoustic profile for the hearing-impaired population. The need for a test battery that can describe auditory capability in the spectral and temporal domain, including the effect of rapid changes in intensity level, would be most helpful. The continued development of tests that reflect the nature of auditory distortion and the residual integrity of the auditory nervous system,

particularly with regard to suprathreshold complex signals such as speech, is needed. This prognostic test battery is essential if there is to be a response to a comment that Killion (1982) made at the first Vanderbilt conference when he summed up technological advances by stating that the question would no longer be what *can* a hearing aid be designed to do but rather what *should* a hearing aid be designed to do.

Further study of psychoacoustic paradigms is still a major research need in order to characterize the impaired ear and develop a prognostic test battery to evaluate the processing capacity of the ear under conditions of hearing-aid use. A psychoacoustic profile might help us to categorize auditory problems and explain why individuals with similar pure tone audiograms and discrimination ability can respond so dissimilarly to amplification. Ultimately, these alterations in performance characteristics of the impaired ear must be related to signal processing capabilities in hearing aid design.

The search for underlying factors that can account for results and can be used to plan auditory rehabilitative strategies is a paramount consideration to answer the question of what a hearing aid should be designed to do. It is conceivable that a set of electroacoustic characteristics could be individually planned to compensate for such things as poor frequency resolving power, spread of masking and temporal masking effects, restricted dynamic ranges, and growth of loudness considerations. It appears that signal processing technology will provide such capability.

Clearly, there must be a set of psychoacoustic studies on impaired ears to provide a mandate for the subsequent design of hearing aids. Until this causal relationship regarding the nature of hearing impairment and its ultimate effect on perception is determined, efforts to utilize fully the developing technology will remain elusive.

Programmable hearing aids deserve additional reference at this juncture because these devices, which permit the programming of a set of characteristics into a hearing aid for a potential user, beg the question of how hearing aids should be designed to function for the user. Such programmable devices require an a priori determination of a set of characteristics unique to a patient. This scenario is vastly different from the one in practice today whereby the ITE manufacturer determines electroacoustic characteristics from an audiogram. A survey conducted in 1988 (Hedges 1989) indicated that over 80% of the custom ITE orders consisted of audiograms sent to the manufacturer. For many clinical practitioners, the philosophy of hearing aid selection will have to change dramatically to incorporate a sense of responsibility for determining electroacoustic characteristics rather than an evaluation of characteristics that some other person has deemed to be appropriate based on an audiogram.

At present, hearing aid technology has developed more rapidly than the ability to evaluate its benefits. If these technological advances are to become part of the rehabilitative armamentarium, it will be essential for technical researchers and skilled clinical practitioners to develop the methodology necessary for determination of appropriate characteristics based on an in depth study of prognostic indicators of auditory deficit.

Low Frequency Response: Quality and Masking Effects

Perhaps a good example of a continuing dilemma regarding the application of technology to auditory deficit can be illustrated by considering the current state of the art for providing low frequency amplification. Danaher and Pickett (1975) published what became a benchmark article in which low frequencies were shown to be effective maskers of high frequencies and hearing-impaired persons were found to suffer from upward spread of masking. As a result, some professionals advocated limited or no amplification of the low frequencies.

A number of multifactor analysis studies relating hearing aid characteristics to ratings of quality reported that low-frequency response was the salient factor for quality judgment; that is, listeners prefer hearing aids with more low-frequency response (Punch 1978; Punch et al. 1980). Other studies reported that moderate amounts of low-frequency response enhanced quality without degrading speech intelligibility (Punch and Beck 1986). And still others reported that this preference for low-frequency response was present for comfort level settings but was not maintained at higher input levels. The now so-called upward spread of masking phenomenon was frequently cited as an explanation for deleterious results, although subjects reported that the response with more low frequency was simply too loud at high input levels and as a result, annoying, in contrast to the pleasantness reported at comfort level settings (Tecca and Goldstein 1984). Does the presence of low frequencies result in an upward spread of masking effect at high input levels or is it simply a perception of excessive loudness that is annoying? Low frequencies were

implicated as well because much of the spectral content of noise is heavily weighted with low frequencies. Many prescription fitting formulae advocate some restriction of the amount of low-frequency amplification for this reason.

Adaptive Frequency Response Circuits

In the mid 1980s, while many studies were in progress, a technological breakthrough occurred whereby special circuits became available that purported to reduce or eliminate background noise. Appropriate electroacoustic analysis has shown that effective noise reduction was achieved by reducing the amount of low-frequency amplification with increasing input levels. Results from clinical trials as well as anecdotal reports have been equivocal. Clearly, the benefits of this type of circuit were overstated; but the research literature, leaving so many unanswered questions regarding low frequencies and upward spread of masking problems, does not provide a foundation for candidacy determination, indications for use, expected benefit, and appropriate clinical evaluation methods. These circuits, while no longer generating the wholesale enthusiasm among clinical practitioners or consumers they once did, seem to help some of the people some of the time under the right set of conditions. It is difficult to determine for whom and when these conditions will occur. As a consequence, clinicians are often advised to fit the adaptive frequency response circuits because they certainly can't hurt and they might help. Some recent attempts to characterize the upward spread of masking phenomenon in an impaired ear as a precursor to an evaluation of the effectiveness of this noise reduction technology provide an example of the approach that is needed to determine technical suitability on an individual basis (Crain, Van Tasell, and Fabry 1990).

Professional hearing care in the 1990s will require accountability regarding the effectiveness of an expensive device like a hearing aid. A special research need underlying clinical service delivery will be the development of methods to assess the performance characteristics of circuitry that purports to achieve a certain goal. In the area of adaptive frequency response or noise reduction circuitry it is probable that clinicians will be able to determine the nature of spectral response change. Without guidance from an organized and systematic research effort, the likelihood of resolving these issues is small.

The lack of effectiveness of hearing aids in

background noise continues to be the major negative factor associated with hearing aid use. While it now seems naïve to have expected some simple adjustment in the spectral input to one microphone to provide the solution, experience with these approaches has taught us that there are ways to control some deleterious effects. The unpredictable acoustic environment with its varying input level and reverberant conditions is a major limiting factor as well. Signal processing techniques should compensate for the acoustic environment in general as well as the speech signal in particular. Hearing aid users want to hear both the soft and the loud speech at a comfortable listening level without continually adjusting volume controls. While compression generally is recognized as an effective way to control the distortion and the saturation sound pressure level of a hearing aid, sophisticated uses of compression techniques deserve further study. Engineering solutions, such as multiple microphone arrays, perhaps in conjunction with wireless technologies, should be evaluated. Improvement in conventional fitting methods as well as the application of new techniques should remain of paramount importance.

Two significant events occurred during the 1980s that hastened changes in the selection and evaluation of hearing aids. The ITE hearing aid became the most widely used type of fitting, responsible for 80% of the sales in the United States. Custom fitting of the aid, either by manufacturers or by audiologists, was by a prescribed set of characteristics. This accelerated the renewed interest in the use of prescription fitting approaches. At about the same time, the use of probe-tube instrumentation permitted direct verification of these electroacoustic characteristics of the hearing aid on the user. Data about hearing-aid performance, heretofore available only on couplers, could now be measured on the ear.

Hearing Aid Selection and Evaluation

At the first Vanderbilt conference, Studebaker (1982), in his overview on hearing aid selection and evaluation methods, commented that the situation was much like a political revolution with the old methods being down and out and many new approaches competing for recognition. The speech-recognition-based comparative hearing aid evaluation approach advocated by Carhart (1946) came under indictment because it did not differentiate among hearing aids during the clinical trial, and

it did not predict successful hearing-aid use in an individual's real world communicative environment. As an alternate to the empirically determined speech-discrimination-based approach, a number of investigators advocated the use of procedures that specified amplification characteristics appropriate to compensate for individual hearing-loss characteristics, in short, a rationale for selection of electroacoustic characteristics based on some measure(s) of the auditory abilities of a prospective user (Skinner et al. 1982; McCandless and Lyregaard 1983; Byrne and Dillon 1986). Byrne (1982) judiciously pointed out that such a procedure should have a theoretical basis and should be accompanied by an empirical evaluation. Many such prescription fitting formulae have been developed without the emergence of a universally accepted single method. Use of any of these approaches should be preceded by careful study of its theoretical rationale to judge whether it will achieve the amplification goal desired for the potential user. The most meaningful result of all of these efforts has been the emphasis on the issue of audibility. Placement of the conversational level long-term speech signal in the audible range for the user has become a fitting goal. Such an approach has high face validity because this spectrum audibility method has been shown to relate to intelligibility of the speech signal (Levitt 1982).

A body of literature has developed over the last decade emphasizing the importance of loudness discomfort level and its relation to maximum power considerations. Disregard for the tolerance issues of a user will almost certainly preclude successful use of amplification, particularly outside of that quiet sound room where the fitting takes place.

In summary, prescription fitting formulae have provided a method of determination of electroacoustic characteristics. They pertain to the audibility of conversational level speech in large part, and provide a first order approximation of the linear frequency response. Sullivan et al. (1988), in a comparison of four prescription fitting formulae, found that subjective preference for quality and clarity, as well as speech recognition ability, differed as a function of the intensity level of the speech signal, thus reminding us once again that any fitting rationale must account for the varying nature of acoustic signals.

Probe-tube real-ear measures have emerged as an essential clinical tool for direct verification of the amplification characteristics of a hearing aid. The prognostic value of the individual open ear frequency response, the real ear unaided response (REUR), has been studied and individual corrections for gain and SSPL advocated (Punch, Chi, and Patterson 1990). It is hoped that research efforts to date can assist in the development of a clinical protocol for probe-tube real-ear measures. A key question is what will the probe-tube benchmark be? Under what conditions should it be the target in situ or insertion response? How much deviation from the desired response is permitted? What should happen if the manufacturer has provided the matrix requested on the 2-cm³ coupler but the resulting real-ear response is not the desired response? Should there be an empirical validation of this prescription fitting/real ear assessment procedure, and if so, what should it be? Clearly, there is a need to determine how to use these data most effectively to achieve the desired goal. The selection of an appropriate task for an empirical clinical evaluation is a complex issue. Frustration with speech-recognition-based techniques resulted in the development of alternate approaches such as judgments of quality, relative intelligibility, and clarity. Many approaches to obtaining performance indices for these subjective factors have been advocated. It is time to take a critical look at the myriad speech tests and clinical evaluation techniques to determine how each can best be used to evaluate perception and communication performance. The question of which speech tasks are most useful as prognostic indicators of performance must be addressed. Criteria for changes in performance must be developed as well. Is the expanded use of confidence intervals (Thornton and Raffin 1978) to all tests appropriate to indicate performance change? Should norms for test performance be developed such as was done for the Minimal Auditory Capabilities (MAC) test (Owens et al. 1985)? Is there a way to judge aided speech performance in relation to best personal score, perhaps in relation to PB max? The compelling issue is whether speech materials should be used for the empirical trial and, if so, how they should be used. It is hoped that ensuing research efforts can address these questions, for they are essential to clinical service delivery needs.

Hearing Aid Benefit and Satisfaction

Ultimately, the success of a hearing aid will not be fully determined in the clinic or the laboratory. Information about performance with a hearing aid in everyday life will be the deciding factor for an individual, and such performance provides the most effective way to find out how much a hearing aid helps. For this reason, the self-report method has been widely used, ranging in practice from a technique of informal questioning to the use of objective methods of reporting change in communication abilities. Currently, research efforts for self-reporting instruments continue to progress. Demorest (1985), among others, has written about the conceptual and methodological issues relating to the assessment of hearing-aid benefit. It is evident that there is a science of self-reporting that must be fully developed for the clinical purpose of empirical validation. It should be used as a research tool as well to query hearing aid users about the effectiveness of amplification in various situations. Progress will be made by finding out from successful hearing aid users how hearing aids function in the everyday environment and where hearing aids do not help. There is growing recognition that inherently personal and individual factors, many of a psychosocial nature, influence how much a person will be helped. Awareness of these intrinsic variables has led to a renewed interest in developing counseling programs that address coping strategies. The likelihood of hearing aid satisfaction is increased when a fitting is accompanied by a thoughtful counseling and rehabilitation strategy that has been designed to account for subjective needs.

As hearing care professionals, it is necessary that we acknowledge the limitations of a personal hearing aid. In many situations it will be very helpful, but in some situations it will be of limited benefit. We have a responsibility to our patients to recognize these limitations and offer alternatives. The increasing availability of assistive listening devices is welcome and should be considered in the initial stages of determination for amplification either as an adjunct to a personal hearing aid or an alternative. A personal hearing aid will have another function, that is, to act as a coupling device either through direct audio input or the use of the telecoil. The passage of the ADA makes this issue even more important because accessibility is expected to be achieved through coupling of group ALD systems to personal hearing aids. Consideration of the many factors involved in the fitting and use of such devices is required and clinical protocols for selection and evaluation must be developed. Alternate technologies that can substitute for auditory deficits will become increasingly available and should be part of the clinical practitioner's knowledge base for hearing loss remediation.

In my estimation, the future is bright. We are poised on the threshold of significant changes in the technology and the clinical service delivery of hearing aids and, in particular, the role of the audiological profession as a leader in the hearing aid dispensing arena.

References

Americans with Disabilities Act 1990. Public law 101-336, 42 United States Code 12204. Buildings and Facilities, Title 36, Code of Federal Regulations.

American Association of Retired Persons. 1989. *Hearing Aids*. Product report. Washington, DC: AARP.

Burnett, E.D., and Beck, L.B. 1987. A correction for converting 2-cm³ coupler responses to insertion responses for custom in-the-ear nondirectional hearing aids. *Ear and Hearing* 8:89S–94S.

Byrne, D. 1982. Theoretical approaches for hearing aid selection. In *The Vanderbilt Hearing Aid Report: State of the Art-Research Needs*, eds. G. Studebaker and F. Bess. Upper Darby, PA: Monographs in Contemporary Audiology.

Byrne, D., and Dillon, H. 1986. The national acoustic laboratories' (NAL) new procedure for selecting the gain and frequency response of a hearing aid. *Ear and Hearing* 7:257–65.

Carhart, R. 1946. Tests for selection of hearing aids. *Laryngoscope* 56:780–94.

Crain, T.C., Van Tasell, D.V., and Fabry, D.A. 1989. Aided masking patterns with an adaptive frequency response hearing aid. Paper presented at the meeting of the American Speech-Language-Hearing Association in St. Louis, MO.

Danaher, E.M., and Pickett, J.M. 1975. Some masking effects produced by low frequency vowel formants in persons with sensorineural hearing loss. *Journal of Speech and Hearing Research* 18:261–71.

Demorest, M. 1985. Techniques for measuring hearing aid benefit through self report. In *Symposium on Hearing Technology: Its Present and Future*, ed. J.M. Pickett. Washington: Gallaudet Press.

FDA hearing aid guidelines. 1977. *Federal Food, Drug, and Cosmetic Act*. Federal Register 42:9286–96.

Gates, G.A., Cooper, J.C., Kannel, W.B., and Miller, N.J. 1990. Hearing in the elderly: The Framingham cohort, 1983–1985. Part I. Basic audiometric test results. *Ear and Hearing* 11:247–56.

Handbook of Hearing Aid Measurement. 1989. Available from the Government Printing Office, Washington, DC: Department of Veterans Affairs.

Hedges, A. 1989. Personal communication.

Kates, J.M. 1988. Acoustic effects in in-the-ear hearing aid response: Results from a coupler simulation. *Ear and Hearing* 9:119–32.

Kates, J.M. 1990. A test suite for hearing aid evaluation. *Journal of Rehabilitative Research and Development* 27.

Killion, M.C. 1982. Transducers, earmolds, and sound quality considerations. In *The Vanderbilt Hearing Aid Report: State of the Art-Research Needs*, eds. G. Studebaker and F. Bess. Upper Darby, PA: Monographs in Contemporary Audiology.

Killion, M.C., and Monser, E.L. 1980. Coupler response

for flat insertion gain. In *Acoustic Factors Affecting Hearing Aid Performance*, eds. G. Studebaker and I. Hochberg. Baltimore: University Park Press.

Levitt, H. 1982. Speech discrimination ability in the hearing impaired: Spectrum considerations. In *The Vanderbilt Hearing Aid Report: State of the Art-Research Needs*, eds. G. Studebaker and F. Bess. Upper Darby, PA: Monographs in Contemporary Audiology.

McCandless, G.A., and Lyregaard, P.E. 1983. Prescription of gain/output (POGO) for hearing aids. *Hearing Instruments* 34:16–20.

Owens, E., Kessler, D., Raggio, M., and Schubert, E. 1985. Analysis and revision of the minimal auditory capabilities (MAC) battery. *Ear and Hearing* 6:280–87.

Punch, J.L. 1978. Quality judgments of hearing aid processed speech and music by normal and otopathologic listeners. *Journal of the American Audiological Society* 3:179–88.

Punch, J.L., and Beck, L.B. 1986. Relative effects of low-frequency amplification on syllable recognition and speech quality. *Ear and Hearing* 7:57–62.

Punch, J.L., Chi, C., and Patterson, J. 1990. A recommended protocol for prescriptive use of target gain rules. *Hearing Journal* 41:13–17.

Punch, J.L., Montgomery, A.A., Schwartz, D.M., Walden, B.E., Prosek, R.A., and Howard, M.T. 1980. Multidimensional scaling of quality judgments of speech signals processed by hearing aids. *Journal of the Acoustical Society of America* 68:458–66.

Schum, D.J. 1986. Inter-subject variability effects on coupler to real ear correction curves. *Hearing Instruments* 37:25–26.

Shaw, E.A.G. 1974. Transformation of sound pressure from the free field to the eardrum in the horizontal plane. *Journal of the Acoustical Society of America* 56:1848–61.

Skinner, M.W., Pascoe, D.P., Miller, J.D., and Popelka, G.R. 1982. Measurements to determine the optimal placement of speech energy within the listener's auditory area: A basis for selecting amplification characteristics. In *The Vanderbilt Hearing Aid Report: State of the Art-Research Needs*, eds. G. Studebaker and F. Bess. Upper Darby, PA: Monographs in Contemporary Audiology.

Studebaker, G.A. 1982. Hearing aid selection: An overview. In *The Vanderbilt Hearing Aid Report: State of the Art-Research Needs*, eds. G. Studebaker and F. Bess. Upper Darby: Monographs in Contemporary Audiology.

Studebaker, G.A., and Bess, F.H. 1982. *The Vanderbilt Hearing Aid Report: State of the Art-Research Needs*. Upper Darby, PA: Monographs in Contemporary Audiology.

Sullivan, J.A., Levitt, H., Hwang, J., and Hennessey, A. 1988. An experimental comparison of four hearing aid prescription methods. *Ear and Hearing* 9:22–32.

Tecca, J., and Goldstein, D. 1984. Effects of low-frequency hearing aid response on four measures of speech perception. *Ear and Hearing* 5:22–29.

Thornton, A., and Raffin, J.M. 1978. Speech discrimination scores modeled as a binomial variable. *Journal of Speech and Hearing Research* 21:507–518.

Telecommunications for the Disabled Act. 1982. Public Law 97-410, amended in 1988. Section 3, Title VI of the Communications Act of 1934, 47 U.S.C. 601.

PART I
Prescriptive Procedures
for Present-Day Hearing Aids

CHAPTER 2
Prescribing Gain Characteristics of Linear Hearing Aids

Larry E. Humes

The conventional "linear" analog electroacoustic hearing aid has been the predominant type of hearing instrument selected by audiologists for individuals with sensorineural hearing loss since the field of audiology came into existence. The term "linear" is somewhat of a misnomer, however, in that none of these devices operate linearly *throughout* their entire range of operation. Nonetheless, this adjective is required today to distinguish those instruments that operate linearly over a wide range of intensities from those that are intentionally nonlinear over much of their operating range. Although the size of these instruments has been reduced enormously and the quality of their electroacoustic characteristics improved considerably over the past several decades, the linear analog instrument has remained the predominant type of hearing aid delivered to hearing impaired persons throughout this time.

Throughout the history of audiology, the audiologist has been confronted with the problem of selecting the most appropriate aid for a patient from a set of commercially available instruments. In the 1940s, when there were fewer instruments in both number and variety, audiologists developed a means of selecting the most appropriate hearing aid for a patient from those available. The method, developed by Carhart (1946) and referred to as the *comparative method*, remained as the primary method of hearing aid selection used by audiologists well into the 1980s (Burney 1972; Smaldino and Hoene 1981a, 1981b). The rationale behind this approach was influenced largely by the Harvard Report (Davis et al. 1946) and the Medresco Report (Radley et al. 1947). Essentially, both of these landmark reports suggested that most hearing-impaired listeners performed best with hearing instruments having either a flat or gently sloping (+ 6 dB/octave) frequency response regardless of the individual's audiometric configuration. Assuming this to be true, the task of the audiologist became one of determining which of several electroacoustically similar instruments was

most appropriate for the user. The comparative approach advocated by Carhart (1946) was an extensive battery of tests that included tests of functional gain for speech, loudness discomfort, speech recognition in quiet, and speech recognition in noise. The instrument yielding the best performance across the battery of tests was the one recommended for the patient.

In the decades that have passed since the development of the comparative approach, several problems have been identified with this method. First, the assumption that individual patients differing in audiometric configuration did not require individualized electroacoustic characteristics for their hearing aids was not supported by research subsequent to the Harvard and Medresco Reports (Braida et al. 1980; Byrne 1983; Skinner 1988). Second, the reliability, and to some extent the validity, of the comparative approach were questioned (Shore, Bilger, and Hirsh 1960; Resnick and Becker 1963; Walden et al. 1983). Walden et al. (1983) identified and examined systematically five key assumptions underlying the comparative approach and found them all to be violated when the method was used with several electroacoustically similar instruments. The comparative approach was found to be inadequate as a means of hearing aid *selection*. The impact of this research is evident in more recent surveys of clinical practices among audiologists in this country. According to Martin and Morris (1989), for example, by the end of the 1980s only about 15% of the audiologists in this country relied on the comparative approach as their primary means of selecting a hearing aid, which is down considerably from the 80% to 85% who indicated they were using this approach earlier in that same decade (Smaldino and Hoene 1981a, 1981b).

Alternatives to the comparative approach to hearing aid selection were explored by audiologists as early as the 1960s, but it wasn't until the mid-1970s that several well-defined alternatives became

available. For the most part, the alternatives that began to emerge during this period were theoretically
based prescriptive methods (Byrne and Tonisson
1976; Berger, Hagberg, and Rane 1977; Pascoe 1980;
McCandless and Lyregaard 1983). Although differing in detail and approach, most of these methods,
and the ones that ensued, shared a common objective of selecting an instrument that amplified
conversational speech in order to optimize speech
understanding without sacrificing the wearer's listening comfort.

New prescriptive methods continued to be developed in the late 1970s and 1980s. By the mid-
1980s, at least ten such methods could be identified
(Humes 1986), and some have been developed
since. Some of the methods developed earlier,
moreover, have been revised or updated and currently are in their second or third versions (Byrne
and Dillon 1986; Cox 1988; Schwartz, Lyregaard,
and Lundh 1988). Martin and Morris (1989) indicated that 70% of the audiologists they surveyed
used a prescriptive method of hearing aid selection,
either alone or in combination with another approach. Prescriptive approaches clearly have replaced the comparative method as the preferred

method of hearing aid selection among audiologists
in this country.

But which of the numerous prescriptive methods available should one use to select a hearing aid
for a patient? Until the mid-1980s, there were no attempts to answer this question. Developers of new
prescriptive methods seemed content to describe
their rationale and the details of their method without comparing the results of their prescription to
those from other methods. One of the most basic
approaches to this issue would be to determine first
if the numerous methods available all converged on
the same set of response characteristics for a given
group of patients. That is, were there redundancies
among the dozen or so methods such that, in the
extreme case, they all produced identical results?
There are numerous ways, however, in which the
prescriptions might produce "identical results." For
example, all of the methods might prescribe the
same amount of average or overall gain. This outcome is illustrated by the top two frequency-gain
curves in figure 1. Note, however, that these two
methods prescribed markedly different relative frequency responses. On the other hand, the bottom
frequency response prescribed by method A (solid

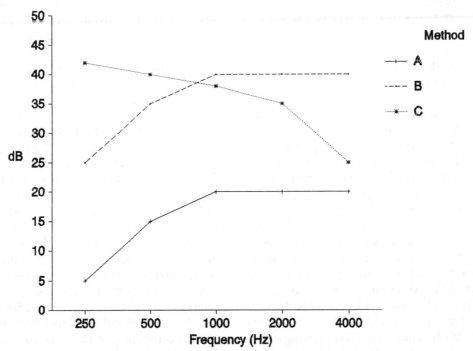

Figure 1. Comparison of three hypothetical sets of gain prescriptions made by methods
A, B, and C. Note that the top two responses, from methods B and C, are matched for
overall gain, but not relative frequency response. On the other hand, the frequency responses prescribed by methods A (solid line) and B (dashed line) are equivalent, but their
overall gain values differ substantially.

line) in figure 1 is a perfect match to that of method B (dashed line), but the average or overall gain is grossly mismatched for these two methods. When comparing the results of several prescriptive methods, comparisons should be made for both overall gain and relative frequency response.

In an effort to explore the similarities and differences among prescribed response characteristics, Byrne (1987) compared the prescribed frequency responses from six threshold-based methods. Eight different hearing losses were considered in this evaluation: two degrees of loss (mild and severe-to-profound) for each of four audiometric configurations (flat, rising, moderately sloping, and steeply sloping). Confined primarily to a descriptive analysis, Byrne (1987) viewed the resulting frequency responses to be quite different across the six prescriptive procedures. To evaluate these same data more quantitatively for this review, two measures of relative frequency response and one measure of overall gain were calculated from the prescriptions depicted in figures 2 through 5 of Byrne (1987). The two frequency-response measures were the low-frequency slope in dB/octave (gain at 1000 Hz minus gain at 250 Hz, divided by 2) and the high-frequency slope in dB/octave (gain at 4000 Hz minus gain at 1000 Hz, divided by 2). The measure of overall gain was simply the average gain for 500, 1000 and 2000 Hz.

Pearson product-moment correlation coefficients calculated for each of the possible pairs of prescription methods across the eight hypothetical subjects were all greater than 0.95 for both high-frequency slope and average gain. For low-frequency slope, however, the correlations were slightly lower with a range of 0.63 to 0.98 and a mean correlation of 0.87. All of the correlations less than 0.8 for low-frequency slope involved one of the prescription methods, the original half-gain rule suggested by Lybarger (1944). This method consistently yielded a low-frequency slope that was not strongly related to the low-frequency slopes prescribed by the other methods. In general, then, the six threshold-based prescriptive procedures included in this evaluation are closely related. That these response characteristics are correlated across prescription methods is not surprising given that no known method prescribes *less* gain for *more* hearing loss. Thus, at least moderately strong positive correlations across prescription methods were expected. The magnitude of the observed correlations, however, was quite strong, frequently exceeding 0.95.

The mean low-frequency slopes, high-frequency slopes, and average gain values prescribed by each

method are shown in figure 2. A repeated-measures analysis of variance (ANOVA) was performed on the data in each panel to examine the effects of hearing aid selection method on each response measure. The ANOVAs revealed a significant effect ($p < .01$) of prescriptive method for all three response measures. Post hoc testing revealed that

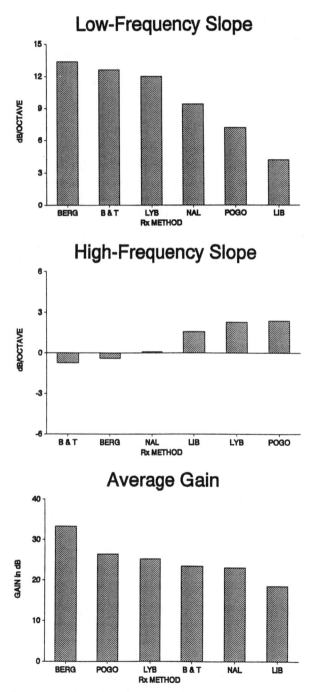

Figure 2. Mean low-frequency slopes, high-frequency slopes, and average gain values prescribed by six different threshold-based prescriptive (Rx) methods.

only two of the possible fifteen paired contrasts were signficant for the high-frequency slope parameter. The high-frequency slopes prescribed by the POGO method were significantly greater than those prescribed by the Berger and Byrne and Tonisson methods. For average gain and low-frequency slope, the post hoc analyses could be summarized by noting that the values prescribed by the Berger method were significantly greater than those of the other methods, and those prescribed by the Libby procedure were significantly lower than the others.

A cluster analysis was performed as another means of assessing the degree of similarity among these six prescriptive methods. Briefly, cluster analysis seeks to group "subjects" into clusters according to the similarity of values for several variables used to define the clusters. In this case, the "subjects" to be clustered were the six prescriptive methods. The variables used to define the clusters were the low-frequency slope, the high-frequency slope, and the average gain. When cluster analysis was performed using squared standardized Euclidean distances for each of the eight audiometric configurations, two distinct clusters of similar methods were observed. The revised NAL (NAL-R) (Byrne and Dillon 1986), the original NAL (Byrne and Tonisson 1976), the POGO (McCandless and Lyregaard 1983), and the original Lybarger (1944) methods were members of one cluster, whereas the Berger (Berger, Hagberg, and Rane 1977) and Libby (1985) methods were members of the other. This was not the case, however, for the steeply sloping audiometric configuration. For this configuration, the methods could not be clustered into fewer than three clusters, and the methods belonging to each cluster changed for the two magnitudes of hearing loss.

Another way in which the redundancy of various prescriptive methods could be evaluated with respect to prescribed response characteristics would be to ask whether the use of different methods resulted in the selection of a different, most closely matching hearing aid for the patient. Using this approach, Humes (1986) evaluated seven audiometric configurations and ten prescriptive methods. Following the generation of a prescription for each audiometric configuration by each method, a data base of over 400 hearing aid responses was searched, and the four instruments most closely matching the prescription were identified. If all ten prescriptive methods selected the same four hearing aids for a given configuration, then all ten would have to be considered to be equivalent in a practical clinical sense, even if a statistically sig-

nificant difference existed among their response characteristics. On the other hand, if a total of 40 different hearing aids had been identified from the data base for a given audiometric configuration, then no overlap among methods would be implied (4 different hearing aids per method × 10 methods = 40 unique fittings). Figure 3 illustrates the outcome for the seven audiometric configurations: three sloping (S1, S2, S3), three flat (F1, F2, F3), and one rising (R3). For the most part, with the exception of the very mild sloping hearing loss (S1), about 20 to 30 different hearing aids were identified by the various methods for each configuration, indicating a significant degree of overlap among the methods evaluated. On the other hand, it was clear that the methods were not identical. In that case, only four different hearing aids, the same four, would have been identified by all of the prescriptive methods.

These results from Humes (1986), together with the preceding analyses of the results from Byrne (1987), suggest that although there is considerable similarity and overlap among existing prescriptive methods in terms of prescribed response characteristics, the methods certainly are not identical. One might ask, then, are the observed differences of any practical consequence? That is, do the different methods actually realize different outcomes in terms of some criterion performance measure? Although the benefit to be derived from amplification is not confined solely to the improvement in understanding speech when using amplification, this is clearly the primary objective of the amplification device. Do existing prescriptive procedures result in different degrees of improvement in understanding speech?

Humes (1986) attempted to answer this question theoretically by making use of the Articulation Index (French and Steinberg 1947; ANSI 1969). Briefly, the Articulation Index (AI) is an acoustical index that is monotonically related to speech intelligibility. A hearing aid yielding a higher AI can be expected to yield a higher speech-intelligibility score for the same patient. This premise has been validated recently by several investigators (Rankovic 1988; Fabry and Van Tasell in press; Humes 1991). Thus, for hypothetical patients for whom gain prescriptions could be established and AI values calculated, one could compare the expected speech-recognition performance of various prescriptive methods by comparing their calculated AI values. Humes (1986) found that eight of the ten prescriptive methods evaluated yielded equivalent speech-intelligibility estimates using the AI. In addition, if provision were made for adjustment of the volume

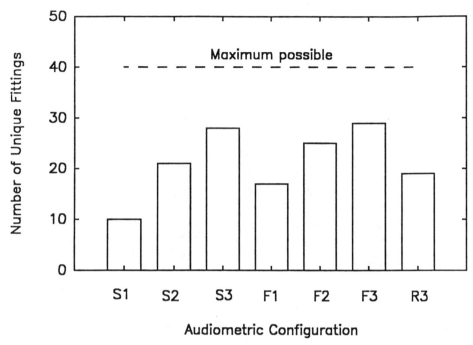

Figure 3. Summary of results from Humes (1986) illustrating the number of unique hearing aids selected by ten different prescriptive methods when applied to seven different audiometric configurations: three degrees of sloping loss (S1, S2, S3), three degrees of flat loss (F1, F2, F3), and one rising, low-frequency loss (R3). Each of the ten prescriptive methods identified the four most closely matching hearing aids from a large data base. If all ten methods selected a different set of four hearing aids from the data base, then the maximum number of unique fittings (40) would have resulted.

control to a point midway between the prescribed "use" gain and full-on gain, then all ten methods optimized speech intelligibility.

Byrne (1986) directly compared the speech-recognition performance of 14 ears listening through systems adjusted for three or four different frequency responses. Actual hearing aids were not used. Rather, a ⅓-octave equalizer was used to shape the frequency response of the system so as to match the gain characteristics prescribed by each of six different methods. The methods included one threshold-based procedure, one method based on Loudness Discomfort Levels (LDLs), and four techniques based on Most Comfortable Levels (MCLs). The primary difference among the MCL methods was the bandwidth of the stimuli used to measure MCL. Despite a goal of 84 unique responses (6 responses for each of 14 ears), a total of only 44 unique responses was produced. Many of the methods converged on the same response. In addition, many of the "unique" responses that remained were very similar for at least 4 of the 14 ears. Thus, despite efforts to produce different or unique responses deliberately for each listener, the various methods resulted in very similar response characteristics about

half of the time. This observation is consistent with the considerable degree of overlap in prescribed response characteristics among prescriptive methods noted previously.

Regarding speech-recognition performance, Byrne (1986) found that mean performance did not vary across the various prescriptive methods. Figure 4 contains a plot of these data and reveals the high degree of similarity in group performance across methods. In addition, of the 60 possible individual comparisons among scores from different responses, only 10 were found to be significant. Thus, on both a group and an individual basis, the results of Byrne (1986) suggest equivalence of speech-recognition performance across prescriptive methods.

Sullivan et al. (1988) also examined performance differences among various prescriptive hearing aid selection methods. A digital filter was used to simulate the responses prescribed by four prescriptive methods: (1) the half-gain rule (Lybarger 1944); (2) the original NAL method (Byrne and Tonisson 1976); (3) the C.I.D. MCL-based method (Skinner et al. 1982); and (4) an adaptive protocol (Levitt et al. 1987). Word-recognition

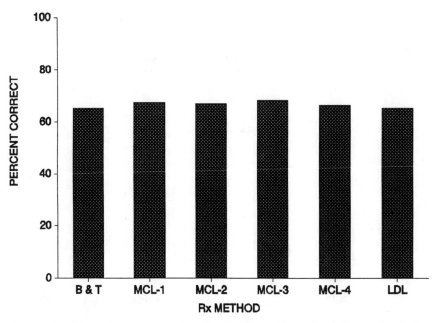

Figure 4. Mean nonsense-syllable identification scores from Byrne (1986) for each of six different prescriptive methods. There are no statistically significant differences among the means.

scores were obtained from each listener and for each frequency response at each of three output levels: two fixed sound pressure levels and one corresponding to the listener's MCL. Figure 5 displays the mean speech-recognition scores across the four methods for the MCL output level. The mean scores are very similar, ranging from a minimum of 60% for the adaptive method to a maximum of 70% for the original National Acoustics Laboratories (NAL) procedure. Post hoc testing by Sullivan et al. (1988) revealed that the response prescribed according to the adaptive method yielded performance significantly poorer than the other three responses, whereas that prescribed by the original NAL method resulted in scores that were significantly better than those obtained with the other three methods. This ordering of performance from best to worst across prescriptive method, however, varied with output level. At the lowest output level, an ordering completely opposite that shown in figure 4 was observed, with the original NAL response yielding the poorest performance and the adaptive protocol producing the best. As noted by Sullivan et al. (1988), the similarity of performance across prescriptive methods at the MCL setting was largely due to the similarity in frequency response that resulted for the four methods at this output setting. This similarity again confirms the considerable degree of overlap among prescribed frequency responses noted earlier in this chapter.

Finally, Humes and Hackett (1990) compared the speech-recognition results from 12 listeners wearing hearing aids. The hearing aids were adjusted to optimize the match between measured insertion gain and that prescribed by the revised NAL method, the updated Prescription of Gain Output (POGO) method, and the revised MSU method. Regarding the frequency responses, Humes and Hackett (1990) found significant differences among the three methods in *prescribed* frequency response, but not in *obtained* frequency response. Despite the use of electroacoustically flexible behind-the-ear instruments with readily modified earmolds and our best efforts to match the prescription, the slight but significant differences in prescribed frequency response were not preserved in the obtained responses. The biggest disparity between prescribed and obtained gain occurred at 4000 Hz and was most often observed for listeners with steeply sloping hearing loss. Under these conditions, the obtained gain was less than that prescribed. Similar findings have been reported recently by Cox and Alexander (1990).

Regarding speech-recognition performance in both quiet and noise, Humes and Hackett (1990) found no significant differences in performance among the instruments selected by each of the methods. The mean results are shown in figure 6. Note that all three prescriptive methods result in similar amounts of benefit being derived from am-

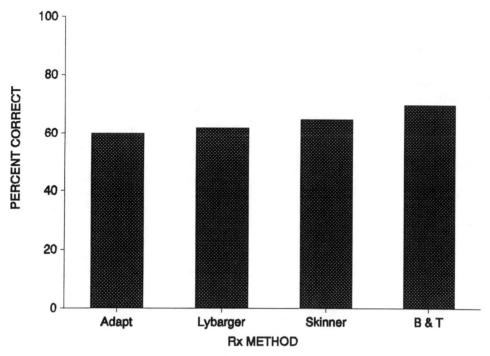

Figure 5. Mean word-recognition scores obtained for the NU-6 materials presented at Most Comfortable Loudness (MCL) by Sullivan et al. (1988).

plification with the largest improvements occurring in quiet. Results from individual subjects were consistent with the mean data in that most individuals did equally well with all three hearing aids. The results of Humes and Hackett (1990) from actual hearing aids confirm the laboratory findings of Sullivan et al. (1988). As Sullivan et al. (1988) stated, "The most striking result . . . is that no single prescriptive method emerged as being clearly superior" (p. 29).

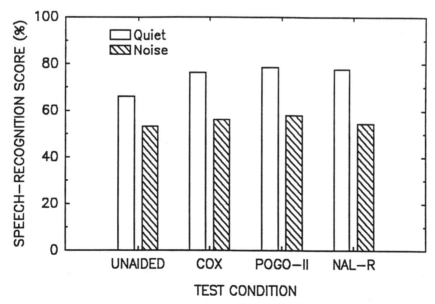

Figure 6. Mean speech-recognition scores obtained by Humes and Hackett (1990) in quiet (unfilled bars) and noise (striped bars) in the unaided condition and in three aided listening conditions. For the three aided conditions, the listener wore a hearing aid selected according to one of three prescriptive methods (Cox or MSU, POGO-II, and NAL-R).

Several recent studies, therefore, have indicated that many contemporary prescriptive hearing aid selection methods do not differ in regard to aided speech-recognition performance. Other performance measures, however, have been suggested as targets for optimization aside from speech-recognition scores. Humes (1986), for example, compared a wide variety of prescriptive methods in terms of their ability to specify frequency-gain characteristics most closely matching those actually preferred by hearing aid users. Byrne (1986) and Sullivan et al. (1988) both obtained ratings of speech intelligibility and speech quality in addition to their measures of speech recognition. In general, prescriptive methods tended to be somewhat less redundant with regard to these other measures of hearing aid performance. That is, a particular prescriptive method appeared to yield superior results compared to alternative methods for a given subject and listening condition. The response producing the best results, however, varied considerably across subjects *and* across listening conditions within a given subject. More research into the reliability and validity of rating methods, however, is needed before they can be considered as viable alternative measures of listener performance.

Frequently, the progress made in an area of clinical audiology is determined, in part, by the technology available. This certainly has been the case with prescriptive hearing aid selection methods. The advent of clinically feasible probe-tube microphone systems and the availability of powerful, yet inexpensive, microcomputers largely has facilitated the move to prescriptive approaches to hearing aid selection. The rapid and reliable measurement of real-ear gain using probe-tube microphones has made it clinically feasible to fit and fine-tune a hearing aid to match a prescribed response. Functional gain, an alternative and more widely available measure of real-ear gain, lacks the reliability (Humes and Kirn 1990) and efficiency (Humes, Hipskind, and Block 1988) to make it a practical alternative in the hearing aid fitting and fine-tuning process.

It is my impression, however, that audiologists have become preoccupied with the confirmation of prescribed insertion gain and frequently have lost sight of the prescriptive method's underlying theory. Consider the POGO prescriptive formula. Theoretically, this method attempts to restore normal perception of stimuli at levels corresponding to most comfortable loudness. Based on an average relationship between threshold and MCL at several frequencies, it has been found that providing real-ear gain equal to one-half the hearing loss will accomplish this goal for frequencies above 500 Hz. For an individual with a flat 40 dB HL hearing loss, for example, POGO would require 20 dB of gain above 500 Hz to accomplish this objective. After the prescription has been generated, the audiologist orders the appropriate aid and fine tunes the response to obtain a good match to the desired target gain. A good match between prescribed and obtained real-ear gain, however, does *not* indicate that the *theoretical objectives* of the method have been accomplished. There are numerous averages included in prescriptive fitting methods, including average real-ear-to-coupler corrections for both 2-cc and 6-cc couplers and average threshold-to-MCL relationships. A perfect match between prescribed and obtained insertion gain can be obtained for a given patient without coming close to realizing the theoretical objective of the method. In the case of the POGO method, for example, the patient simply may have MCLs that differ considerably from those of the "average" person with similar hearing loss. Efforts have been made in recent years to shift the focus from matching the prescribed gain to accomplishing the desired theoretical objectives (Seewald, Ross, and Stelmachowicz 1987; Cox and Alexander 1990). The technology exists, for example, to measure the real-ear sound pressure levels corresponding to MCL at several frequencies and then to adjust the gain characteristics of the aid to confirm the amplification of a speech-like signal to those values. Thus, the fine-tuning process can be carried out in terms of matching the theoretical objective directly, rather than matching the gain that should be required to accomplish that objective.

Audiologists also have been preoccupied with real-ear gain measurements at the expense of other hearing aid evaluation techniques. Too frequently, the hearing aid fitting process ends with the fine-tuning of gain, as though the lack of sufficient gain was the patient's chief complaint when first arriving at the clinic. Rather, most hearing aid candidates arrive at the clinic with a chief complaint of not being able to hear and understand speech. An evaluation of the aid's performance with speech audiometry is essential, even if a perfect match between prescribed and obtained gain is observed. Although the comparative method lacks the reliability to *select* the best aid from a restricted set of electroacoustically similar instruments, the battery of speech-audiometry tests comprising the comparative test battery can provide helpful information about the benefit received from amplification (Jerger 1987; Humes 1988). Carhart (1946) noted that the comparative test battery not only served the purpose of selecting the most appropriate device for the patient (which would be disputed today), but also defined the patient's problem more fully. Moreover, when used as a hearing aid *evaluation* tool, the reliability of the individual tests in the comparative test battery can be improved by increasing the number of items or trials in each test. Because the clinician is only making these measurements on one instrument, rather than on three or four similar instruments, the time "cost" to the clinician associated with a greater number of tests items is not too great.

References

ANSI S3.5-1969. *The American National Standard Method for the Calculation of the Articulation Index.* New York: ANSI.

Berger, K.W., Hagberg, E.N., and Rane R.L. 1977. *Prescription of Hearing Aids: Rationale, Procedure and Results.* Kent, Ohio: Herald Publishing House.

Braida, L.D., Durlach, N.I., Lippmann, R.P., Hicks, B.L., Rabinowitz, W.M., and Reed, C.M. 1980. Hearing aids—A review of past research on linear amplification, amplitude compression, and frequency lowering. *ASHA Monograph* 19.

Burney, P.A. 1972. A survey of hearing aid evaluation procedures. *Asha* 14:439–44.

Byrne, D. 1983. *Theoretical Prescriptive Approaches to Selecting the Gain and Frequency Response of a Hearing Aid.* Upper Darby, PA: Monographs in Contemporary Audiology.

Byrne, D. 1986. Effects of frequency response characteristics on speech discrimination and perceived intelligibility and pleasantness of speech for hearing-impaired listeners. *Journal of the Acoustical Society of America* 7:257–65.

Byrne, D. 1987. Hearing aid selection formulae: Same or different? *Hearing Instruments* 38(1):5–11.

Byrne, D., and Dillon, H. 1986. The National Acoustic Laboratories' (NAL) new procedure for selecting the gain and frequency response of a hearing aid. *Ear and Hearing* 7:257–65.

Byrne, D., and Tonisson, W. 1976. Selecting the gain of hearing aids for persons with sensorineural hearing impairment. *Scandinavian Audiology* 5:51–59.

Carhart, R. 1946. Selection of hearing aids. *Archives of Otolaryngology* 44:1–18.

Cox, R.M. 1988. The MSUv3 hearing instrument prescription procedure. *Hearing Instruments* 39(1):6–10.

Cox, R.M., and Alexander, G.C. 1990. Evaluation of an in-situ output probe-microphone method for hearing aid fitting verification. *Ear and Hearing* 11:31–39.

Davis, H., Hudgins, C.V., Marquis, R.J., Nichols, R.H., Jr., Peterson, G.E., Ross, D.A., and Stevens, S.S. 1946. The selection of hearing aids. *Laryngoscope* 56:85–115.

Fabry, D.A., and Van Tasell, D.J. In press. Evaluation of an articulation-index based model for predicting the effects of adaptive frequency response hearing aids. *Journal of Speech and Hearing Research*.

French, N.R., and Steinberg, J.C. 1947. Factors governing the intelligibility of speech sounds. *Journal of the Acoustical Society of America* 19:90–119.

Humes, L.E. 1986. An evaluation of several rationales for selecting hearing aid gain. *Journal of Speech and Hearing Disorders* 51:272–81.

Humes, L.E. 1988. And the winner is . . . *Hearing Instruments* 39(7):24–26.

Humes, L. 1991. Understanding the speech-understanding difficulties of the hearing impaired. *Journal of the American Academy of Audiology* 2:59–69.

Humes, L.E., and Hackett, T. 1990. Comparison of frequency response and aided speech-recognition performance for hearing aids selected by three different prescriptive methods. *Journal of the American Academy of Audiology* 1:101–108.

Humes, L.E., and Kirn, E.U. 1990. The reliability of functional gain. *Journal of Speech and Hearing Disorders* 55:193–97.

Humes, L.E., Hipskind, N.M., and Block, M.G. 1988. Insertion gain measured with three probe-tube systems. *Ear and Hearing* 9:108–112.

Jerger, J. 1987. On the evaluation of hearing aid performance. *ASHA* 29(9):49–51.

Levitt, H., Sullivan, J.A., Neuman, A.C., and Rubin-Spitz, J.A. 1987. Experiments with a programmable master hearing aid. *Journal of Rehabilitation Research and Development* 24:29–54.

Libby, E.R. 1985. State-of-the-art hearing aid selection procedures. *Hearing Instruments* 36(1):30–38, 62.

Lybarger, S.F. 1944. U.S. patent application SN 543, 278; July 3.

McCandless, G.A., and Lyregaard, P.E. 1983. Prescription of gain/output (POGO) for hearing aids. *Hearing Instruments* 35(1):16–21.

Martin, F.N., and Morris, L.J. 1989. Current audiologic practices in the United States. *Hearing Journal* 42(4):25–44.

Pascoe, D. 1980. Clinical implications of nonverbal methods of hearing aid selection and fitting. *Seminars in Speech, Language and Hearing* 1:217–29.

Radley, W.G., Bragg, W.L., Dadson, R.S., Hallpike, C.S., McMillan, D., Pocock, L.C., and Littler, T.S. 1947. *Hearing Aids and Audiometers. Report of the Committee on Electroacoustics.* London: His Majesty's Stationery Service.

Rankovic, C.M. 1988. An application of the articulation index to hearing aid fitting. Ph.D. diss., University of Minnesota, Minneapolis.

Resnick, D.M., and Becker, M. 1963. Hearing aid evaluation: A new approach. *ASHA* 5:695–99.

Schwartz, D.M., Lyregaard, P.E., and Lundh, P. 1988. Hearing aid selection for severe-to-profound hearing loss. *Hearing Journal* 41(2):13–17.

Seewald, R.C., Ross, M., and Stelmachowicz, P.G. 1987. Selecting and verifying hearing aid performance characteristics for young children. *Journal of the Academy of Rehabilitative Audiology* 20:25–37.

Shore, I., Bilger, R.C., and Hirsh, I.J. 1960. Hearing aid evaluation: The reliability of repeated measurements. *Journal of Speech and Hearing Disorders* 25:152–67.

Skinner, M.W. 1988. *Hearing Aid Evaluation.* Englewood Cliffs, New Jersey: Prentice Hall.

Skinner, M.W., Pascoe, D.P., Miller, J.D., and Popelka, G.R. 1982. Measurements to determine the optimal placement of speech energy within the listener's auditory area: A basis for selecting amplification characteristics. In *The Vanderbilt Hearing Aid Report* eds. G.A. Studebaker and F.H. Bess. Upper Darby, PA: Monographs in Contemporary Audiology.

Smaldino, J., and Hoene, J. 1981a. A view of the state of hearing aid fitting practices. Part I. *Hearing Instruments* 32(1):14–15, 58.

Smaldino, J., and Hoene, J. 1981b. The nature of common hearing aid fitting practices. Part II. *Hearing Instruments* 32(2):8–11, 43.

Sullivan, J.A., Levitt, H., Hwang, J., and Hennessey, A. 1988. An experimental comparison of four hearing aid prescription methods. *Ear and Hearing* 9:22–32.

Walden, B., Schwartz, D.M., Williams, D.L., Holum-Hardegen, L.L., and Crowley, J.M. 1983. Test of the assumptions underlying comparative hearing aid evaluations. *Journal of Speech and Hearing Disorders* 48:264–73.

CHAPTER 3
Clinical Implications of Prescriptive Formulas for Hearing Aid Selection

Gene W. Bratt and Carol A. Sammeth

Over the past fifteen years there has been a proliferation of formulas developed for prescribing the gain and frequency response of hearing aids. The use of prescriptive procedures for selective amplification in hearing aids now has obtained widespread acceptance, virtually replacing the older Carhart (1946) approach that employed comparative evaluations with speech threshold and intelligibility testing.

The majority of available formulas for frequency response prescription use the pure-tone audiogram as the basis for target calculation (e.g., McCandless and Lyregaard 1983; Berger, Hagberg, and Rane 1984; Libby 1986; Byrne and Dillon 1986), even though the stated goal of the procedure may be to achieve audibility, to maximize the articulation index score, or to amplify speech bands to most comfortable loudness level. Other formulas require additional measurement of comfortable and uncomfortable loudness levels on the assumption that these values cannot be predicted adequately from pure-tone thresholds (e.g., Shapiro 1976; Skinner et al. 1982; Tyler 1986; Cox 1985a). Most recently, versions of some established formulas have been proposed for use with more severely impaired patients (Schwartz, Lyregaard, and Lundh 1988; Byrne, Parkinson, and Newall 1990). This chapter is not intended as a review of available prescription formulas and their differences, as this is covered in greater detail by Humes (this volume, Chapter 1). Rather, our purpose is to discuss some of the practical issues involved in the clinical application of prescriptive approaches for selection of frequency response characteristics in hearing aids.

Current Fitting Practices

The appeal of prescription formulas is that they have a stated scientific rationale and some degree of empirical validation, they are relatively simple and quick to implement, and they generate measurable targets in the dispensary. Unfortunately, it has been our observation that the very ease of implementing a prescriptive approach sometimes has led to oversimplification in fitting practice. In preparation of this chapter, for example, we surveyed five major manufacturers of custom in-the-ear (ITE) hearing aids and found that reportedly between 80% and 95% of ITE hearing aid orders currently are accompanied by technical data consisting of only the pure-tone audiogram. The remaining 5% to 20% of orders specified a particular frequency response, either with a matrix number or with 2-cc coupler full-on gain values as prescribed by a formula approach. The majority of dispensers, therefore, apparently presume that the manufacturer, armed only with the pure-tone audiogram, will consistently tailor the characteristics of the hearing aid in a manner that will result in an optimal fitting for the patient.

It certainly is possible that some clinicans may select a specific manufacturer because the fabrication strategies of the company are fully known; that is, the manufacturer uses a threshold-based approach that is acceptable to the clinician, and consequently the audiogram alone is submitted. The major drawback of this approach is that it does not allow incorporation of probe-tube microphone measurement of an individual's real ear unaided response (REUR) into prescribed gain calculation, as discussed later in this chapter. Clearly, the use of matrix or 2-cc coupler information places responsibility for the fitting more squarely in the hands of the audiologist.

It also is possible that the clinician who sends

The authors wish to thank the following individuals for assistance with collection of the data presented in this article: Dr. Barbara Peek of the Department of Veterans Affairs Medical Center, Nashville, TN, and Susan Amberg, Blake Lazenby, Susan Logan, and Andrea Williams, all of the Bill Wilkerson Center in Nashville. This work was supported by Veterans Administration funded project #C307-RA.

in only the audiogram assumes that the resulting frequency response characteristic will be at least grossly appropriate for the patient, and that he or she can subsequently evaluate and modify the response with potentiometers and venting after the hearing aid is fitted to the patient's ear. Unfortunately, there are indications that not all dispensers verify the obtained frequency response characteristic or evaluate its appropriateness for the individual patient. For example, some of the results of a recent survey of hearing aid fitting practices at VA audiology facilities are displayed in figure 1 (Hedges 1989). While 80% of the facilities responding to the questionnaire reported that they always check hearing aid output by listening to the hearing aid, presumably through a hearing aid stethoscope, less than 25% reported *always* accomplishing electroacoustic analysis of the hearing aid prior to fitting. Electroacoustic measurements were obtained only *sometimes* in nearly two-thirds of the facilities. When asked if the patient *always* is evaluated with the hearing aid fitted on his or her ear prior to issuance, 40% reported always using soundfield threshold measurements and 27% reported always using real ear probe-tube microphone measurements. These numbers indicate that, at best, about one-third of the respondents do not routinely analyze by frequency the performance of the hearing aid fitted on the patient's ear.

There is no reason to believe that practices outside of the VA system are substantially different. The recent results of an annual survey of dispensing practices (Cranmer 1990) reported, in fact, that approximately 20% of respondents do not use any form of testing after fitting an aid to the ear.

These numbers are disconcerting because they suggest that a significant number of clinicians have established no theoretical goal for fitting, and consequently have little motivation for measuring the outcome of a fitting. Given the wealth of clinical and research literature available regarding issues in frequency response selection, a fitting approach that would rely entirely on the manufacturer for decision making, with failure to verify or evaluate the results of the fitting, is not acceptable.

Recent results of a study by Angeli, Seestadt-Stanford, and Nerbonne (1990) also indicate that blind confidence in the internal consistency of hearing aid manufacturers is not warranted. These researchers ordered two hearing aids from each of five manufacturers by sending an identical audiogram at two different times. As shown in figure 2, the difference between the two aids from a given manufacturer could be quite large. Manufacturer B, for example, provided two hearing aids that differed in high-frequency average full-on gain by 11 dB, even though the prescription for each aid was derived from the same audiogram. These results

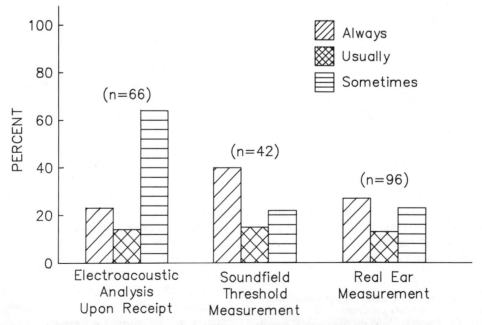

Figure 1. Results of a survey of VA audiology facilities by Hedges (1989), giving the percentage of respondents who reported *always, usually,* and *sometimes* accomplishing the indicated measurements of hearing aid performance.

are not to be construed as an indictment of the hearing aid manufacturers, most of whom performed quite consistently across the measures depicted in figure 2; rather, they simply illustrate that inconsistencies can occur.

In Nashville, Tennessee, at the Audiology and Speech Pathology Service, Department of Veterans Affairs Medical Center, and at the Bill Wilkerson Center, we have developed an approach to the selection and fitting of hearing aids, particularly with regard to the shaping of frequency response, that has the following four-point rationale:

1. Hearing aid fittings should be designed to achieve a goal that has a scientific basis and empirical validation, with measurable targets articulated in terms of 2-cc coupler and real ear insertion gain (REIG).
2. Individual rather than averaged data should be incorporated into the target calculation and fitting whenever possible.
3. Hearing aid performance should be verified in terms of 2-cc coupler and REIG or functional gain.
4. Prescribed targets should be considered only preliminary goals, with final fitting characteristics dictated by measurement of aided responses to speech or speech-like stimuli, and by the individual needs and desires of the patient.

Each clinician must assume the responsibility for determining the specific prescriptive approach to be used, and thus the goal to be achieved in the fitting. Most of the prescriptive techniques that currently are available for hearing aid fitting appear to provide an acceptable theoretical basis for the fitting of amplification. Although there are significant differences in the amount of prescribed gain under various formulas, particularly for steeply sloping audiograms (Humes 1986; Byrne 1987), there have been, to date, few evaluative studies regarding the relative success of one formula approach compared with another. As a first step in evaluating the success of our fitting strategy, we examined our ability to achieve prescribed gain and frequency response when fitting analog ITEs (Sammeth et al. 1989).

Ability to Achieve Prescribed Gain With Analog ITES

To evaluate the degree of fitting accuracy (or, conversely, the fitting error) that can be expected using prescription formulas, we collected data on hearing aid fittings for 90 adult ears demonstrating the average audiogram shown in figure 3. All subjects were fitted with custom analog ITE hearing aids from a major manufacturer who worked closely with us to achieve the desired frequency response. Target gain

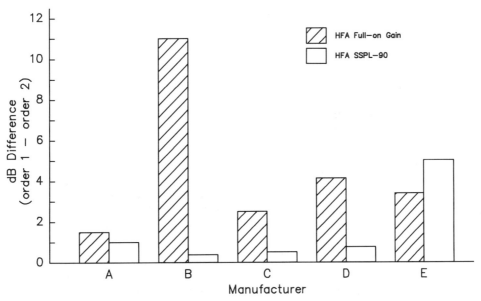

Figure 2. The difference in high-frequency average gain and SSPL-90 for two custom ITE hearing aids ordered with identical audiograms from each of five manufacturers. Adapted from Angeli, Seestadt-Stanford, and Nerbonne (1990), with permission.

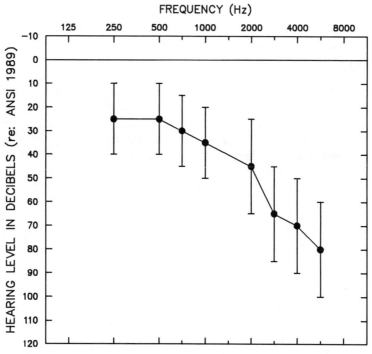

Figure 3. Means and standard deviations of hearing levels for the 90 ears fitted with ITE hearing aids using the revised NAL prescription formula.

and frequency response were calculated for each ear using the revised National Acoustic Laboratories (NAL) formula developed by Byrne and Dillon (1986). The manufacturer was given the calculated full-on 2-cc coupler values (which, in this study, were based on average real-ear-to-coupler correction factors); in other words, the patient's audiogram was not given. For maximum flexibility in fitting the frequency response, each hearing aid was ordered with both a tone control and output potentiometer (peak clipping), and with variable venting inserts.

Electroacoustic and probe-tube microphone measurements were made with a Fonix model 6500 test system. When a hearing aid arrived from the manufacturer, the clinician first adjusted the trimpots as necessary to achieve the closest possible match to the prescribed (target) 2-cc coupler full-on gain values. These "best-fit" values were compared to the target 2-cc coupler values to examine the degree of fitting error that occurred. Subsequently, the hearing aid was fitted to the patient's ear using probe-tube microphone measurement of REIG. Trimpots and/or venting were again adjusted as necessary to achieve the closest possible match to target REIG values. These "best-fit" REIG values were compared to the target REIG values to exam-

ine the degree of fitting error that occurred with the hearing aid on the patient's ear.

For illustrative purposes, 35 of the 90 cases have been selected randomly for depiction in scatterplot form in figure 4. Data from 2-cc coupler measurements are shown in figure 4A. Each datum point represents the difference between actual and target gain, with a positive value indicating that the gain fit was greater than that which had been prescribed. Notice that too much gain frequently was given in the low and mid frequencies, and too little gain in the high frequencies. These data are very similar to those of Bratt et al. (1987), who used a similar investigative protocol with 122 hearing aids not included in this study.

Figure 4B illustrates the data for REIG measurement from the same 35 ears. Fitting generally was accurate within + or − 5 dB of target through 2000 Hz, but target was achieved in only three of the 35 ears at 4000 Hz. Of course, the desired insertion gain at 4000 Hz could have been achieved in some cases by turning up the overall gain, but this would result in excessive gain in the midfrequency range. This pattern of overfitting the mid-frequencies and underfitting the high frequencies probably stems from the juxtaposition of the high frequency amplification needs of the majority of our patients with

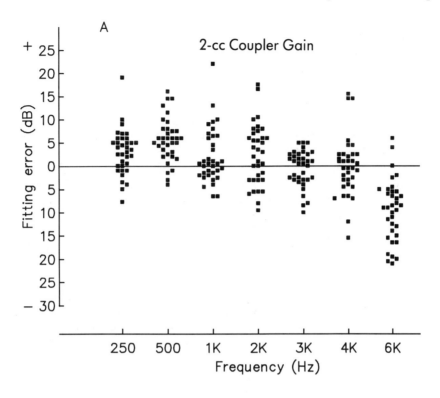

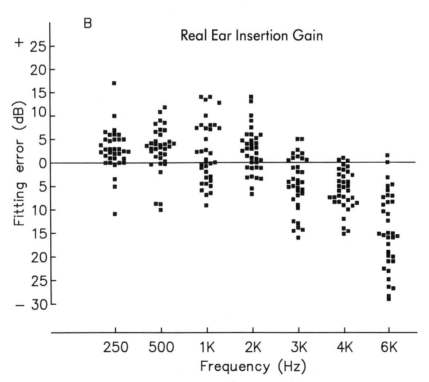

Figure 4. Scatterplot of fitting error for 35 of the 90 ears fitted using the revised NAL formula. Each datum point represents the difference between prescribed gain and that which was actually fitted, at each frequency. Figure 4A shows data for 2-cc coupler full-on gain measurement, and figure 4B shows data for real ear insertion gain measurement.

the well-known tendency for analog circuitry to peak in the 2000 to 3000 Hz region.

To determine if the degree of fitting accuracy achieved was greater with one prescription approach than with another, we also fitted 20 hearing aids using the Prescription of Gain/Output (POGO) formula (McCandless and Lyregaard 1983; Lyregaard 1986) and 20 hearing aids using the Memphis State formula developed by Cox (Cox 1985a, 1988). In figure 5A, the mean of the absolute differences in 2-cc coupler fitting error under each of these prescriptive approaches is compared with that obtained for the 90 ears fitted with the NAL formula. Shown in figure 5B is the mean absolute fitting error under each formula using REIG measurements. Overall, there appears to be relatively little difference in mean fitting error among the three formulas with either measurement procedure.

Finally, we were interested in how much difference there is in prescribed gain curves among these three prescription formulas. To examine this issue,

we selected 15 ears that represented a range of audiometric configurations and degrees of hearing loss, and, for each ear, calculated prescribed REIG gain curves with each of the three formulas (NAL, POGO, and the Memphis State University/Cox procedure). Then we calculated the absolute differences between the prescribed gain values for each individual ear at each frequency.

Shown in figure 6 are the means of the differences between the formulas in prescribed REIG. Although differences for some audiograms were found to exceed those for others, the overall mean differences shown here are relatively small, except at the highest frequencies where POGO tended to prescribe greater gain than the other two procedures. Recall, however, that we were often unable to obtain sufficient gain at these high frequencies with any of the formulas (see figure 4). In fact, when the mean prescribed REIG differences between the formulas (figure 6) are compared with the mean degree of REIG fitting error found under

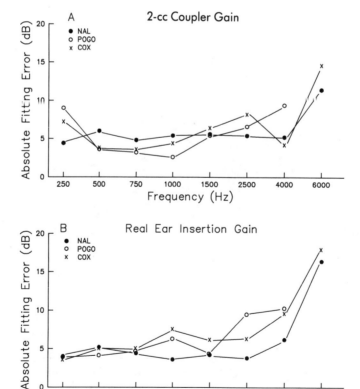

Figure 5. The degree of fitting error under each of the three prescription gain formulas used. Data shown are the means of the absolute differences between prescribed gain and that which was actually fitted, at each frequency. Figure 5A shows data for 2-cc coupler full-on gain measurement, and figure 5B shows data for real ear insertion gain measurement.

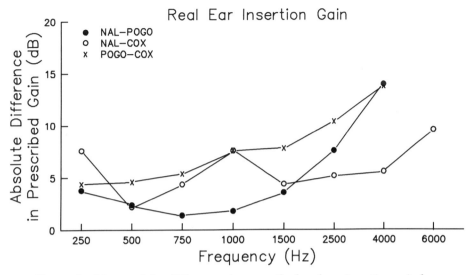

Figure 6. Means of the differences in prescribed real ear insertion gain between the three prescription gain formulas for 15 ears representing a range of audiometric configurations and degrees of losses.

each formula (figure 5B), it can be seen that the formula differences generally are not much larger than the mean fitting error. Based on these data, there does not seem to be a strong rationale for using any one of these three formulas over another, at least when fitting analog ITEs.

If a manufacturer supplies a hearing aid that is too deviant from the target values ordered, it would be reasonable to send it back with instructions that the manufacturer attempt to match the order more accurately. A problem arises in clinical practice, however, in that it is neither time- nor cost-efficient to return too many hearing aids upon receipt, particularly when it is suspected that the manufacturer can do no better on subsequent tries. To make the situation worse, none of the published formulas, to our knowledge, specifically answers the question of how much fitting error can be tolerated before the principles driving the method are violated. We can, however, evaluate the effect of various acceptance criteria, specified in terms of fitting error, on the percentage of hearing aids that we would have to return to the manufacturer.

Figure 7A illustrates for 2-cc coupler measurements the percentage of hearing aids that would be accepted for a given degree of fitting error (in dB). Two functions are shown, each representing a different frequency range. To accept 90% of the hearing aids as received from the manufacturer, an error of more than 15 dB would have to be tolerated at one frequency or more in the frequency range of 250 to 4000 Hz. To accept 50% of the hearing aids, a fitting error of 10 dB would need to be tolerated at one or

more frequency in this range. Narrowing the frequency window by excluding 250 and 4000 Hz does not make much difference. Figure 7B illustrates acceptance data for REIG measurements, which are similar.

It certainly would be desirable to approximate more closely coupler and REIG prescriptions, and we expect to be able to achieve greater fitting flexibility in the future, particularly when programmable digital and digital-hybrid circuitry becomes more widely available. We confined our data presentation in this report to ITEs because, like the national average (Mahon 1989; Cranmer 1990), they constitute 80% or more of our fittings. It is notable that Humes and Hackett (1990) achieved only slightly greater accuracy in fitting with the use of more flexible behind-the-ear hearing aids.

Even with the magnitude of fitting error we found, however, we are not discouraged from using a prescriptive approach for fitting analog ITE hearing aids. While we have presented data on the degree of fitting error when using prescriptive formulas, we do not believe that complete accuracy in fitting to a target curve is necessarily crucial, nor that it should be the final goal. Most of the developers of prescriptive approaches clearly specify that the target curve should be considered as only a starting point in the fitting of a linear frequency response (e.g., McCandless and Lyregaard 1983; Byrne and Dillon 1986; Cox 1985b). While recognizing the limitations of the prescriptive approach, we believe each of these prescription formulas will provide a reasonable first approximation, which

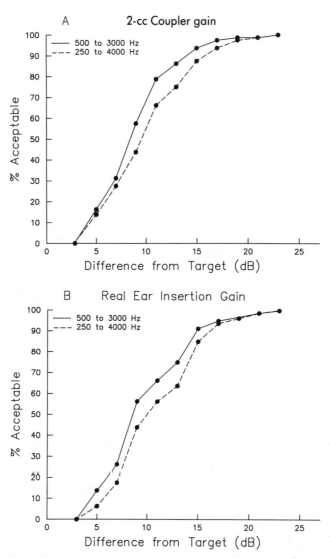

Figure 7. The percentage of 90 hearing aids fitted using the revised NAL formula which would be accepted for a given degree of fitting error in dB. Two functions are shown, representing a wider and narrower range of measurement frequencies. Figure 7A shows data for 2-cc coupler full-on gain measurement and figure 7B shows data for real ear insertion gain measurement.

should be followed by individualization of the frequency response and gain.

Individualizing the Frequency Response

There are a number of reasons why the best frequency-gain function for an individual patient might deviate from that prescribed by a formula. First, the majority of formula approaches are based on averaged data for several fitting parameters, including real-ear-to-coupler corrections and MCL/ UCL estimates. An individual patient may deviate substantially from any of these averages. In addition, while most of the prescriptive approaches are based only on audiometric threshold and loudness measurements, it is well known that patients may differ widely in suprathreshold, psychoacoustic, and speech discrimination abilities. Following a reasonable approximation to a target then, there is a clear need to evaluate an individual patient's performance and to "fine tune" the fitting.

Recall that the second and third points in our fitting rationale stated that individual rather than averaged data should be incorporated into the target calculation whenever possible, and that verification of the response of the hearing aid on the patient's ear is imperative. Hearing aid characteristics are routinely specified in the coupler so that the clinician and the manufacturer can communicate with each other for purposes of quality control, but the 2-cc coupler was never meant to, nor does it, closely represent the frequency-gain function of a hearing aid on the human ear (e.g., Cox 1979; Seewald, Ross, and Spiro 1985). There is also a significant degree of individual variability across human ears, so that an individual's real-ear-to-coupler correction factor may differ significantly from the average (e.g., Bratt 1980; Feigin et al. 1989). The use of REIG measurement obtained with a probe-tube microphone system, or of behaviorally measured functional gain, is necessary to give the dispenser an indication of actual performance of the hearing aid in the listener's ear.

One means of individualizing the hearing aid fitting, which we recently have begun to use, is the incorporation of probe-tube microphone measurements into the calculation of the target 2-cc coupler gain curve. The goal of this approach as implemented by Mueller (1989) is to account for the difference between an individual patient's real ear unaided response (REUR) and the average REUR. Because most prescription formulas calculate desired 2-cc coupler gain based on averaged data, the use of individual measurement may reduce fitting error for those patients with atypical REURs and, thus, reduce the number of hearing aids returned to the manufacturer for frequency response modification. Shown in figure 8 (adapted from Mueller 1989) is an example of a patient whose REUR is larger in the mid–high frequency range than is the average response from KEMAR. Consequently, greater gain will be needed in this frequency region in order to overcome the insertion loss produced when this ear is occluded with the hearing aid. When ordering the hearing aid, these difference values can be added to the formula-prescribed 2-cc coupler gain, thus maximizing the likelihood of achieving REIG. A similar approach is described by Punch, Chi, and Patterson (1990).

The final point in our fitting rationale was that prescribed targets should be considered preliminary, with final fitting characteristics dictated by individual responses to speech or speech-like stimuli. While a detailed discussion of the issues involved in evaluating and "fine tuning" the hearing aid are beyond the scope of this report, we want to review briefly some of the factors that we routinely consider in a hearing aid fitting. The primary goal in

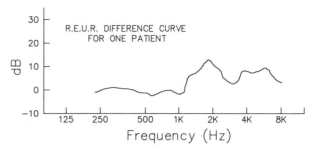

Figure 8. The difference between one individual patient's real ear unaided response and the KEMAR average Adapted from Mueller (1989), with permission.

amplification is to obtain maximal speech intelligibility, particularly in those listening environments where the patient reports having the most difficulty. The first step in evaluating the frequency response should be objective or subjective measurement of the patient's speech understanding ability in quiet and/or in various types of noise with appropriate signal-to-noise ratios. We routinely use the Speech-in-Noise (SPIN) test (Kalikow, Stevens, and Elliot 1977; Bilger et al. 1984) because it provides us with an indication of functioning when contextual cues are, and are not, available. This comparison is very useful in counseling the patient regarding expected hearing aid benefit.

Speech intelligibility cannot, however, be the only factor that is evaluated. Too often, a patient with excellent aided-speech recognition ability rejects his or her hearing aid because of unpleasant sound quality or loudness discomfort. Punch and Beck (1980) have suggested that, while speech intelligibility is dependent primarily upon mid- to high-frequency energy, sound quality correlates best with increased low-frequency gain. If a patient complains of poor sound quality, it certainly may be appropriate to adjust the frequency response to provide more low-frequency gain, as long as good speech understanding is not sacrificed, for instance, due to an excessive upward spread of masking or to amplification of low-frequency environmental noise.

Clinical considerations in output limiting and the use of advanced signal processing algorithms are discussed in other chapters in this volume, but it is important to emphasize that the linear frequency response is not entirely independent of other parameters in the hearing aid fitting. Even with linear peak-clipping aids, an output potentiometer often does not function independently of the tone control trimpot. For patients with severe loudness recruitment or those who frequently must function in a noisy environment, the use of such features as adaptive signal processing (ASP), automatic gain control (AGC) circuits, or directional microphones may be indicated. Unfortunately, none of the available prescriptive approaches provides much guidance in the fitting of adaptive, nonlinear hearing aids. With these devices, then, it is even more important to evaluate an individual's performance and satisfaction with the hearing aid, and to implement follow-up protocols.

Finally, it deserves mention that several of the new digital-hybrid hearing aids offer the potential for more than one fixed frequency response—user-selectable with a pushbutton or switch (see Sammeth 1990, for a review). The clinician may choose to approximate a target frequency response in one of the listening modes and to program either more low-frequency or more high-frequency gain in other modes, depending on the listening environments experienced by the patient and the trade-off necessary between speech clarity and sound quality.

In summary, we believe that prescriptive techniques offer the best approach to the selection of hearing aids at the current state of the art. Even though variability shown in utilizing current analog circuitry may weaken somewhat the impact of the prescriptive approach, it probably does not negate its validity. Small differences between target curves prescribed with each approach may not be achievable, but the result is a frequency response that is "in the ballpark," i.e., that provides an appropriate starting point for fitting. Verification of hearing aid output in the coupler and in the real ear is essential, because it cannot be assumed that what is received from the manufacturer is what is intended for the patient, particularly when average real-ear-to-coupler correction factors are used. Finally, achieving the prescribed target should not be considered the ultimate goal of the fitting process. Rather, it should be considered as a preliminary step, with subsequent adjustment made based upon evaluation procedures with attention to the patient's individual needs.

References

Angeli, G.M., Seestadt-Stanford, L., and Nerbonne, M.A. 1990. Consistency among/within manufacturer regarding electroacoustic properties of ITE instruments. *Hearing Journal* 43(3):23–26.

Berger, K.W., Hagberg, E.N., and Rane, R.L. 1984. *Prescription of Hearing Aids: Rationale, Procedures and Results* (4th Ed). Kent, OH: Herald.

Bilger, R.C., Nuetzel, J.M., Rabinowitz, W.M., and Rzeczkowski, C. 1984. Standardization of test of speech perception in noise. *Journal of Speech and Hearing Research,* 27:32–48.

Bratt, G.W. 1980. Hearing aid receiver output in occluded ear canals in children. Ph.D. diss., Vanderbilt University, Nashville.

Bratt, G.W., Peek, B.F., Bacon, S.P., and Logan, S.A. 1987. Variance from prescribed frequency response in custom ITE hearing aids. Paper read at the annual convention of the American Speech-Language-Hearing Association, November 1987, New Orleans.

Byrne, D. 1987. Hearing aid selection formulae: Same or different? *Hearing Instruments* 38(1):5–11.

Byrne, D., and Dillon, H. 1986. The National Acoustic Laboratories (NAL) new procedure for selecting the gain and frequency response of a hearing aid. *Ear and Hearing* 7(4):257–65.

Byrne, D., Parkinson, A., and Newall, P. 1990. Hearing aid gain and frequency response requirements for the severely/profoundly hearing impaired. *Ear and Hearing* 11(1):40–49.

Carhart, R. 1946. Tests for the selection of hearing aids. *Laryngoscope* 56:780–94.

Cox, R.M. 1979. Acoustic aspects of hearing aid—ear canal coupling systems. *Monographs in Contemporary Audiology* 1(3).

Cox, R.M. 1985a. ULCL-based prescriptions for in-the-ear hearing aids. *Hearing Instruments* 4:12–14.

Cox, R.M. 1985b. A structured approach to hearing aid selection. *Ear and Hearing* 6:226–39.

Cox, R.M. 1988. The MSU hearing instrument prescription procedure. *Hearing Instruments* 39(1):6,8,10.

Cranmer, K.S. 1990. Hearing instrument dispensing—1990. *Hearing Instruments* 41(6):4,6 12.

Feigin, J.A., Kopun, J.G., Stelmachowicz, P.G., and Gorga, M.P. 1989. Probe-tube microphone measures of ear-canal sound pressure levels in infants and children. *Ear and Hearing* 10:254–58.

Hedges, A. 1989. Personal communication.

Humes, L.E. 1986. An evaluation of several rationales for selecting hearing aid gain. *Journal of Speech and Hearing Disorders* 51:272–281.

Humes, L.E., and Hackett, T. 1990. Comparison of frequency response and aided speech-recognition performance for hearing aids selected by three different prescriptive methods. *Journal of American Academy Audiology* 1:101–108.

Kalikow, D.N, Stevens, K.M., and Elliott, L.L. 1977. Development of a test of speech intelligibility in noise using sentence materials with controlled word predictability. *Journal of the Acoustical Society of America* 61(5): 1337–1351.

Libby, E.R. 1986. The ⅓–⅔ insertion gain hearing aid selection guide. *Hearing Instruments* 37:27–28.

Lyregaard, P.E. 1986. On the practical validity of POGO. *Hearing Instruments* 37(5):12–14,16,147.

Mahon, W.J. 1989. 1989 U.S. hearing aid sales summary. *Hearing Journal* 42(12):9–12.

McCandless, G.A. and Lyregaard, P.E. 1983. Prescription of gain/output (POGO) for hearing aids. *Hearing Instruments* 34(1):16–17,19–21.

Mueller, G. 1989. Individualizing the ordering of custom hearing instruments. *Hearing Instruments* 40(2):18,20,22.

Punch, J. and Beck, E. 1980. Low-frequency response of

hearing aids and judgments of aided speech quality. *Journal of Speech and Hearing Disorders* 45:325–35.

Punch, J., Chi, C., and Patterson, J. 1990. A recommended protocol for prescriptive use of target gain rules. *Hearing Instruments* 41(4):12,14,16,18–19.

Sammeth, C. 1990. Current availability of digital and digital-hybrid hearing aids. *Seminars in Hearing* 11(1): 91–100.

Sammeth, C., Bess, F., Bratt, G., Peek, B., Logan, S., and Amberg, S. 1989. The Vanderbilt/Veterans Administration hearing aid selection study: Interim report. Poster presentation at the annual meeting of the American Speech-Language-Hearing Association, November 1989, St. Louis.

Seewald, R.C., Ross, M., and Spiro, M.K. 1985. Selecting amplification characteristics for young hearing-impaired children. *Ear and Hearing* 6:48–55.

Schwartz, D.M., Lyregaard, P.E., and Lundh, P. 1988. Hearing aid selection for severe-to-profound hearing loss (POGO II). *Hearing Journal* 41(2):13–17.

Shapiro, I. 1976. Hearing aid fitting by prescription. *Audiology* 15:163–173.

Skinner, M.W., Pascoe, D.P., Miller, J.D., and Popelka, G.R. 1982. Measurements to determine the optimal placement of speech energy within the listener's auditory area: A basis for selecting amplification characteristics. In *The Vanderbilt Hearing Aid Report* eds. G.A. Studebaker and F.H. Bess. Upper Darby, PA: Monographs in Contemporary Audiology.

Tyler, S. 1986. Adjusting a hearing aid to amplify speech to the MCL. *Hearing Journal* August:24–27.

CHAPTER 4
Output Limiting and Speech Enhancement

David A. Preves

The purpose of this chapter is to review several techniques for output limiting and speech enhancement in hearing aids. The primary goal of output limiting is to keep the saturation sound pressure level (SSPL90) of a hearing aid below the loudness discomfort level (LDL) of the hearing aid wearer. Secondary goals are to provide automatic level adjustment and to improve speech intelligibility, if possible, via the output limiting process. Methods of output limiting include peak clipping, compression or automatic gain control, and adaptive high-pass filtering. Speech intelligibility improvement may be obtained by reducing the amplification of environmental noise, by enhancing the speech signal, or by a combination of both. Some of the output limiting methods traditionally used in hearing aids also enhance the speech signal, at least in terms of increasing the amplitude of consonants relative to the amplitude of vowels (table I). Theoretically, consonant-vowel-ratio (CVR) enhancement is expected to improve speech intelligibility, but relatively little work has been done to substantiate this theory. Improving CVR by increasing consonant level to audibility may be more important to speech perception than enhancing CVR itself (e.g., Freyman and Nerbonne 1989)

Techniques primarily intended for speech enhancement rather than for output limiting include signal expansion as well as high-pass filtering, with and without infinite amplitude clipping. Methods for reducing environmental noise and improving signal-to-noise ratio (S/N) are discussed elsewhere in this volume. Other speech enhancement techniques that will not be discussed are changing the duration of speech segments, spectral sharpening of formants to increase peak-to-valley differences, and manipulation of the shape of the short-term speech spectrum (Williamson and Punch 1990).

Most of the currently available output limiting

and speech enhancement techniques have been implemented in hearing aids with analog circuitry or with programmable-digital-control of analog circuitry. On the other hand, many of the techniques specifically intended for speech enhancement such as consonant/vowel ratio manipulation have been systematically studied primarily with digital algorithms in nonhearing aid implementations (e.g., Montgomery and Edge 1988; Harasaki and Ozawa 1983; Ohde and Stevens 1983). While digital techniques for improving the CVR provide exquisite control over the levels of individual consonants and vowels as compared to that provided by analog circuitry, these algorithms, due to their complexity, may not be currently packagable in cosmetically-appealing, headworn hearing aids.

Assessing CVR for
Output Limiting/Speech Enhancement

The consonant/vowel and vowel/consonant nonsense syllables in the nonsense syllable test (NST) lists (Resnick et al. 1975) provide a convenient means for assessing the effects of different circuitry on CVR. Several tape-recorded nonsense syllables were digitized in our laboratory with a Spectrum Signal Processing DSP32c System Board in an NEC 386 computer using Hypersignal Workstation software. Ratios of the root mean square (RMS) levels of the consonant and vowel (CVR) in each unprocessed or hearing aid-processed nonsense syllable were determined with DADiSP software. CVRs for processed syllables were assessed for various hearing aid circuits on Knowles Electronic Manikin for Acoustic Research (KEMAR). Three NST syllables /iθ/, /ta/, and /is/ were arbitrarily selected for this chapter to demonstrate changes in CVR with different types of output limiting circuitry: two frequently confused voiceless fricatives, both paired with one vowel in the initial position (/iθ/, /is/), and a voiceless stop paired with another vowel in the fi-

The author is grateful to Brian Woodruff and James Newton of Argosy Electronics for their assistance in implementing and evaluating the circuitry used herein and for their comments on this chapter.

Table I. Several Techniques for Output Limiting and Consonant/Vowel Ratio (CVR) Improvement

	Output limiting	Consonant/vowel ratio improvement
Fixed high-pass filtering	x	x
Adaptive high-pass filtering	x	x
Peak clipping	x	x
High-pass filtering with infinite amplitude clipping	x	x
Gain control with SSPL90 tracking gain	x	
Whole-range syllabic compression	x	x
Compression limiting	x	x
Slow acting AVC	x	
Compression together with high-pass filtering and expansion	x	x

nal position (/ta/). Time segments used for all of the CVR calculations were consistently 257/258, 47/279, and 192/349 ms for /iθ/, /ta/, and /is/, respectively across all conditions. Figure 1 shows the time waveforms for the three syllables directly measured from the tape recording of the NST lists from the Graduate Center for Speech and Hearing Sciences at the City University of New York. From column b in table II, CVRs derived from the time waveforms in figure 1 are −17 dB, −9 dB, and 0 dB for /iθ/, /ta/, and /is/, respectively. This indicates, for example, that the vowel in the unprocessed /iθ/ on the tape is at a 17 dB higher sound pressure level (SPL) than the consonant. The influence of the KEMAR open ear response on the spectra of the three syllables was determined. To facilitate this measurement, the three syllables were reproduced in sound field within a Tracoustics audiometric booth via a Grason Stadler GSI-10 audiometer. The effect of the unaided KEMAR response on the CVRs for the three syllables is seen in column c of table II: relative to the CVRs on the tape, CVRs in the KEMAR open ear were 2 dB poorer, 6 dB better, and 6 dB poorer for /iθ/, /ta/, and /is/, respectively. These decrements in CVR for /iθ/ and /is/ may have been due to vowel energy increasing from peaks in the Manikin Frequency Response occurring at or near one or more vowel formants.

High-Pass Filtering

Although high-pass filtering is not typically thought of as an output limiting technique, sharply sloping high-pass filters can produce enough attenuation to limit the maximum low-frequency signal processed through the hearing aid (figure 2). High-pass filtering alone can produce an increase in speech intelligibility because most of the information-bearing content of speech occurs in the high frequencies (e.g., French and Steinberg 1947 showed that less than a 10% reduction in articulation index would result from virtually eliminating the speech signal below 800 Hz via high-pass filtering). Because of the low-frequency attenuation, consonant amplitude is enhanced relative to vowel amplitude, and an improvement in speech intelligibility in noise may result (Thomas and Ohley 1972). For vowels, high-pass filtering followed by amplification will increase the amplitude of higher formants relative to the amplitude of the first formant. Thomas and Ohley state that a speech signal is obtained that contains more intelligibility information per unit of speech energy than the original speech signal.

Column d in table II shows the CVRs for the three NST syllables provided by a linear in-the-ear (ITE) hearing aid with 2-pole high-pass filter (HPF) having its cutoff frequency adjusted via a low-frequency tone potentiometer to 2 kHz. The hearing aid was mounted on KEMAR, and the CVRs reflect the aided SPL delivered at the KEMAR "eardrum." By 2-pole high-pass filtering, CVRs improved by 2, 7, and 6 dB for /iθ/, /ta/, and /is/, respectively relative to that for the unaided KEMAR condition. As expected, the amount of CVR enhancement is quite dependent on the high-pass filter order and type. The 2-pole filter employed above was a Butterworth design. CVRs were also determined for a 2-pole high-pass Chebychev filter, which produced a steeper slope than the Butterworth filter. Using a 2-pole Chebychev high-pass filter, CVRs improved further for two of the three syllables (by 6, 9, and 6 dB for /iθ/, /ta/, and /is/, respectively) relative to that for the unaided KEMAR condition.

A fixed amount of high-pass filtering is typically implemented in analog hearing aid circuitry by using a ski-slope microphone response and/or tailoring resistor and capacitor values. Several studies have demonstrated that both normal-hearing and hearing-impaired persons associate better sound quality of speech processed by hearing aids with increased low-frequency gain in the hearing aid (e.g., Punch and Beck 1986; Punch et al. 1980).

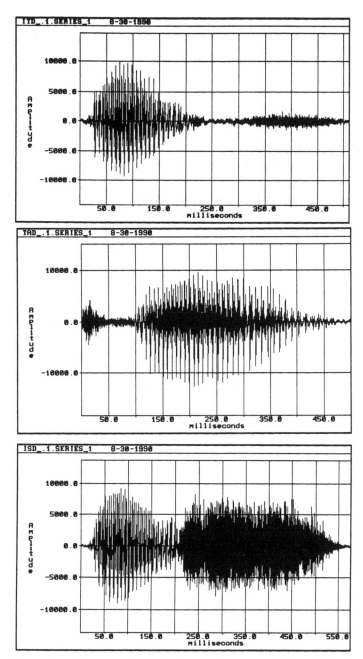

Figure 1. Time waveforms for three nonsense syllables obtained directly from the CUNY tape recording of the NST lists. Top /iθ/; middle /ta/; and bottom /is/.

Table II. Consonant/Vowel Ratios for Three Nonsense Syllables from NST Lists (Reznick et al. 1975)

(a) Syllable	(b) From Tape	(c) KEMAR (unaided)	(d) 2-pole HPF 2kHz fc	(e) Adaptive 4-pole HPF Man. II	(f) Diode clipping Genn. 505	(g) 2-pole HPF/ Infinite clip/ modulated	(h) Syllabic Compress Genn. 512
/iθ/	−17 dB	−19 dB	−17 dB	−18 dB	−13 dB	−12 dB	−11 dB
/ta/	−9	−3	4	0	0	5	4
/is/	0	−6	0	−4	−4	2	−2

dB SSPL90 and Frequency Response Curves

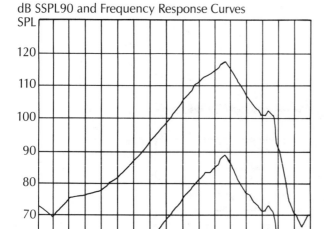

Peak SSPL90: 117 dB SPL @ 3,000kHZ
HFA SSPL90: 104 dB SPL
HFA full on gain: 15 dB
Ref test gain: 14 dB
Frequency Range (F1): 0.620 kHz–(F2): 7,220 kHz

Figure 2. Example of low-frequency output limiting provided by high-pass filtering. Top curve–SSPL90; bottom curve–frequency response. Data per ANSI S3.22–1982.

Although effective in improving the CVR, too little low frequency amplification often elicits comments of "tinny sound quality" from hearing aid wearers. To alleviate this, a variable amount of low-frequency attenuation can be achieved by utilizing screwdriver-actuated tone trimmers or user-adjustable low-frequency tone controls to vary the cutoff frequency or filter order manually.

To provide hearing aid wearers the perception of better sound quality in quiet environments but reduced low-frequency response in noisy backgrounds, an automatically variable amount of low-frequency attenuation has been implemented with voltage-controlled high-pass filters. These adaptive filters increase their cutoff frequency as the level of the input signal increases (e.g., Iwasaki 1981; Kates 1986; Preves and Sigelman 1986). The higher the cutoff frequency, the more the low-frequency attenuation. Recent reports suggest that this type of processing may alleviate upward spread of masking (e.g., Zurek and Rankovic 1990). In addition to reducing the low-frequency gain to suppress background noise, some amount of output limiting is achieved at frequencies below the high-pass filter cutoff frequency (i.e., if the cutoff frequency is allowed to reach higher frequencies in the hearing aid passband at very high input levels, an automatic

gain control [AGC] like effect results with nearly the entire frequency range being attenuated). Figure 3 depicts how the electrical frequency response of a 4-pole adaptive high-pass filter in such a system changes as the input level of a steady-state, shaped noise is raised in 5 dB steps.

Table II, column e gives CVRs provided for the three NST syllables by an ITE hearing aid having a 4-pole, Butterworth adaptive high-pass filter on KEMAR. The three NST syllables were presented at 75 dB SPL. With a 55 dB SPL noise input signal, the adaptive high-pass filter cutoff frequency was preset to 200 Hz, providing maximum low-frequency response as shown in figure 3. The HFA gain of the hearing aid per ANSI S3.22 was 30 dB. CVRs were −18 dB, 0 dB, and −4 dB for /iθ/, /ta/, and /is/, respectively. Because it had maximum low-frequency response at low input SPLs, the hearing aid with 4-pole high-pass filter adapting and removing some low-frequency energy provided 1 dB, 4 dB, and 4 dB poorer CVRs for /iθ/, /ta/, and /is/, respectively, than the fixed 2-pole high-pass filter with 2 kHz cutoff frequency at 75 dB input SPL. However, this still represents a 1 dB, 3 dB, and 2 dB improvement in CVR relative to the unaided KEMAR condition (column b). In fitting sloping high-frequency losses with a hearing aid with such an adaptive high-pass filter, the cutoff frequency of the adaptive filter for low input SPLs would normally be pre-set to a higher cutoff frequency than 200 Hz. Under these

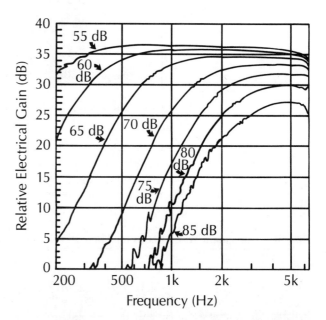

Figure 3. Electrical frequency responses of Argosy Manhattan II adaptive high-pass filter with speech-shaped noise input levels varying in 5 dB steps from 55 dB to 85 dB SPL.

conditions, a further improvement in CVR from this adaptive high-pass filtering technique could be expected.

Peak Clipping

While peak clipping for output limitation usually is implemented in the power output stage of the amplifier, it also may occur unintentionally in other sections of the amplifier if they saturate at lower levels than the output stage. Every hearing aid amplifier has a particular portion of its circuitry that saturates from signal swing limitations at a lower level than other parts of the amplifier. This feature sometimes is used deliberately in preamplifier and signal processing stages to prevent succeeding sections of the amplifier from being overdriven with large signal excursions.

Peak clipping in the amplifier output stage essentially uses the saturation mechanism caused by the inability of the combination of the power output amplifier, battery, and receiver to produce a larger output signal in response to a larger input signal. Saturation occurs because of a limited headroom ceiling (Preves 1990). Headroom is the difference in decibels between the combination of peak input level and gain and the level at which peak clipping occurs (Preves and Woodruff 1990). Inadequate headroom is produced within many linear (nonadaptive) hearing aids that have a low SSPL90 combined with a high gain, causing saturation at high input levels. Because speech and many environmental noises have significant crest factors, hearing aids with linear amplifiers can be driven easily into saturation by even moderate input levels (Frye 1987). Due to inadequate headroom, many linear hearing aids saturate via peak clipping at levels significantly lower than the loudness discomfort level of the hearing aid wearer, producing an unnecessarily low saturation sound pressure level. This problem no doubt has influenced the results of several studies that have employed actual hearing aids to evaluate the effects of various output limiting techniques on speech perception.

Although peak clipping is thought of in a positive sense for limiting the saturation sound pressure level below the loudness discomfort level, it does have an undesirable side effect: because it is a saturation phenomenon, it generates distortion components (Walker and Dillon 1982). Distortions of hearing aid processed signals in adverse signal-to-competing-noise listening conditions cause complaints of poor sound quality and lack of clarity (Agnew 1988). These common complaints may be a direct result of the hearing aid operating in saturation. Saturation via peak clipping creates additional harmonic and intermodulation distortion components that decrease the signal-to-noise ratio (S/N) of signals processed by the hearing aid. Artificial formants may be produced in the processed speech signal output from the hearing aid at multiple frequencies or at difference frequencies of the distortion components (Linblad 1987). These distortions sometimes make the processed speech sound quality so poor and the listening experience so annoying and fatiguing that, in noisy environments, hearing aids are turned off or even removed. It is these distortions that may lead to outright rejection of hearing aids. Reducing the saturation sound pressure level via peak clipping without reducing gain in a linear hearing aid amplifier reduces the headroom and causes saturation to occur at lower input levels.

The type of distortion components introduced by peak clipping depends to a large extent on how clipping is performed. The level at which peak clipping occurs can be made variable in most amplifiers by introducing diodes, resistors, and/or transistors (Keller 1984). One of the simplest forms of peak clipping that achieves a variable output limiting level is implemented with different resistor values in series with the receiver in a class A output stage. This technique usually results in asymmetrical peak clipping with some attendant gain reduction and produces both even and odd harmonics. Whereas resistor clipping produces a strident sound, diode peak clipping generally produces symmetrical peak clipping with little or no accompanying gain reduction. Diode peak clipping results mainly in odd harmonics and has been called soft peak clipping because it usually sounds less harsh than resistor peak clipping (figure 4). The literature is mixed on how asymmetrical and symmetrical peak clipping affect intelligibility. Licklider (1946) states that neither type of peak clipping resulted in a significant reduction in intelligibility even with an "infinite" amount of clipping, whereas Krebs (1972) and Keller (1984) maintain that even harmonics are more detrimental to speech intelligibility than odd harmonics.

Table II, column f shows CVRs provided on KEMAR for the three NST syllables by an ITE hearing aid with 30 dB HFA gain and 100 dB SSPL90 having a Gennum 505 circuit with full diode clipping activated for the output stage. The low-frequency response slope of the hearing aid was approximately the same as that of the hearing aid with the

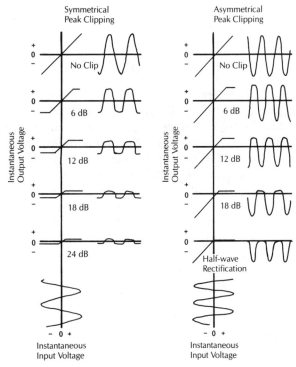

Figure 4. Examples of asymmetrical and symmetrical peak clipping (after Licklider 1946).

2-pole high-pass filter. For these tests, the syllables were presented at 75 dB SPL. The CVRs were −13 dB, 0 dB, and −4 dB for /iθ/, /ta/, and /ls/, respectively, which is 6 dB, 3 dB, and 2 dB better, respectively, than the unaided KEMAR condition CVRs (column c).

High-Pass Filtering with Infinite Amplitude Clipping

Infinite amplitude clipping should be distinguished from peak clipping. Infinite amplitude clipping is not simply asymmetrically or symmetrically lopping off the tops of high level signals with 5 or 10 dB of peak clipping. Infinite amplitude clipping results in even the very lowest levels of a signal between its zero crossings being amplified to the rails or to the limits of the circuitry. Thus, this processing scheme essentially is a zero crossing detector, producing a constant amplitude output signal having the same zero crossings as the input signal waveform. This phenomenon occurs over nearly an infinite range of input signal amplitudes, down to the threshold of the zero crossing detector comparator, essentially independent of how small the input signal amplitude is. Because this type of processing results in a signal expansion at low input levels and signal com-

pression at high input levels, it has the effect of significantly narrowing the dynamic range of a signal. Thus, this output limiting/CVR enhancement technique may be suitable for fitting persons with recruiting ears that have narrow dynamic ranges.

As early as 1948, Licklider and Pollack showed that infinite amplitude clipping preceded by high-pass filtering improved speech intelligibility in white noise for normal hearing subjects. They used a single pole high-pass filter having a 16 kHz cutoff frequency prior to clipping. The white noise was added after clipping. This result was later replicated by Thomas and Niederjohn (1970) who optimized the high-pass filter for highest intelligibility in varying levels of white noise to a second order design with an 1100 Hz cutoff frequency (figure 5). These authors point out that the power level of the speech signal can be increased up to 14 dB by high-pass filtering and infinite amplitude clipping. Similar results were found at statistically significant levels for hearing-impaired listeners by Thomas and Sparks (1971) using the same processing scheme as Thomas and Niederjohn. It is important to note that for all of

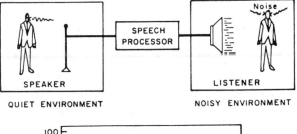

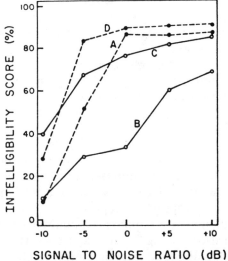

Figure 5. The intelligibility of normal and processed speech in noise. A–high-pass filter, infinitely clipped; B–unmodified speech; C–high-pass filtered, amplitude normalized; D–high-pass filtered (after Niederjohn 1979).

these studies, the modified speech was presented to the listeners at the same level as the unmodified speech.

Niederjohn (1979) suggested, based upon data obtained in several studies, that (1) the high-pass filter/clipper process results in greater speech intelligibility than high-pass filtering alone at higher signal-to-noise ratios, and (2) high-pass filtering alone results in greater speech intelligibility at lower signal-to-noise ratios. According to Niederjohn, this follows because at higher S/Ns it is more important to emphasize low amplitude, unvoiced speech events relative to the higher amplitude voiced speech events than to emphasize higher frequency energy relative to lower frequency energy. Such emphasis would pull low amplitude speech sounds out of the noise. The amplitude of voiced speech will generally be greater than that of the noise anyway. However, at low S/N, attenuating low frequency energy so that high-frequency energy is emphasized is of greater significance.

Qualitatively, this procedure for output limiting and CVR enhancement may be explained as follows. High-pass filtering makes the amplitude of the vowels and consonants more nearly equal by attenuating some of the low-frequency, vowel, first formant energy. Infinite amplitude clipping amplifies the remaining high-frequency consonant energy to the maximum level allowed by the circuitry. Thereafter, the processed signal is more resistant to additive noise. Additionally, high-pass filtering ensures that any distortion products produced will lie mainly in a frequency range above the passband of the hearing aid (Thomas and Ravindran 1974).

In a hearing aid application, noise would be additive with the speech source, rather than at the listener after the clipping occurs as in the above referenced studies. In one of the few studies of infinite amplitude clipping with white noise added prior to the clipper, Thomas and Ravindran (1974) showed that intelligibility improved for hearing-impaired persons with this processing as compared to linear amplification over a range of signal-to-noise ratios (figure 6).

Although high-pass filtered and infinitely clipped speech with white noise added prior to clipping may be more intelligible for hearing-impaired persons, it has a poor sound quality in a quiet environment and is difficult to listen to for long periods of time. As a refinement of the procedure that improves sound quality, Licklider and Pollack (1948) and Thomas and Sparks (1971) added a 20 kHz sine wave modulation and Thomas and Niederjohn (1970) added a 47 kHz sine wave modulation to the

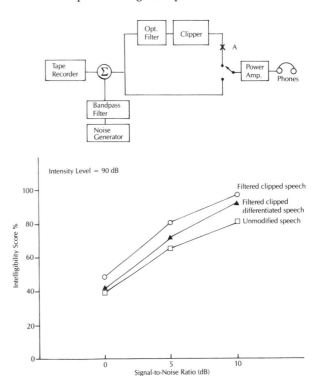

Figure 6. Intelligibility scores in 90 dB SPL of white noise for unmodified speech and for high-pass filtered/ infinitely clipped speech as a function of signal-to-noise ratio. Band-limited white noise added prior to processing. Optimum filter is a 2-pole high-pass with 1100 Hz cutoff frequency (after Thomas and Ravindran 1974).

speech waveform prior to infinite clipping (figure 7). This has the effect of producing a pulse width modulation waveform similar to that used in a class D hearing aid output stage described by Carlson (1988). Licklider and Pollack point out that if the modulation waveform amplitude is comparable to that of the speech waveform amplitude, the infinite clipping/zero crossing detector effect is reduced substantially, resulting in nearly linear processing if the modulation waveform is removed from the clipper output by low-pass filtering. Originally, just enough modulation was added to keep the level of the background noise down in the silent periods between the speech signals. (If the modulation amplitude is comparable to the background noise amplitude, the background noise remaining during the silent periods of speech will be processed nearly linearly rather than being amplified to the highest levels permitted by the amplifier.)

Visser (1987) and Meyers (1988) of Extrema Systems Inc. state that without this added sine modulation, the distortion is so bad that the Licklider and Pollack technique cannot distinguish between sinusoidal and triangular input waveforms. To alleviate

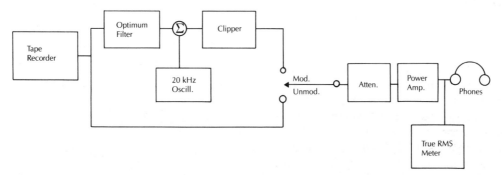

Figure 7. Block diagram showing a 20 kHz oscillator added prior to infinite amplitude clipping to suppress background noise in the silent periods of speech (after Thomas and Sparks 1971).

this problem, Visser advocates a similar technique to that of Licklider and Pollack with a wideband Gaussian noise substituted for the modulating sinusoid (figure 8). To date, there is little published data to be found on speech intelligibility with this modified filtering-clipping technique.

An ITE hearing aid having 30 dB HFA gain and 105 dB HFA SSPL90 was constructed with low-

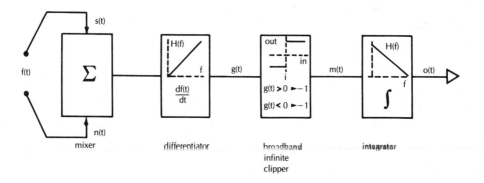

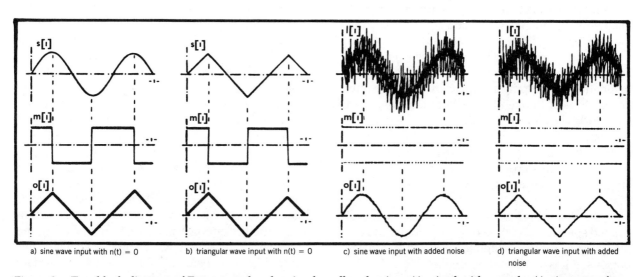

a) sine wave input with n(t) = 0   b) triangular wave input with n(t) = 0   c) sine wave input with added noise   d) triangular wave input with added noise

Figure 8. Top: block diagram of Extrema coder showing broadband noise n(t) mixed with speech. A): time waveform output for a sinusoid input (top) to a high-pass filtered/infinitely clipped system without noise added; middle is clipper output; lower is integrator output. B): same as A) but for a triangle input; note integrator outputs (lower graphs) for sinusoid and triangle are identical. C): same as A) but with noise added to input (top). D): same as B) but with noise added to input (top). Note that integrator output (lower graph) differentiates sinusoid and triangle correctly with noise added to input. (Reprinted, by permission, from Visser [1987], *Official Proceedings of International Speech Tech '87*, Media Dimensions, Inc., 42 East 23 Street, New York, NY 10010. 212-533-7481.)

frequency response approximating that for the 2-pole high-pass filter and diode peak clipping conditions. A 50 kHz triangular modulation was added to the audio signal after the 2-pole high-pass filter and prior to the clipper as in the Licklider and Pollack approach. The amount of infinite amplitude clipping was adjusted by listening tests while varying the level of the 50 kHz modulation. Typical time waveforms for this system are shown in figure 9 as the modulation level is varied. Each of the three charts has one cycle of a 10 kHz sinusoid representing the audio signal to be processed shown in the

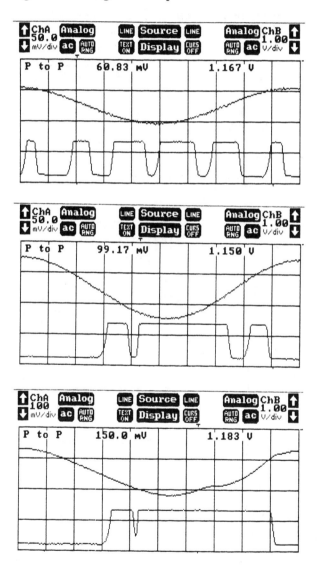

Figure 9. Waveforms from the high-pass filter/clipper system with added sine wave modulation as the modulation level is varied. Upper trace in each—10 kHz sinusoid audio signal; lower trace in each—clipper output. Top chart—linear processing (modulation amplitude larger than audio signal). Middle chart—modulation amplitude equal to audio amplitude. Bottom chart—nearly pure infinite clipping or zero-crossing detector mode.

upper trace and the clipper output shown in the lower trace. The top chart represents linear processing via pulse-width modulation when the modulation amplitude is larger than the audio signal (100 mv versus 60 mv). When integrated, the high frequency modulation signal is filtered out and the clipper output is a sinusoidal audio waveform, but inverted from the top trace. For this amount of modulation, linear processing will be maintained for sinusoidal inputs up to 80 mv. The middle chart represents the condition for modulation amplitude equal to audio amplitude. This is quasilinear/quasizero crossing detector, with less modulation and more of the inverted sinusoid visible in the clipper output. The bottom chart represents nearly pure infinite clipping or zero crossing detection with the clipper output being an almost perfect inversion of the sinusoid and with essentially no carrier present. The final amount of infinite clipping was derived empirically by trading off reasonable sound quality with the sensation of significant consonant emphasis. This setting resulted in linear amplification for a 4 kHz sinusoid at input levels up to 74 dB SPL and infinite amplitude clipping above this level. Because of the 2-pole high-pass filter prior to the clipper, the input level was higher for lower frequencies before the onset of infinite clipping. Table II, column g shows that the CVRs provided by this hearing aid were −12 dB, 5 dB, and 2 dB for /iθ/, /ta/, and /is/, respectively, which is 7 dB, 8 dB, and 8 dB better, respectively, than the unaided KEMAR condition CVRs (column c). The net result from adding the modulation and clipping was a 5 dB, 1 dB, and 2 dB further increase in CVRs for /iθ/, /ta/, and /is/, respectively, relative to that for the same 2-pole high-pass filter alone.

Notwithstanding the clear and substantive results of the older investigations of Licklider, Niederjohn, Thomas, and others, many of the subsequent studies have reached different conclusions regarding whether peak clipping for *hearing aids* reduces speech intelligibility as compared to AGC or linear processing. The lack of agreement in the literature may have resulted from several factors, including (1) not specifying the type and amount of clipping technique used (i.e., asymmetrical or symmetrical and whether peak clipping or infinite amplitude clipping was used), (2) not restoring the overall RMS signal level following clipping to equal that of the signal or signals it is being compared to, (3) not specifying whether any high-pass filtering was employed prior to clipping, and (4) utilizing laboratory instrumentation for the evaluations that had infinite headroom compared to the headroom provided by hearing aid components with their low voltage batteries.

Output Limiting with the Hearing Aid Gain Control

Linear amplification may not be ideal for persons with recruitment or a tolerance problem. Because high gain must be provided in order to make the weaker high-frequency sounds audible, more intense sounds may become too loud to the point of being intolerable. A variable amount of output limiting that does not introduce distortion can be achieved under control of the hearing aid wearer by utilizing a circuit in which the gain control reduces SSPL90 as it reduces gain. With this type of circuit, SSPL90 and gain track each other and change in the same relationship together as the gain control on the hearing aid is turned up and down. Figure 10 shows an example of such a hearing aid circuit (Argosy Manhattan II) in which HFA gain and HFA SSPL90 per ANSI S3.22 track each other as the gain control is rotated. Gain and SSPL also track each

other for input compression hearing aids as the gain control is rotated. This simple technique of output limiting is not expected to provide speech enhancement. To the contrary, it may detract from speech intelligibility when the gain control is turned down to avoid discomfort from high input levels, especially in background noise.

Compression or Automatic Gain Control

Lowering the gain of a hearing aid also may be accomplished automatically with compression. Compression, like peak clipping, has been used in input stages of hearing aid amplifiers to reduce the level excursions presented to succeeding amplifier sections. Unlike peak clipping, however, it accomplishes this without introducing harmonic distortion. However, compression systems have a finite

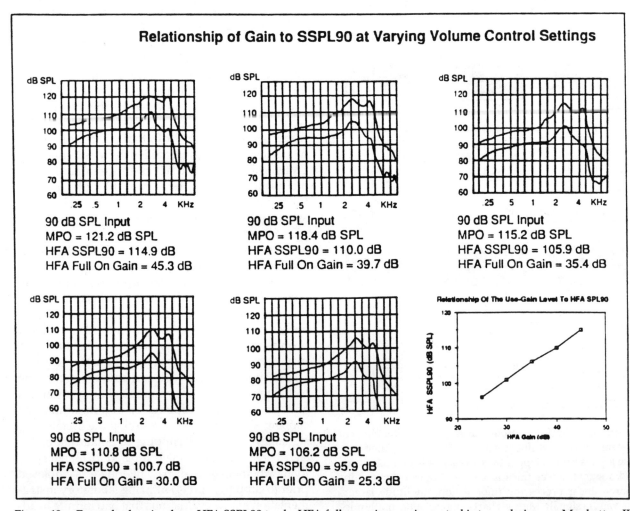

Figure 10. Example showing how HFA SSPL90 tracks HFA full-on gain as gain control is turned. Argosy Manhattan II ITE hearing aid on HA-1 2 cc coupler.

dynamic range of input levels they can function over, especially with the limited headroom available in hearing aid circuitry; when the input level becomes so high as to permit the signal to exceed the range of the compressor, saturation occurs. Nielsen (1972) points out that compression may be thought of as that part of the input/output characteristic between gain and saturation (figure 11).

Compression has been studied for use in hearing aids for about 40 years (e.g., see Braida et al. 1979; Walker and Dillon 1982). During this time there have been numerous studies examining whether compression is superior to linear processing and how varying compression ratio, compression threshold, and attack and recovery times affect speech intelligibility. Some researchers have produced conflicting data in comparing compression to linear processing and while attempting to optimize compression parameter values. Among the possible reasons for this lack of consensus are (1) comparing results for subjects with different types of auditory system pathologies, different hearing loss configurations, and different dynamic ranges; (2) studying the effects of varying compression parameters with different types of recorded speech stimuli, some being precompressed during recording; (3) comparing data from hearing aids having different attack and recovery times, different compression ratios, and different AGC kneepoints; and (4) comparing results from studies employing actual hearing aids to those utilizing laboratory equipment having comparatively infinite headroom. The general inconclusiveness about compression has led researchers and clinicians to continue to ask whether it is appropriate to use AGC in hearing aids for persons with reduced dynamic range (e.g., King and Martin 1984; Peterson, Feeney, and Yantis 1990). Adding a confounding factor to these inconsistencies, the trade literature is contaminated with much

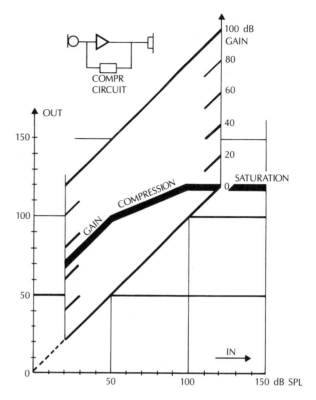

Figure 11. Compression as that portion of the input/output characteristic between gain and saturation (Nielsen 1973).

jargon, making it difficult to identify which type of compression is being used. At times in this literature, peak clipping aids have been said to have compression.

Walker and Dillon (1982) describe two categories of compression—single channel and multi-channel —and further, three distinct types of compression: compression limiting, whole-range syllabic compression, and slow acting automatic volume control (AVC). Their classification system is shown in table III.

Table III. Classification Scheme for Compression Hearing Aids (After Walker and Dillon 1982)

	Low Compression Threshold		High Compression Threshold	
	LOW CR*	HIGH CR*	LOW CR	HIGH CR
Short time constants	Whole range syllabic compression	Whole range syllabic compression	—	Compression limiting
Long time constants	Slow acting automatic volume control	Slow acting automatic volume control	—	—

*CR = compression ratio

Whole-Range Syllabic Compressors

Whole-range syllabic compression may be particularly useful in mapping the entire dynamic range of input signals into the dynamic range of an impaired auditory system that exhibits recruitment. Syllabic compressors generally have a low-compression threshold, a low-compression ratio, and short time constants. Niederjohn and Grotelueschen (1976) studied the effects on speech intelligibility, in high levels of competing noise, of high-pass filtering followed by automatic amplitude normalization (syllabic compression). They hypothesized that, unlike infinite amplitude clipping, compression does not introduce harmonic distortion and so may result in better processed sound quality. They employed a compressor with rapid attack and release times (8 ms) so as not to interfere with the transient characteristics of speech. Additionally, they pointed out that because of its quick response time, the compressor would produce an attenuation of high-level vowel energy which would tend to increase the CVR. They found significant intelligibility advantages for high-pass filtering followed by amplitude normalization compared to unprocessed speech and to high-pass filtering followed by infinite amplitude clipping. Bustamente and Braida (1987) also found that, depending on the amount of pre-compression high-frequency emphasis, intelligibility of vowels or consonants would be enhanced. They concluded that high-pass filtering preceding single channel, wideband syllabic compression provides an advantage over linear amplification for lower input level signals but not for higher input level signals. Vargo (1977) found better speech intelligibility for high-pass filtering and compression as compared to linear processing only at 10 dB SL presentation level, but not at 20 or 30 dB SL. Dreschler (1988a) indicated that syllabic compression equalizes levels between successive sounds, thus bringing up consonant levels. This is especially valuable for persons with severely reduced dynamic ranges. He concluded that for better speech perception, the compression threshold should be set below the mean presentation level. In another study, the same author found that the advantage of syllabic compression in compensating for a reduced dynamic range may be lost in noisy backgrounds (Dreschler, Eberhardt, and Melk 1984).

Although syllabic compression has considerable intuitive face validity for compensating the reduced dynamic range of hearing-impaired persons, it is not routinely employed in a high percentage of hearing aid fittings. Several researchers have shown little if any benefit when comparing syllabic compression to linear amplification. Walker and Dillon (1982) and Dreschler (1988b) speculate that the benefits of recruitment compensation may be nullified in effect by temporal distortions from the compressor attack and recovery times and its alterations of the normal intensity cues of speech. The effectiveness of syllabic compressors as output limiters is somewhat questionable because of their low compression ratios. For this reason, King and Martin (1984) recommended that syllabic compressors employ lower compression thresholds so that louder sounds do not exceed the listener's loudness discomfort level.

Compression Limiters

A compression limiter generally employs a much higher compression ratio than the syllabic compressor and may thus be a more effective limiter in terms of controlling the peak output SPL from a hearing aid. Compression limiters frequently are used in place of peak clippers in hearing aids to limit SSPL90 without producing harmonic distortion. Because compression limiting is only active at high signal levels, it may provide output limitation with some CVR enhancement without significantly altering the dynamics of conversational speech signals compared to the effect of a syllabic compressor (Caraway and Carhart 1967; Walker and Dillon 1982). Studies evaluating compression limiting systems have in general produced more positive results than those that evaluated syllabic compressors. In one of the first uses of compression, Edgardh (1952) recommended a compression limiter for hearing-impaired listeners to equalize the dynamic differences between consonant and vowel levels. In this thoughtful article, the author speculated as to whether the resulting abnormal amplification of respiratory sounds would have a disturbing effect on the listener and whether the size of the circuitry required could be small enough for hearing aid packaging. Peterson, Feeney, and Yantis (1990) concluded from recordings of processed speech through a single channel AGC hearing aid that AGC improves speech perception of low-intensity high-frequency fricatives and stops in quiet, in comparison to linear amplification for those hearing-impaired listeners with significantly reduced dynamic ranges. However, they found that this advantage was not shown for listeners with larger dynamic ranges. They also concluded that the single channel AGC hearing aid produced poorer speech perception, as compared to linear amplification, for low-intensity, high-frequency fricatives and stops in cafeteria babble at a single SNR. The compression threshold for the hearing aid employed in their study was set at 60 dB SPL so that it was always compressing for the 75 dB SPL speech signal utilized. While this situation might be categorized as an example of syllable compression, the compression ratio was 10:1, more typical for output limiters, and the recovery time of the compression circuit was 180 ms. This recovery time is much slower than that suggested in most studies for syllabic compressors so as to prevent the AGC time constants from affecting the dynamics of the speech signal.

Recently, to compensate for a reduced dynamic range while also providing output limiting, some compression amplifiers employ both syllabic compression and compression limiting. Table II, column h shows CVRs obtained for such a circuit (Gennum 512 compression amplifier) in an ITE hearing aid on KEMAR. HFA gain was 30 dB and HFA SSPL90 was 101 dB for this hearing aid. The aid was operating as a syllabic compressor for input levels above 50 dB SPL and the threshold for compression limiting was 85 dB SPL. Attack time was 6 ms and recovery time was 48 ms. The low-frequency response of this hearing aid was similar to that provided by the ITE hearing aid with 4-pole adaptive high-pass filter. CVRs were -11 dB, 4 dB, and -2 dB for the three nonsense syllables /iθ/, /ta/, and /is/, respectively. Thus, CVRs improved by 8 dB, 7 dB, and 4 dB for /iθ/, /ta/, and /is/, respectively, relative to those for the unaided KEMAR condition.

Slow Acting AVC

Slow acting automatic volume control (AVC) systems are useful in limiting maximum output while preventing harmonic distortion from peak clipping saturation. Although this type of compression commonly is used in cassette tape recorders for keeping the signal level fairly constant, it has not been widely used in hearing aids. In a hearing aid application, this feature may reduce the need for hearing aid wearers to adjust the gain control over a wide range of environmental input levels. There is scant research in the compression literature as to the viability of employing slow acting AVC in hearing aids. King and Martin (1984) showed that slow acting AGC with a 1-second recovery time with a high compression threshold was preferred by listeners over AGC circuits with a faster recovery

time. They also point out that the exact compression ratio is not critical, except for persons with very restricted dynamic ranges.

Output Compression (AGC$_o$) and Input Compression (AGC$_i$)

There are several salient differences between these two types of compression systems. Most of these involve how the compressor interacts with gain control as shown in the following exhibit.

	AGC$_o$	AGC$_i$
Gain control location	Gain control located before AGC level sensor	Located after AGC level sensor
Effect of gain control on compression threshold	Threshold varies with gain control setting	Threshold doesn't vary with gain control setting
Effect of gain control on SSPL	SSPL doesn't vary with gain control setting	SSPL varies with gain control setting
Notes	Effect of tone controls may be reduced by AGC	Maps dynamic range of input into dynamic range of listener; often used with peak clipping circuit for independent control of SSPL

With low compression ratios, it is not atypical for input AGC to reduce input signal dynamic range from 30 dB to 7–8 dB (Dreschler 1988a). Dreschler, Eberhardt, and Melk (1984) were not able to find a difference in speech reception threshold in quiet or in noise between a linear hearing aid and two AGC$_o$ and two AGC$_i$ hearing aids. In this study, to cover all bases, evaluations were performed both with the gain controls fixed and with the subjects adjusting the gain controls for the AGC hearing aids. Likewise, King and Martin (1984) found no preference between AGC$_o$ and AGC$_i$ as long as the AGC$_o$ compression threshold was suitable for each individual. Dillon and Walker (1983) recommend either AGC$_o$ or AGC$_i$ for whole-range syllabic compressors, AGC$_o$ for compression limiters, and AGC$_i$ for slow acting AVC systems.

Multichannel Compressors

To eliminate the problem of single channel compressors in which gain across the entire frequency range is reduced by a low-frequency noise, a multiband compressor having independent AGC circuits for each frequency band has been utilized. Such a system is thought to be superior to a single band compressor, especially for severely hearing-impaired persons with extreme loudness recruitment (Villchur 1973; Waldhauer and Villchur 1988). With multichannel compression, low-frequency noise theoretically would cause gain reduction only in the low-frequency band(s) and the weaker high-frequency components of speech, critical for good speech intelligibility, would continue to be maximally amplified (Kates 1986). In addition, severe loudness recruitment in the high frequencies may be compensated for by a separate high-frequency band compressor (Goldberg 1982; Laurence, Moore, and Glasberg 1983).

Several reports have documented the benefits of multichannel compression hearing aids over single channel and linear hearing aids (Yanick 1976; Mangold and Leijon 1981; Goldberg 1982; Laurence, Moore, and Glasberg 1983; Moore and Glasberg 1986; Moore 1987; Moore and Glasberg 1988). There also are studies that have generally failed to demonstrate significant improvements in speech intelligibility in noise using multichannel AGC systems over single channel AGC and linear amplification hearing aids (Barfod 1976; O'Loughlin 1980; Abramovitz 1980; Lippman, Braida, and Durlach 1981; Byrne and Walker 1982; Nabelek 1983).

Bustamante and Braida (1987) compared three approaches to syllabic compression: single channel wideband, multichannel with 16-bands, and principal components. The authors controlled two short-term principal components: overall level and spectral tilt. It was thought that control of these components would greatly reduce the range of speech level variations without reducing the peak/valley structure of the short-term speech spectrum. They found that over a 10 to 15 dB range of input levels, multiband compression did not provide higher intelligibility than either carefully shaped linear amplification or wideband compression (from single channel compression and first principal component compression); manipulating the second principal component, spectral tilt, degraded speech intelligibility relative to linear amplification, possibly due to reduced spectral differences between weak fricatives.

High compression ratios with multichannel

AGC may degrade the relative intensity cues required to identify stops or fricatives (De Gennaro, Braida, and Durlach 1986; Plomp 1988). The problems with interference of the speech signal by syllabic compressors may apply even more strongly to fast-acting multichannel AGC (King and Martin 1984). The optimal time constants for multiband compression in hearing aids are still debatable in terms of whether the circuit should react to and correct for the rapid level changes of speech—a kind of deliberate distortion of the speech signal in itself— or whether the natural temporal and spectral cues of speech should be preserved (Braida et al. 1982; Plomp 1989). Fast-acting multichannel compressors with many independent compression bands reduce the natural amplitude contrasts in the speech signal (Plomp 1988). Therefore, Plomp contends that longer compressor time constants be used with multichannel AGC. However, Villchur (1989) reminds us that Licklider and Pollack (1948) showed that speech was perfectly intelligible after infinite amplitude clipping, working with a signal with no amplitude contrasts. Villchur states that although multichannel AGC decreases the peak-to-valley level differences within speech, the audibility of weaker components of speech such as consonants may be preserved after compression. He concluded that only field experience with 2-channel compression will prove the viability of multichannel AGC.

Frequency-Dependent Compression

Although not a true multichannel compression system, a single channel AGC system with frequency-dependent compression provides a restricted amount of control over compression threshold by frequency. Frequency-dependent compression usually refers to a type of input compression in which the compression threshold changes as a function of frequency. In most implementations of single channel compressors, a greater low-frequency SPL than high-frequency SPL is required to cause a gain reduction in the high frequencies. This pseudomultichannel AGC effect is achieved by making the compression threshold higher in the lower frequencies than in the higher frequencies. This feature is easily provided with a high-pass filter near the front end of the amplifier. This filter may take the form of a fixed low-frequency slope in the preamplifier, a variable tone control, or a high-pass microphone response. Virtually every hearing aid that incorporates a tone control prior to the AGC sensor in the forward path of the hearing aid has frequency-dependent compression (Walker and Dillon 1982).

Recently, frequency-dependent compressors have been developed with the high-pass filter in the AGC feedback loop (Killion 1988). These systems have higher compression thresholds for low-frequency energy than for high-frequency energy (Walker and Dillon 1982). However, they also exhibit a pseudomultichannel AGC effect by lowering high-frequency gain more than low-frequency gain when the input signal level is increased (Killion, Staab, and Preves 1990; Dillion 1988).

Employing Expansion and Compression Together

Whereas compression tends to keep the hearing aid output signal at a constant level or at least reduces the difference between different levels in the input signal, expansion does the opposite. Expansion magnifies the differences between signals and does not attempt to hold the signal at a constant level. This type of processing may be useful in improving S/N compared to linear processing for low level signals (Villchur 1973; Dillon 1989).

There are few studies in the literature that evaluate the use of expansion in hearing aids. Yanick and Drucker (1976) concluded that a combination of expansion and compression was superior to both compression and linear amplification. Walker, Byrne, and Dillon (1984) evaluated speech intelligibility for a 6-channel expander/compressor for a small group of subjects (figure 12). The expander operated mainly on low-level energy in the high-frequency channels. They concluded that expansion degraded low-level speech intelligibility, or, at best, did not change it as compared to linear 6-channel frequency shaping. Most notably, expansion failed to improve intelligibility of very low-level final consonants. Perhaps the outcome of this study was influenced by the degradation of the speech signal resulting from automatically manipulating the gain simultaneously in 6 bands. As a follow-up study, it may be worthwhile to evaluate an expander/compressor system with fewer channels.

Conclusion

This chapter has reviewed several output limiting techniques, some of which also provide consonant/vowel ratio (CVR) enhancement. Most of the techniques involving high-pass filtering and compression achieve CVR enhancement by attenuating

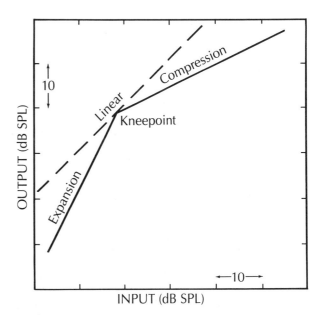

Figure 12. Input/output transfer functions of linear and expansion/compression processing (Walker, Bryne, and Dillon 1984).

vowel energy without a significant accompanying attenuation of consonant energy. Thus, the resulting signal, when amplified, has a higher CVR. A few of the output limiting/CVR enhancement methods, such as high-pass filtering with infinite amplitude clipping and compression/expansion, appear to increase consonant energy while attenuating vowel levels. Further investigation is needed to determine whether these CVR enhancements result in improved speech perception in both quiet environments and in competing noise. Specifically, further research is needed to determine whether making consonants audible as a result of improving CVR is more significant than improving the CVR itself.

References

Abramovitz, R. 1980. Frequency shaping and multiband compression in hearing aids. *Journal of Communication Disorders* 13:483–88.

Agnew, G. 1988. Hearing instrument distortion: What does it mean for the listener? *Hearing Instruments* 39(10):10–20.

ANSI S3.22-1982 Specification of hearing aid characteristics: American National Standards Institute. New York.

Barfod, J. 1976. Multi channel compression hearing aids, Report 11, The Acoustics Lab., Tech. Univ. of Denmark.

Braida, L., Durlach, N., Lippman, R., Hicks, B., Rabinowitz, W., and Reed, C. 1979. Hearing aids—A review of past research on linear amplification, amplitude compression, and frequency lowering. *ASHA Monograph No. 19.* Rockville, MD.

Braida, L., Durlach, N., De Gennaro, S., Peterson, P., and Bustamante, D. 1982. Review of recent research on multiband amplitude compression for the hearing impaired, *The Vanderbilt Hearing Aid Report*, eds. G. Studebaker and F. Bess, Upper Darby, PA: Monographs in Contemporary Audiology.

Bustamante, D., and Braida, L. 1987. Principle component—Amplitude compression for the hearing impaired. *Journal of the Acoustical Society of America* 82(4):1227–1242.

Byrne, D., and Walker, G. 1982. The effects of multichannel compression and expansion amplification on perceived quality of speech. *Australian Journal of Audiology* 4(1):1–8.

Caraway, B., and Carhart, R. 1967. Influence of compressor action on speech intelligibility. *Journal of the Acoustical Society of America* 41(6):1424–1433.

Carlson, E. 1988. An output amplifier whose time has come. *Hearing Instruments* 39(10):30–32.

DeGennaro, S., Braida, L., and Durlach, N. 1986. Multiband syllabic compression for severely impaired listeners. *Journal of Rehabilitative Research and Development* 23:17–24.

Dillon, H. 1988. Compression in hearing aids. In *Handbook of Hearing Aid Amplification, V. 1* ed. R. Sandlin Boston: College-Hill Press.

Dillon, H. 1989. U.S. Patent #4,803,732. 1989. Hearing aid amplification method and apparatus.

Dillon, H., and Walker, G. 1983. Compression—input or output control? *Hearing Instruments* 34(9):20–22.

Dreschler, W. 1988a. The effect of specific compression settings on phoneme identification in hearing-impaired subjects. *Scandinavian Audiology* 17:35–43.

Dreschler, W. 1988b. Dynamic-range reduction by peak clipping or compression and its effects on phoneme perception in hearing-impaired listeners. *Scandinavian Audiology* 17:45–51.

Dreschler, W., Eberhardt, D., and Melk, P. 1984. The use of single-channel compression for the improvement of speech intelligibility. *Scandinavian Audiology* 13:231–36.

Edgardh, B. 1952. The use of extreme limitation for the dynamic equalization of vowels and consonants in hearing aids. *Acta Otolaryngology* 40:376–86.

French, N.R., and Steinberg, J.C. 1947. Factors governing the intelligibility of speech sounds. *Journal of the Acoustical Society of America.* 19:90–119.

Freyman, R., and Nerbonne, G. 1989. The importance of consonant-vowel intensity ratio in the intelligibility of voiceless consonants. *Journal of Speech and Hearing Research* 32:524–35.

Frye, G. 1987. Crest factor and composite signals for hearing aid testing. *Hearing Journal* 40(10):15–18.

Goldberg, H. 1982. Signal processors: application to the hearing-impaired. *Hearing Aid Journal* 35(4):23–27.

Harasaki, H., and Ozawa, S. 1983. Hearing aid using an emphasized speech for hearing-impaired subjects. Paper read at 106th Annual Meeting of the Acoustical Society of America, San Diego.

Iwasaki, S. 1981. Automatic noise suppression in hearing aids. *Hearing Aid Journal* 13:10–11.

Kates, J. 1986. Signal processing for hearing aids. *Hearing Instruments* 36(2):19–22.

Keller, F. 1984. Peak clipping. *Hearing Instruments* 35(4):24–26.

Killion, M. 1988. An "acoustically invisible" hearing aid. *Hearing Instruments* 39(10):44.

Killion, M., Staab, W., and Preves, D. 1990. Classifying automatic signal processors. *Hearing Instrument* 41(8):24.

King, A., and Martin, M. 1984. Is AGC beneficial in hearing aids? *British Journal of Audiology* 18:31–38.

Krebs, D. 1972. Output limiting and related harmonic distortion. Paper read at Oticongress 2, Copenhagen.

Laurence, R., Moore, B., and Glasberg, B. 1983. A comparison of behind-the-ear high-fidelity linear hearing aids and two-channel compression aids, in the laboratory and in everyday life. *British Journal of Audiology,* 17:31–48.

Licklider, J. 1946. Effects of amplitude distortion upon the intelligibility of speech. *Journal of the Acoustical Society of America* 18(2):429–434.

Licklider, J., and Pollack, I. 1948. Effects of differentiation, integration and infinite peak clipping upon the intelligibility of speech. *Journal of the Acoustical Society of America* 20:42–51.

Linblad, A.C. 1984. Influence of nonlinear distortion on speech intelligibility: Hearing-impaired listeners. *Report TA # 116.* Karolinska Institute, Stockholm: Dept. of Technical Audiology.

Lippmann, R., Braida, L., and Durlach, N. 1981. Study of multichannel amplitude compression and linear amplification for persons with sensorineural hearing loss. *Journal of the Acoustical Society of America* 69:524–31.

Mangold, S., and Leijon, A. 1981. Multichannel compression in a portable programmable hearing aid. *Hearing Aid Journal* 34(6):29–32.

Meyers, R. 1988. Extrema Coding: Perception-based signal processing. *Speech Technology* 4(3):68–73.

Montgomery, A., and Edge, R. 1988. Evaluation of two speech enhancement techniques to improve intelligibility for hearing-impaired adults. *Journal of Speech and Hearing Research* 31:386–93.

Moore, B. 1987. Design and evaluation of a two-channel compression hearing aid. *Journal of Rehabilitation Research and Development* 24(4):181–92.

Moore, B., and Glasberg, B. 1986. A comparison of two-channel and single-channel compression hearing aids. *Audiology* 25:210–26.

Moore, B., and Glasberg, B. 1988. A comparison of four methods of implementing automatic gain control (AGC) in hearing aids. *British Journal of Audiology* 22:93–104.

Nábèlèk, I. 1983. Performance of hearing-impaired listeners under various types of amplitude compression. *Journal of the Acoustical Society of America* 74(3):776–91.

Niederjohn, R. 1979. Speech processing for improved intelligibility in high noise levels. *Proceedings of Conference on Auditory and Hearing Prosthetics Research* In V. Larson, and D. Egolf, R. Kirlin, and S. Stiles New York: Grune & Stratton.

Niederjohn, R., and Grotelueschen, J. 1976. The enhancement of speech intelligibility in high noise levels by high-pass filtering followed by rapid amplitude compression. *IEEE Transactions of Acoustics, Speech and Signal Processing* ASSP-24 (4):277–82.

Nielsen, T.E. 1972. Information about various methods of output limitation. Oticongress 2, Copenhagen.

Ohde, R., and Stevens, K. 1983. Effect of burst amplitude on the perception of stop consonant place of articulation. *Journal of the Acoustical Society of America* 74(3): 706–714.

O'Loughlin, B. 1980. Evaluation of a three channel compression amplification system on hearing-impaired children. *Australian Journal of Audiology* 2:1–9.

Peterson, M., Feeney, P., and Yantis, P. 1990. The effect of automatic gain control in hearing-impaired listeners with different dynamic ranges. *Ear and Hearing* 11(3): 185–94.

Plomp, R. 1988. The negative effect of amplitude compression in multichannel hearing aids in the light of the modulation-transfer function. *Journal of the Acoustical Society of America* 83:2322–2327.

Plomp, R. 1989. Reply to "Comments on 'The negative effect of amplitude compression in multichannel hearing aids in the light of the modulation-transfer function' " [*Journal of the Acoustical Society of America* 86:425–27 (1989)]. *Journal of the Acoustical Society of America* 86(1): 428.

Preves, D. 1990. Expressing noise and distortion with the coherence measurement. *ASHA* 32, June/July:56–59.

Preves, D., and Sigelman, J. 1986. A new signal processor for ITE hearing aid fittings. *Hearing Instruments* 37(10): 52–59.

Preves, D., and Woodruff, B. 1990. Some methods of improving and assessing hearing aid headroom. *Audecibel* 39(3):8–13.

Punch, J., and Beck, L. 1986. Relative effects of low frequency amplification on syllable recognition and speech quality. *Ear and Hearing* 7(2):57–62.

Punch, J., Montgomery, A., Schwartz, D., Walden, B., Prosek, R., and Howard, M. 1980. Multidimensional scaling of quality judgments of speech signals processed by hearing aids. *Journal of the Acoustical Society of America* 68(2):458–66.

Resnick, S., Dubno, J., Hoffnung, S., and Levitt, H. 1975. Phoneme errors on a nonsense syllable test. *Journal of the Acoustical Society of America* Suppl. 1, 58 S114.

Thomas, I., and Niederjohn, R. 1970. The intelligibility of filtered-clipped speech in noise. *Journal of Audio Engineering Society* 18:299–303.

Thomas, I., and Ohley, W. 1972. Intelligibility enhancement through spectral weighting. *Proceedings of the 1972 Conference on Speech Communication and Processing*:360–63.

Thomas, I., and Ravindran, A. 1974. Intelligibility enhancement of already noisy speech signals. *Journal of the Audio Engineering Society* 22(4):234–36.

Thomas, I., and Sparks, D. 1971. Discrimination of filtered-clipped speech by sensorineural hearing impaired subjects. *Journal of the Acoustical Society of America* 49:1881–1887.

Vargo, S. 1977. Influence of high pass filtering on the intelligibility of amplitude-compressed speech. *Journal of the American Audiological Society* 5(3):163–67.

Villchur, E. 1973. Signal processing to improve speech intelligibility in perceptive deafness *Journal of the Acoustical Society of America* 53, 6:1646–1657.

Villchur, E. 1989. Comments on "The negative effect of amplitude compression in multichannel hearing aids in the light of the modulation-transfer function" [*Journal of the Acoustical Society of America* 83:2322–2327 (1988)]. *Journal of the Acoustical Society of America* 86(1): 425–27.

Visser, A. 1987. The Extrema coding signal processing. *Proceedings of the International Speech Tech '87:* New York: Media Dimensions.

Waldhauer, F., and Villchur, E. 1988. Full dynamic range multiband compression in a hearing aid. *Hearing Journal* 41(9):29–32.

Walker, G., and Dillon, H. 1982. Compression in hearing aids: an analysis, a review and some recommendations. *National Acoustics Laboratories Report No. 90.* Canberra: Australian Government Publishing Service.

Walker, G., Byrne, D., and Dillon, H. 1984. The effects of multichannel compression/expansion amplification on the intelligibility of nonsense syllables in noise. *Journal of the Acoustical Society of America* 73(3):746–57.

Williamson, M., and Punch, J. 1990. Speech enhancement in digital hearing aids. In *Seminars in Hearing* ed. C. Sammeth. NY: Thieme.

Yanick, P. 1976. Effects of signal processing on the intelligibility of speech in noise for subjects possessing sensorineural hearing loss. *Journal of the American Auditory Society* 1:229–238.

Yanick, P., and Drucker, D. 1976. Signal processing to improve intelligibility in the presence of noise for persons with ski-slope hearing impairment. *IEEE Transactions of Acoustics Speech, and Signal Processing* 24:507–512.

Zurek, P., and Rankovic, T. 1990. Potential benefits of varying the frequency-gain characteristic for speech reception in noise. Paper read at 119th Meeting of the Acoustic Society of America, May 1990, State College, PA.

CHAPTER 5

Clinical Assessment of Output Limiting and Speech Enhancement Techniques

Wayne O. Olsen

Of the topics discussed by Preves (this volume, Chapter 4), I have selected three for brief comments here. The three issues are: (1) "headroom," (2) potential methods for clinical assessment of signal processing hearing aids, and (3) possible use of questionnaires for evaluation of performance of special circuitry in hearing aids. Methods for the evaluation of such units and for determination of hearing aid performance and benefit are the subject of other chapters in this book, too, but my focus is primarily on methods for clinical assessment.

Headroom

Concern about the upper output limits and distortion products encountered when hearing aids reach saturation levels was discussed by Preves (this volume, Chapter 4) as part of the "headroom" problem. Distorted sound output in response to input levels exceeding 70 dB SPL for a broad band signal such as speech takes on greater significance when one remembers that the hearing aid wearer's own conversational speech exceeds 70 dB SPL at the hearing aid microphone.

Speech having an overall level of 60 dB SPL one meter from the talker will have an overall level of about 75 dB SPL or greater at his or her ear about 15 cm from the front of the mouth. Granted, there is a directivity factor for speech emanating from the mouth of the talker, but the reduction in level below 1000 Hz is minimal at 90° and 135° azimuths according to the data of Dunn and Farnsworth (1939). Figure 1, taken from Dunn and Farnsworth (1939), shows their plots of azimuths relative to the front of the mouth of their talker. According to this plot, the talker's ear would be at about the 135° azimuth. Dunn and Farnsworth completed a large number of measurements of their talker's speech levels in an anechoic chamber at a variety of azimuths,

altitudes, and distances relative to the front of his mouth.

Their data for the 15 cm distance at 90° and 135° azimuths, 0° altitude are plotted in figure 2. The 0 dB reference is their data for 0° azimuth and altitude at a distance of 15 cm. Note that very little reduction in level was observed through 1000 Hz for the 90° and 135° azimuths. The decrease was about 4 dB from 2000 to 8000 Hz at the 90° azimuth and 7 dB to 14 dB at the 135° azimuth.[1] Thus, the low frequency energy of a talker's own conversational level speech can reach his or her ear or hearing aid microphone at levels of 75 dB SPL or greater.

As shown in the previous chapter, levels in excess of 70 dB SPL driving a hearing aid into saturation can cause considerable distortion. Given such distortion, one wonders about a hearing aid wearer's satisfaction with a device that generates considerable distortion in response to his or her own speech production.

Figure 3 shows the frequency response of an ear-level hearing aid measured according to ANSI S3.22–1982 recommendations. Reference test gain setting was only a few dB below full-on gain. This unit provided a relatively flat, broad-frequency response, 27 dB high-frequency-average gain, maximum output of 105 dB SPL, and 2% or less harmonic distortion. Also shown in figure 3 are responses of this hearing aid at the same setting for pseudo-random noise generated by the Frye 6500 test system. Relatively smooth response curves were observed for 60 and 65 dB SPL inputs. Increasing the input to 70 dB SPL resulted in some "breakup" in the response curve. Response to 75 dB SPL and 80 dB SPL inputs yielded jagged response

---

[1]Studebaker (1985) more recently replicated the measurements of Dunn and Farnsworth at 1 meter, 0° altitude, 0° to 270° azimuths in 45° intervals using a real time spectrum analyzer. The results of the two studies at a distance of 1 meter are remarkably similar.

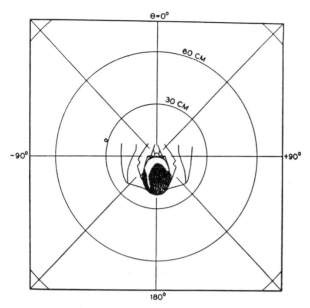

Figure 1. Azimuths at which measurements of speech levels were made by Dunn and Farnsworth. (From Dunn and Farnsworth, 1939, p. 187, with permission.)

curves. Frequency response and harmonic distortion measurements for 70, 75, and 80 dB SPL pure-tone stimuli also shown in figure 3 revealed little harmonic distortion for 70 dB SPL input, but it was in excess of 30% when the input was raised to 75 dB SPL. Distortion approached 60% for 80 dB SPL input.

My listening to this hearing aid as I recited the obligatory phrases, "Joe took father's shoebench out. She was waiting at my lawn." demonstrated a harsh sound quality. Reducing the gain allowed a more pleasant sound to be heard through the hear-

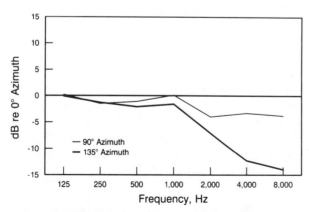

Figure 2. Speech levels as a function frequency at 90° and 135° azimuths re 0° azimuth. (From data of Dunn and Farnsworth 1939.)

ing aid. When the gain was adjusted to a level that sounded more pleasant, the measurement results shown in figure 4 were obtained. Gain was reduced about 10 dB. Response to pseudo-random noise through 75 dB SPL was smooth, but began to break up a little when the input was 80 dB SPL. Harmonic distortion was minimal up to 80 dB SPL input, but increased to about 28% for 85 dB SPL pure-tone signals.

A number of messages present themselves from these observations. One is that even though a hearing aid may seem to function adequately at a reference test gain setting as specified in the ANSI S3.22 test procedure, use of this particular hearing aid at that gain setting probably would not be satisfactory. This unit should be used at a level approximately 10 dB below full-on gain in keeping with the 10 dB "reserve" gain recommended in prescriptive gain formulas for fitting hearing aids.

A second implication here is that when output must be limited so that inputs of 75 dB SPL or slightly higher drive the device into saturation at a "use" gain setting, output limiting other than peak clipping should be considered, even for mild gain hearing aids.

These observations also suggest that even though harmonic distortion values may be relatively low for a given pure tone input, complex noise inputs at the same overall level may reveal "break-up" in the response of the hearing aid. This difference at the same overall input level is related to the 12 dB crest factor in the pseudo-random noise developed by the Frye 6500 system. The recent publication of Stelmachowicz et al. (1990) very nicely reviews differences in hearing aid measurements using different input stimuli.

The results shown in figures 3 and 4, demonstrate that it behooves us to measure our patients' hearing aids at their "use" setting with inputs of at least 75 dB SPL. It was at the urging of a friend, Dianne Van Tasell at the University of Minnesota, that I began to complete measurements of patients' hearing aids at their "use" settings with complex noise inputs increasing in 5 dB steps from 60 to 90 dB SPL. Linear versus AGC or other adaptive control hearing aids are quickly identified even though the make and model are unfamiliar to me. More importantly, observation of "break-up" in the response of a hearing aid such as shown in figure 3 at a "use" gain setting is cause for concern. Unfortunately, I have not recorded the incidence of marked "break-up" at 75, 80, or sometimes even 70 dB SPL inputs, but such observations are not rare.

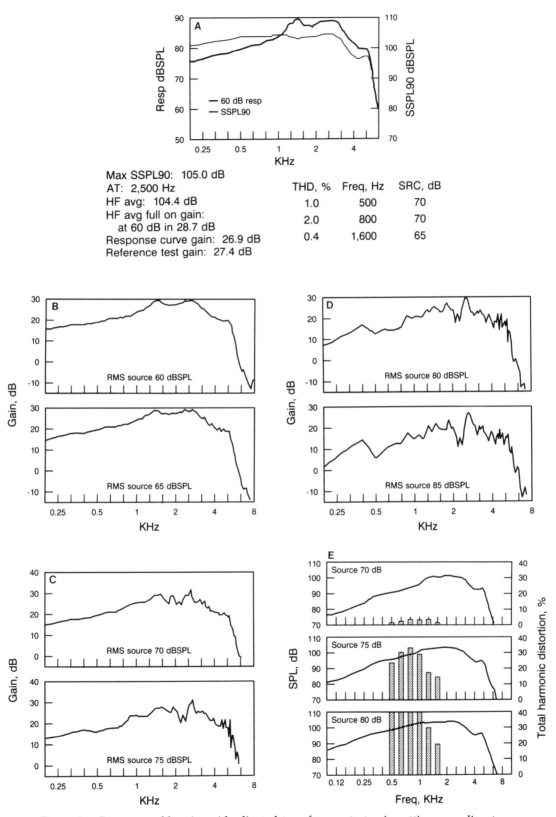

Max SSPL90: 105.0 dB
AT: 2,500 Hz
HF avg: 104.4 dB
HF avg full on gain:
    at 60 dB in 28.7 dB
Response curve gain: 26.9 dB
Reference test gain: 27.4 dB

THD, %	Freq, Hz	SRC, dB
1.0	500	70
2.0	800	70
0.4	1,600	65

Figure 3.   Response of hearing aid adjusted to reference test gain setting according to ANSI S3.22 specifications; response to pseudo-random noise at various inputs; frequency response and harmonic distortion at various input levels.

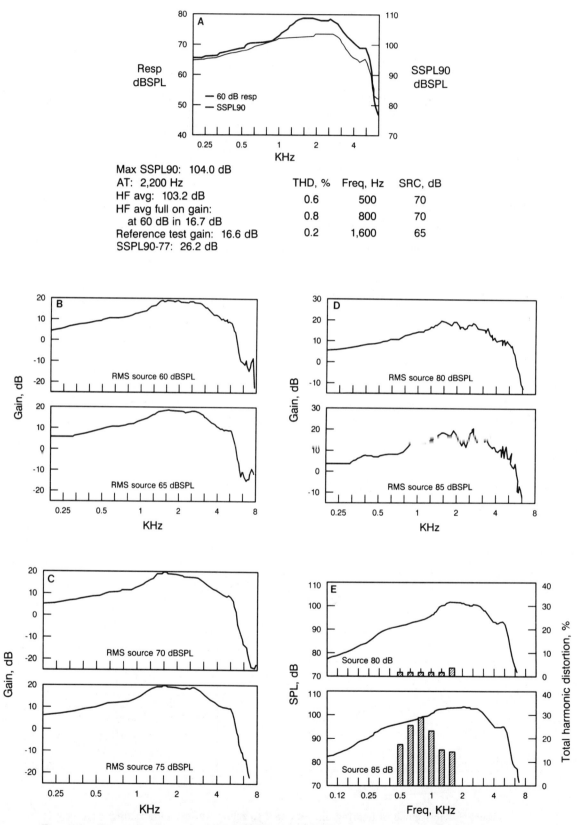

Max SSPL90: 104.0 dB
AT: 2,200 Hz
HF avg: 103.2 dB
HF avg full on gain:
  at 60 dB in 16.7 dB
Reference test gain: 16.6 dB
SSPL90-77: 26.2 dB

THD, %	Freq, Hz	SRC, dB
0.6	500	70
0.8	800	70
0.2	1,600	65

Figure 4.   Response of same hearing aid at lower gain setting; response to pseudo-random noise at various inputs; frequency response and harmonic distortion at various input levels.

Clinical Assessment

Turning now to some possibilities for clinical evaluation of some of the special processing circuits described by Preves, I paraphrase statements in an article by Stein, McGee, and Lewis (1989). They indicate that, to date, the question about these circuits seems to have been global. That is, are such circuits valuable to the hearing-impaired community? They suggest that a more appropriate question might be, specifically who can benefit from these special circuits?

Stein, McGee, and Lewis (1989) suggest use of a single subject experimental design to evaluate such devices. In the single subject experimental design the performance of the patient is compared when the special circuit is off, called condition *A*, and when the circuit is on, condition *B*, followed by a repeat of condition *A*. Figure 5 is derived from the data of these authors; the data show the performance of two patients with two different noise suppression hearing aids. They extended the conditions beyond the usual *ABA* design to include an additional *B* condition followed by a final *A* condition (*ABABA*). The heavy lines mark the performance for the low predictability items of the SPIN test; thin lines are for the high predictability items. The test materials were presented at a signal-to-noise ratio of +8 dB. Improved performance was observed for the noise suppression on *B* condition relative to the noise suppression off *A* condition. The distinction between noise suppression on versus noise suppression off was clearcut for the low predictability items. The ceiling effect was reached for the high predictability test items. Obviously, sufficiently difficult listening situations, precluding

near perfect performance in the *A* control condition, must be used if improvement in the *B* experimental condition is anticipated. The important point is that for these two hearing aid users, improvement in performance for the low predictability items of the SPIN test was observed when the noise suppression circuits of the hearing aids were activated.

It is unlikely that many busy clinics or patients would have the time available for completion of five lists of the SPIN test for an *ABABA* evaluation or even the shorter more usual *ABA* comparisons. However, a test paradigm of this type using less time-consuming procedures could prove valuable.

For those who prefer word recognition scores, use of background competition and 10-word isophonemic word lists, with scoring of each phoneme, might be considered (Boothroyd 1968; Olsen, Van Tasell, and Speaks 1982a; 1982b; 1983; 1986a; 1986b). A 10-word list can be presented in one minute or less. Presentation of two lists of ten words each in condition *A* can be accomplished in about two minutes and allows scoring of the same thirty phonemes twice to provide a quick check on the consistency of the patient's performance. Statistical equivalence of scores across two lists can be ascertained quickly through application of the binomial distribution model to speech recognition scores as described by Thornton and Raffin (1978), Raffin and Schafer (1980), and Raffin and Thornton (1980). If the scores are similar (e.g., within the 95% confidence interval), scores for the two lists can be averaged for condition *A*. If not, more lists can be presented to establish a stable estimate of the patient's performance for that listening condition. The same procedure then can be followed for condition *B* and again for condition *A*. The critical differences established by the binomial distribution model then can be re-applied to determine whether or not the difference in scores for conditions *A* and *B* and for the first *A* and the second *A* reached a predetermined level of statistical significance. Under optimal conditions using two isophonemic word lists per condition, an *ABA* paradigm could be completed in about six minutes.

Another possibility worthy of consideration would be to use the "simple up-down" method described by Levitt (1971) to determine the signal-to-noise ratio for 50% intelligibility of selected speech materials. Figure 6 shows a hypothetical, idealized sample of the up-down procedure described by Levitt (1971). Larger variations of the signal are used for the first four trials to establish a starting point followed by a sufficient number of trials to produce,

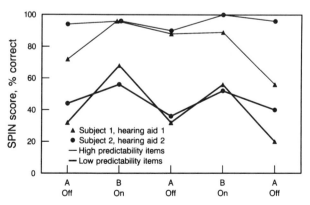

Figure 5. SPIN test results for 2 patients using *ABABA* single subject experimental paradigm; *A*-noise suppression off, *B*-noise suppression on. (From data of Stein, Mcgee, and Lewis 1990.)

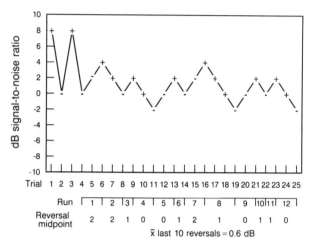

Figure 6. Hypothetical example of measurement of signal-to-noise ratio using up-down method; correct response +, error response −.

in this example, twelve reversals of the signal intensity. In this figure, presentation of 25 items yielded 12 reversals. More or fewer reversals may be used, but averaging the midpoints of the last 10 reversals shown here produced a mean signal-to-noise ratio of 0.6 dB. Standard deviations and confidence intervals for each threshold can be computed to help determine whether or not any observed differences between conditions reach statistical significance. For application with the *ABA* paradigm, the special circuit of the hearing aid would be inactivated for the initial *A* condition, activated for the *B* condition, and inactivated for the final *A* condition.

It has been argued that if the differences between scores for conditions *A* and *B* are so small that they are not readily apparent, they may not be clinically significant either. However, since computer programs are available for control of stimulus presentation, and on-line calculations of means, standard deviations, and confidence intervals for the up-down method, these analyses can be generated at the time of testing.

Obviously, homogeneity of test items is highly desirable for threshold searches using the up-down method in order to reach a predetermined number of reversals or pre-established criterion for stability of threshold response. Two sets of materials that might be considered for *ABA* comparisons using this up-down procedure were described by Van Tasell and Yanz (1987). One set, which relies on low frequency information for intelligibility, is the 11 spondees found to be highly homogeneous by Dubno, Dirks, and Morgan (1984) (drawbridge, eardrum, grandson, northwest, padlock, playground, railroad, sidewalk, toothbrush, woodwork, and

workshop). The second set of words described by Van Tasell and Yanz was made up of eight CVC monosyllables. Each began with a voiceless fricative, used the short, high-frequency vowel [I], and ended with a voiceless stop (hip, hit, hick, sip, sit, sick, ship, thick). The spectra of these stimuli are well described (Van Tasell and Yanz 1987; Van Tasell, Larsen, and Fabry 1988).

Van Tasell and Yanz (1987) successfully used these materials in a closed-message format and the up-down method in demonstrating differences in thresholds in noise for hearing-impaired subjects brought about by differences in the frequency responses of an amplification apparatus. Van Tasell, Larsen, and Fabry (1988) also used these materials in their evaluation of noise suppression circuitry in a hearing aid.

Use of computers for stimulus control and calculation of data gathered with the up-down method, the *ABA* single subject paradigm, and speech materials such as these spondees and monosyllables could prove useful in a clinical setting, such as for evaluating patient performance with noise suppression circuits on and off. Measurement of signal-to-noise ratios for 50% intelligibility with the special circuit inactive, and then with the special circuit active, may provide clinically significant information.

Whether scores from word recognition tests or 50% intelligibility for speech using the up-down method are used, application of single subject experimental design protocols in a clinical setting can, over time, provide important information regarding patient performance with some of the "speech enhancement" circuitry available in current and future hearing aids. Perhaps in this way we can begin to answer the question posed by Stein, McGee, and Lewis (1989) as to who can benefit from use of such special circuit devices.

Hearing Aid Performance/Benefit

Assessing the value of various noise reduction or speech enhancement hearing aid circuits in everyday life settings is another matter. Perhaps some of the questionnaires or inventories designed to assess hearing aid handicap warrant consideration. Reports in the literature describe the use of some of those questionnaires or inventories to assess hearing aid benefit. For example, in 1974 Birk-Nielsen and Ewertsen demonstrated a reduction in perceived handicap with hearing aid use based on comparison of results from the Social Hearing

Handicap Index (Ewertsen and Birk-Nielsen 1973) administered before hearing aid fitting and after three to six months of hearing aid use. Tannahill (1979) reported similar findings from a study using the two 20-item forms of the Hearing Handicap Scale of High, Fairbanks, and Glorig (1964) before and after hearing aid use. More recently, based on administration of the Hearing Handicap Inventory for the Elderly (Ventry and Weinstein 1982) before and after hearing aid use, Newman and Weinstein (1988), Malinoff and Weinstein (1989), and Mulrow, Tuley, and Aguilar (1990) concluded that this 25-item questionnaire could be used successfully to assess hearing aid benefit. Further, Mulrow, Tuley, and Aguilar (1990) suggested that even the 10-item screening version of the Hearing Handicap Index for the Elderly (Weinstein 1986) can satisfactorily detect decrease in perceived hearing handicap associated with hearing aid use. Similarly, Schow and Nerbonne (1982) indicated that improvement in communication associated with hearing aid use can be demonstrated by comparing scores from administration of their 10-item Self Assessment of Communication, and/or Significant Other Assessment of Communication scales prior to and following use of a hearing aid.

Kuk and Tyler (1990) have suggested a different scaling system for listening comfort, speech understanding, speech quality, and noise interference with a given hearing aid arrangement, and for overall liking of the hearing aid. Each of the five items is rated from 0 to 100, with 100 being extremely comfortable, understanding every word, highest quality, no noise interference, and excellent overall liking of the hearing aid. They suggested that this scale might be used in clinical hearing aid evaluations, and that the noise interference item might help evaluate the efficacy of different noise reduction hearing aids.

Whether or not these questionnaires or scales can reveal differences among hearing aids or benefits of innovative hearing aid circuitry in everyday life situations remains to be seen. It should be noted, however, that the scales are available and that computer programs for administering and scoring some of them have been developed and are available commercially. A set of disks for administration and scoring of both forms of the Hearing Handicap Scale (High, Fairbanks, and Glorig 1964), the Hearing Handicap Inventory for the Elderly (Ventry and Weinstein 1982), the Hearing Handicap Inventory for the Elderly Screening Version (Weinstein 1986), the Revised Hearing Performance Inventory (Lamb, Owens, and Schubert 1983), and

the Hearing Aid Performance Inventory (Walden, Demorest, and Hepler 1984) have been prepared by Humes (1988). Because these questionnaires can be computer administered and scored, therefore requiring little time on the part of the clinician, it would seem that these materials await clinical trials and more reports in the literature about their utility.

Very likely the ability of any of these shorter questionnaires or rating scales to reveal differences in the performance of various hearing aid circuits in everyday life situations will be compared to results from the Profile of Hearing Aid Performance (PHAP) reported by Cox and Gilmore (1990). This inventory probably will become the "gold standard." Drawing from reports of inventories such as the Hearing Aid Performance Inventory (Walden, Demorest, and Hepler 1984), the Communication Profile for the Hearing Impaired (Demorest and Erdman 1986, 1987), an article on factors affecting binaural hearing aid use by Chung and Stephens (1986), and other publications, Cox and Gilmore developed and evaluated 100 statements about hearing aid use in various listening situations. Statistical item analyses subsequently made it possible to reduce the inventory to 66 items requiring 20 to 30 minutes to complete in a paper and pencil format. The Profile of Hearing Aid Performance is described in greater detail elsewhere in this book (see Cox, this volume, Chapter 17). The influences of 7 factors or subscales, namely, ease of communication, familiar talkers, background noise, reverberation, reduced cues, aversiveness of sounds, and distortion of sounds are surveyed by the 66 items. The profile is generated by responses to the 66 items on a 7-point scale expressed as: (a) Always (99% of the time), (b) Almost Always (87% of the time), (c) Generally (75% of the time), (d) Half-the-time (50% of the time), (e) Occasionally (25% of the time), (f) Seldom (12% of the time), and (g) Never (1% of the time). Responses to the 66 items can be grouped into the 7 subscales mentioned above, or into 4 scales labelled *Environment A, Environment B, Environment C,* and *Environmental Sound.* Environment A encompasses items describing conversational level speech, availability of visual cues, low background noise, and little reverberation (subscales ease of communication and familiar talkers). Environment B is described as low background noise with conditions of reverberation, or reduced auditory cues due to soft speech levels, or reduced visual cues (reverberation and reduced cues subscales). Environment C reflects noisy conditions with raised speech levels and visual cues available (background noise subscale). Statements on environmental sound deal with sound quality and loudness of environmental sounds (aversiveness of sounds and distortion of sounds subscales).

Cox and Gilmore (1990) suggest that the Profile of Hearing Aid Performance could be used to assess differences in everyday life experiences, comparing hearing aids that differ in some performance feature.

> The hearing impaired individual could use the first fitting for 1–2 weeks and then complete the inventory. The second fitting could then be tried for the same period and the inventory completed again (the time interval used in the test-retest study was chosen with this sort of application in mind). Two fittings that differ in noise reduction strategies, for example, may produce significantly different scores on the BN [Background Noise] subscale and perhaps on other subscales also (Cox and Gilmore 1990, p. 353).

As suggested by Cox and Gilmore, a Profile of Hearing Aid Benefit also can be established if the patient responds to each item twice, one set of responses being based on experiences without hearing aid use, and the other set reflecting performance while wearing the hearing aid(s).

With the availability of computer software for administering, scoring, and graphing responses to the Profile of Hearing Aid Performance, this inventory will be extremely valuable in assessing hearing aid performance in everyday life situations, and in evaluating a variety of innovative hearing aid circuits.

Summary

Given the recent innovations in measurement, fitting, and adjustment of hearing aids, these are truly exciting times for all of us. Quick measurements of hearing aids at their use settings with different types and levels of input stimuli are now possible. New methods for clinical evaluation of special circuits in hearing aids while patients are wearing the devices await application and modification. Questionnaires and inventories have been developed to assess communication problems, hearing aid performance, and hearing aid benefit in everyday life experiences. We now have the tools to learn a great deal about our patients and their use of hearing aids. The time required for administration of many of these new procedures is reaching the point that they may be feasible in busy clinical settings.

References

American National Standards Institute. 1982. *Specification of Hearing Aid Characteristics ANSI S3.22-1982.* New York: Acoustical Society of America.

Birk-Nielsen, H., and Ewertsen, H.W. 1974. Effect of hearing aid treatment. Social Hearing Handicap Index before and after treatment of new patients. *Scandinavian Audiology* 3:35–38.

Boothroyd, A. 1968. Developments in speech audiometry. *Sound* 2:3–10.

Chung, S.M., and Stephens, S.D.G. 1986. Factors influencing binaural hearing aid use. *British Journal of Audiology* 20:129–40.

Cox, R.M., and Gilmore, C. 1990. Development of the Profile of Hearing Aid Performance (PHAP). *Journal of Speech and Hearing Research* 33:343–57.

Demorest, M.E., and Erdman, S.A. 1986. Scale composition and item analysis of the Communication Profile for the Hearing Impaired. *Journal of Speech and Hearing Research* 29:515–35.

Demorest, M.E., and Erdman, S.A. 1987. Development of the Communication Profile for the Hearing Impaired. *Journal of Speech and Hearing Disorders,* 52:129–43.

Dubno, J.R., Dirks, D.D., and Morgan, D. E. 1984. Effects of age and mild hearing loss on speech recognition in noise. *Journal of the Acoustical Society of America* 76:87–96.

Dunn, H.K., and Farnsworth, D.W. 1939. Exploration of pressure field around the human head during speech. *Journal of the Acoustical Society of America* 10:184–99.

Ewertsen, H.W., and Birk-Nielsen, H. 1973. Social Hearing Handicap Index. *Audiology* 12:180–87.

High, W.S., Fairbanks, G., and Glorig, A. 1964. Scale for self-assessment of hearing handicap. *Journal of Speech and Hearing Disorders* 29:215–30.

Humes, L. 1988. HI-5. Bloomington, IN: Venture 4th.

Kuk, F.K., and Tyler, R.S. 1990. Relationship between consonant recognition and subjective rating of hearing aids. *British Journal of Audiology* 24:171–77.

Lamb, T.G., Owens, E., and Schubert, E.D. 1983. The revised form of the Hearing Performance Inventory. *Ear and Hearing* 4:152–57.

Levitt, H. 1971. Transformed up-down methods in psychoacoustics. *Journal of the Acoustical Society of America* 49:467–77.

Malinoff, R.L., and Weinstein, B.E. 1989. Measurement of hearing benefit in the elderly. *Ear and Hearing* 10:354–56.

Mulrow, C.D., Tuley, M.R., and Aguilar, C. 1990. Discriminating responsiveness of two handicape scales. *Ear and Hearing* 11:176–80.

Newman, C.W., and Weinstein, B.E. 1988. The hearing handicap inventory for the elderly as a measure of hearing aid benefit. *Ear and Hearing* 9:81–85.

Olsen, W.O., Van Tasell, D.J., and Speaks, C.E. 1982a. Preparation of isophonemic word list and sentence materials. Paper read at annual convention of Speech-Language-Hearing Association, November, 1982, Toronto.

Olsen, W.O., Van Tasell, D.J., and Speaks, C.E. 1982b. Evaluation of isophonemic word list and sentence materials. Paper read at annual convention of American Speech-Language-Hearing Association, November, 1982, Toronto.

Olsen, W.O., Van Tasell, D.J., and Speaks, C.E. 1983. Further evaluation of isophonemic word list and sentence materials. Paper read at annual convention of American Speech-Language-Hearing Association, November, 1983, Cincinnati.

Olsen, W.O., Van Tasell, D.J., and Speaks, C.E. 1986a. List equivalence of isophonemic word lists. Paper read at annual convention of American Speech-Language-Hearing Association, November, 1986, Detroit.

Olsen, W.O., Van Tasell, D.J., and Speaks, C.E. 1986b. Comparison of scores for words in isolation and in sentence. Paper read at annual convention of American Speech-Language-Hearing Association, November, 1986, Detroit.

Raffin, M.J.M., and Schafer, D. 1980. Application of a probability model based on the binomial distribution to speech discrimination scores. *Journal of Speech and Hearing Research* 23:570–75.

Raffin, M.J.M., and Thornton, A.R. 1980. Confidence levels for differences between speech discrimination scores. *Journal of Speech and Hearing Research* 23:4–18.

Schow, R.L., and Nerbonne, M.A. 1982. Communication screening profile: Use with elderly clients. *Ear and Hearing* 3:135–47.

Stein, L., McGee, T., and Lewis, P. 1989. Speech recognition measures with noise suppression hearing aids using a single-subject experimental design. *Ear and Hearing* 10:375–81.

Stelmachowicz, P.G., Lewis, D.E., Seewald, R.C., and Hawkins, D.B. 1990. Complex and pure-tone signals in the evaluation of hearing-aid characteristics. *Journal of Speech and Hearing Research* 33:380–85.

Studebaker, G.A. 1985. Directivity of the human vocal source in the horizontal plane. *Ear and Hearing* 6:315–19.

Tannahill, J.C. 1979. The Hearing Handicap Scale as a measure of hearing aid benefit. *Journal of Speech and Hearing Research* 44:91–99.

Thornton, A.R., and Raffin, M.J.M. 1978. Speech discrimination scores modeled as a binomial variable. *Journal of Speech and Hearing Research* 21:507–18.

Van Tasell, D.J., and Yanz, J.L. 1987. Speech recognition threshold in noise: Effects of hearing loss, frequency response and speech materials. *Journal of Speech and Hearing Research* 30:377–86.

Van Tasell, D.J., Larsen, S.Y., and Fabry, D.A. 1988. Effects of an adaptive filter hearing aid on speech recognition in noise by hearing-impaired subjects. *Ear and Hearing* 9:15–21.

Ventry, I.M., and Weinstein, B.E. 1982. The hearing handicap inventory for the elderly: A new tool. *Ear and Hearing* 3:128–34.

Walden, B.E., Demorest, M.E. and Hepler, E.L. 1984. Self report approach to assessing benefit derived from amplification. *Journal of Speech and Hearing Research* 27:49–56.

Weinstein, B.E. 1986. Validity of a screening protocol for identifying elderly people with hearing problems. *Asha* 28(5):41–45.

PART II
Advanced Signal Processing of Hearing Aids

CHAPTER 6

Programmable and Automatic Noise Reduction in Existing Hearing Aids

David A. Fabry

One of the greatest challenges faced by hearing aid manufacturers today is to design a wearable device that reduces background noise while also improving speech intelligibility. An often cited indictment of present hearing aids is that they do nothing to alleviate this problem because they amplify *both* speech and noise, and in fact may add some noise of their own.

Recently, hearing aids that employ level-dependent amplification have been heralded as the solution to the background noise problem (Mahon 1987). Unfortunately, there has been a great deal of confusion about what is accomplished by this signal processing, who is a candidate, and how to fit patients properly with these devices. These issues have been complicated further by the introduction of commercially available hearing aids that offer multiple-band compression and storage of multiple-frequency responses. The focus of this chapter is on some of the underlying assumptions related to commercially available "noise reduction" hearing aids, and on whether these assumptions provide realistic expectations for everyday use by hearing-impaired persons.

Signal Processing: The Buzzword

The proliferation of the term *signal processing* in hearing aid advertisements has been remarkable. In fact, the expression has enjoyed such widespread use that it is impossible to generalize performance from one signal processing hearing aid to another. Strictly speaking, *all* hearing aids process some input signals differently from others; even the so-called "linear" hearing aids amplify high-level sounds differently than low and moderate signals (figure 1A). When input sounds exceed some criterion level, peak clipping or output compression prevent uncomfortably loud sounds from reaching the

ear by reducing overall hearing aid gain. Figure 1B shows 2-cc coupler measurements for a conventional hearing aid with 55 dB SPL and 80 dB SPL input signal levels. When below output saturation, gain is added linearly across all frequencies. The fundamental assumption related to the design of conventional amplification systems is that for a selected individual there exists a fixed frequency response that is appropriate for all listening environments. In addition, this theory is the cornerstone on which all prescriptive fitting techniques used for clinical fitting of hearing aids are based. Recently, the simplicity of these fitting strategies has been challenged by *noise reduction* hearing aids that use level-dependent amplification. These devices do not use multiple microphones or complicated processing strategies, and therefore may not represent the latest word in noise reduction strategies, but they are *commercially available* hearing aids.

Level-Dependent Amplification

"Automatic" Noise Reduction

Hearing aids that employ a switchable *noise reduction* mode have been available for several decades (Lybarger 1947). Hearing aids with *automatic* activation of a noise reduction circuit, however, have been available commercially for only the past five to ten years. Although there is a variety of strategies used for noise reduction, for practical purposes these can be broken down into four or five categories. Unfortunately, the terminology used to characterize these groups has not been standardized, despite the efforts of many individuals to develop stock nomenclature. Recently, Killion, Staab, and Preves (1990) developed yet another classification scheme based on the present technology (table I). Those terms will be used in this paper, with the hope that they be-

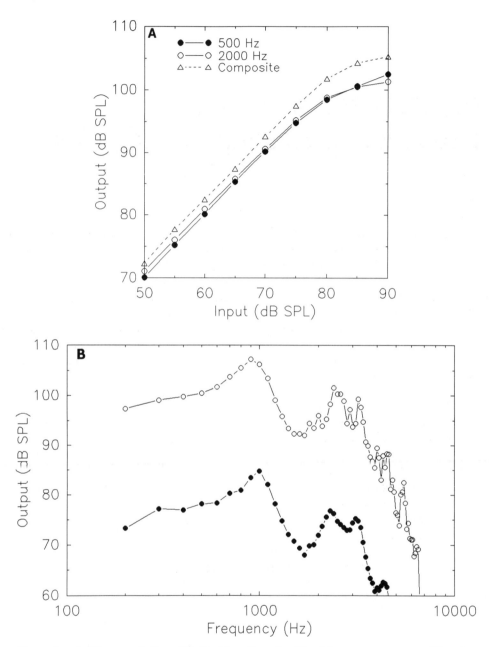

Figure 1.   A. (Top panel): Input/Output functions for "fixed frequency response" hearing aid for 500 Hz (filled circles), 2,500 Hz (open circles), and composite noise (open triangles) signals. B. (Lower panel): Gain-by-frequency values for 55 dB SPL (filled circles) and 80 dB SPL (open circles) "fixed frequency response" hearing aid.

come better known than their predecessors (despite my disdain for cleverly worded acronyms). The focus of this chapter is on those devices that employ level-dependent changes in frequency response (LDFR).

Bass Increases at Low Levels (BILL)   These hearing aids have also been called adaptive frequency response (AFR), automatic signal processing (ASP), and automatic noise reduction (ANR), to name only

a few types. BILL hearing aids comprise the majority of commercially available noise reduction hearing aids. One of the primary differences between these hearing aids and those with conventional ("fixed frequency response" [FFR]) amplification is shown in figure 2A. For BILL hearing aids, nonlinear amplification occurs at levels below output saturation. The net result is that most conventional hearing aids reach output saturation at lower input levels than the BILL device used in this example.

Table I. Classification Scheme for Use with "Automatic Signal Processing" Hearing Aids (As Recommended by Killion, Staab, and Preeves 1990)

I. Automatic Signal Processing (ASP)
  A. Fixed Frequency Response (FFR)
     1. Compression limiting
     2. Wide-range dynamic compression
  B. Level-dependent Frequency Response (LDFR)
     1. Bass Increases at Low Levels (BILL)
        —lows reduced at high levels
     2. Treble Increases at Low Levels (TILL)
        —highs reduced at high levels
     3. Programmable Increases at Low Levels (PILL)
        —either low or highs reduced at high levels

The nonlinear amplification applied by BILL hearing aids is frequency dependent; figure 2B shows the output of one such device, the Manhattan circuit (Sigelman and Preves 1987) measured in the 2-cc coupler for flat-spectrum noise inputs ranging from 50 to 90 dB SPL. This device is a voltage-controlled high-pass filter circuit that is activated at approximately 60 dB SPL and becomes more high pass with increasing levels of background noise by varying the filter slope. Similarly, other high-pass filter BILL hearing aids may change the cutoff frequency of the high-pass filter with increasing background noise level. They may be activated either by the overall level of background noise or by the SPL in specific frequency regions.

Another way that BILL amplification can be achieved is via multiple-band compression. Villchur (1973) was one of the first to extol the virtues of multiple-band compression in hearing aids. Recently, multiple-band compression has been advocated for use in enhancing speech intelligibility in noise (Mangold and Leijon 1979; Moore 1987; Moore and Glasberg 1988; Yund, Simon, and Efron 1987). Typically, input compression is used, and the low-frequency band is activated at lower input SPLs than the high-frequency band(s). The input/output function for a two-channel compression hearing aid is shown in figure 3A. When a 2000 Hz tone is used, the input/output function is similar to the conventional hearing aid's function. When a 500 Hz tone or composite noise is used, however, the function looks very similar to the adaptive high-pass filter hearing aid (figure 2A). Figure 3B shows the effects on frequency response for high-level input signals, with low frequencies attenuated by approximately 20 dB. A wide variety of time constants is used for these devices, but typically fast activation times (10 msec or less) are used in conjunction with slower release times (50–200 msec).

Treble Increases at Low Levels (TILL) Recently, Killion reported on his design of a four-stage compression amplifier to provide high fidelity over a broad range of input levels (Killion 1990). This strategy is similar to one proposed in 1972 by Hyman Goldberg as the "Utopian" hearing aid (Goldberg 1972). This device is based on the premise that hearing-impaired subjects have normal growth of loudness for high-level stimuli; therefore, intense sounds should be "acoustically invisible," and thus not amplified. In contrast to BILL hearing aids, the theory behind TILL hearing aids is that low frequencies should be *reduced* for low-level signals. Goldberg (1972) contended that doing so would improve speech recognition in noise and maintain high fidelity. At first glance, this device appears to be at odds with the amplification provided by BILL hearing aids. However, further inspection reveals some similarities. For example, figure 4 shows hypothetical insertion gain for a K-amp hearing aid and for an adaptive high-pass filter hearing aid as they would be fitted to a patient with high-frequency hearing loss. Although the coupler gain data for the high-pass filter circuit show a sizeable reduction in low-frequency energy with increasing input (figure 2B), these effects would be smaller when a vented earmold is used on a real ear. Although this comparison is for a single type of hearing loss, it reinforces the concept that a primary difference between BILL and TILL hearing aids occurs for low input levels (below 60 dB SPL input levels). Figure 5 shows input/output functions for BILL and TILL hearing aids compared to the open ear and a conventional FFR hearing aid. Both BILL and TILL prevent the hearing aid from reaching output saturation when compared to the conventional device.

"Programmable" Hearing Aids

The newest generation of hearing aids allow the audiologist to program multiple frequency responses and/or multiple-band compression. Although many of these hearing aids are not designed specifically for noise reduction, several manufacturers refer directly to that issue in advertising copy and/or product literature. Hearing aids with programmable memory use digital control of the analog signal, but at present there are no all-digital units in production. For an overview of some of the commercially available programmable hearing aids, see Sammeth (1990). The intention of this chapter is to discuss some fundamental principles of programmable hearing aids as they apply to level-dependent am-

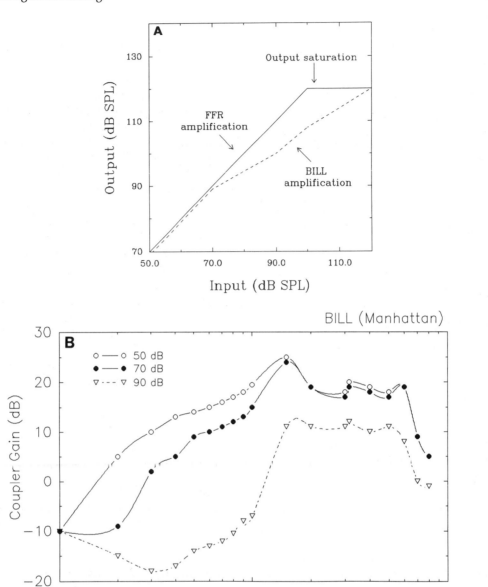

Figure 2.   A. (Top panel): Input/Output functions to composite noise for "fixed frequency response" (FFR) and adaptive high-pass filter "bass increased at low levels" (BILL) type amplification. B. (Lower panel): BILL (Manhattan circuit) response to flat-spectrum noise at input levels ranging from 50 dB SPL (circles) to 90 dB SPL (inverted triangles).

plification. At present, all programmable devices may be divided into two groups that are related to the number of programmable memories available to the hearing aid user.

"Automatic" Programmable Increases at Low Levels (A/PILL)   These devices use multiple-band compression or frequency-dependent compression and allow the user to program various hearing aid characteristics, such as overall gain, low- and high-frequency cutoff, or crossover frequency to arrive at

a *single* frequency response that is programmed into the hearing aid. The simplest of these devices (for example, the Dahlberg Dolphin™ or Audiotone System 2000™) are similar to conventional, fixed-frequency response amplification. Others, like the Siemens Triton or Ensoniq™, may use multiple-band compression programmed into a single frequency response and are similar to BILL noise reduction hearing aids. These devices may be easily fitted using existing prescriptive formulae and conventional evaluation techniques.

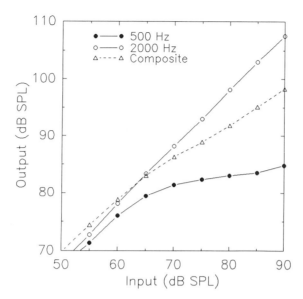

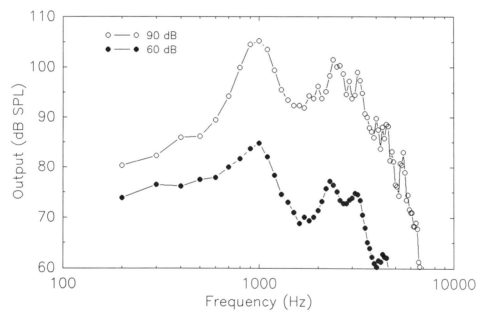

Figure 3.   A. (Top panel): Input/Output functions for multiple-channel compression hearing aid for 500 Hz (filled circles), 2500 Hz (open circles), and composite noise (open triangles) signals. B. (Lower panel): Gain-by-frequency values for 60 dB SPL (filled circles) and 80 dB SPL (open circles) multiple-channel compression hearing aid.

User-Adjustable Programmable Increases at Low Levels (U/PILL)   These hearing aids, such as the 3M Memory Mate™ or Widex Quattro, may use multiple-band compression *plus* different user-selected frequency responses. The number of responses used presently varies from two to eight (table II); the assumption is that users will change frequency responses as they move from one listening environment to another. The fitting strategies used by different manufacturers have not been studied widely, but some offer fitting guidelines that do not appear to be empirically based (for example, see Widex 1989).

The "Orphans"

Some types of hearing aids that have been advocated for use in reducing background noise do not fit neatly into any of the categories proposed by Killion, Staab, and Preves (1990). For example, adaptive compression™ (Gittles and Wilson 1987) changes the recovery time of the compression circuit as a

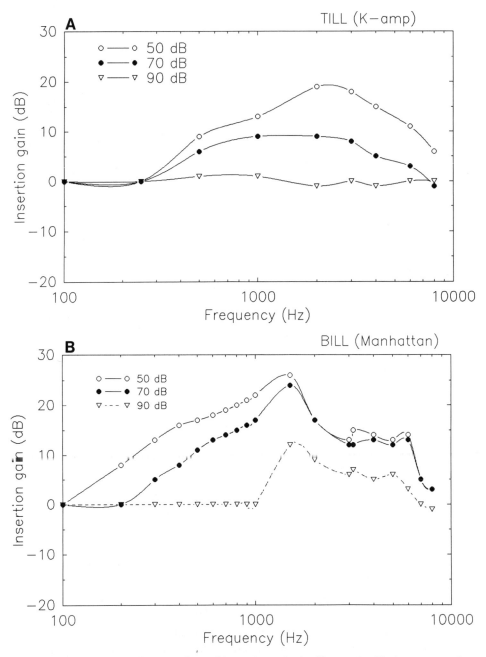

Figure 4.   A. (Top panel): Hypothetical insertion gain for K-amp "treble increases at low levels" (TILL) hearing aid for three input levels (50, 70, and 90 db SPL composite noise) with vented earmold. B. (Lower panel): Hypothetical insertion gain values for "bass increases at low levels" (BILL) hearing aid for three input levels (50, 70, and 90 dB SPL composite noise) with vented earmold.

function of the duration and level of the input signal without necessarily changing the hearing aid's frequency response. The Zeta Noise Blocker™ (Graupe, Grosspietch, and Basseas 1987) changes frequency response adaptively for both low- and high-frequency sounds, so it is somewhat like a PILL hearing aid (but it is not user adjustable) and is also reminiscent of BILL processing strategies.

Assumptions Related to
Noise Reduction Hearing Aids

Although not clearly identified by manufacturers, the rationale for design of many automatic and manual noise reduction hearing aids appears to be based on some or all of the following assumptions:

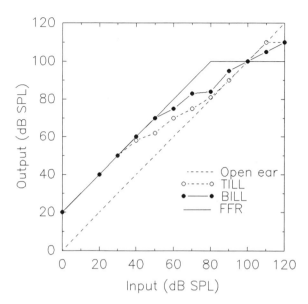

Figure 5. Input/Output functions for open ear (dashed line), FFR (solid line), TILL (open circles), and BILL (filled circles) hearing aids, using composite noise.

1. For a given individual, there is no single frequency response that is optimal for every listening situation. Level-dependent changes in frequency response should occur.
2. Low-frequency, high-amplitude sounds should not be amplified. As stated earlier, BILL and TILL hearing aids appear to be different in principle for low-level sounds. PILL hearing aids can be programmed to reduce low- or high-frequency sounds at low levels. Still, PILL and BILL are just like TILL when they reduce their gain to nil.
3. Nonlinear amplification should be used to prevent the hearing aid from reaching saturation for moderate input signals. Essentially, these devices approach the notion of full dynamic range compression hearing aids.
4. Speech intelligibility will be optimized when you accomplish steps (1) through (3).

Table II. Programmable Hearing Aids, and the Number of User-Selectable Memories for Each Device

	Memories
Audiotone 2000™	1
Dahlberg Dolphin™	1
Ensoniq™	1
PHOX	1 or 2
Resound	2
Siemens Triton 3000	1
3M Memory Mate™	8
Widex Quattro	4

Evaluation of these Assumptions

Is there empirical support for these assumptions in the literature?

Assumption 1 Level-dependent Changes in Frequency Response Are Beneficial

The idea for using level-dependent changes in frequency response has been proposed by Goldberg (1972), Villchur (1973), Skinner (1980), and others. In her review of research on amplification parameters, Skinner (1991) suggested that several frequency responses that optimize listening in different situations should be considered for modern hearing aids. This postulate is consistent with the principles of the Articulation Index (French and Steinberg 1947), which suggests that frequency response should change to maximize speech audibility for different background noises. A recent study by van Dijkhuizen, Festen, and Plomp (1989) examined the effects of rapid changes in the amplitude-frequency response on masked SRT in hearing-impaired subjects. Their results indicated that rapid changes in the frequency response did not cause an increase in masked SRT under certain conditions. Although there is much historical support for the *concept* of level-dependent changes in frequency response, there have been few studies that actually explored the issue outside of the laboratory, in actual hearing aids, because the technology has not been available until recently.

Assumption 2 Low Freqencies Should Be Reduced at High Levels

Several published reports have examined the frequency content of typical, continuous background noise in everyday environments and reported that they contain much low-frequency energy (Klumpp and Webster 1963; Ono, Kanzaki, and Mizoi 1983). In addition, several investigators have shown that high-pass filtering followed by either peak clipping (Thomas and Niederjohn 1970) or rapid amplitude compression (Niederjohn and Grotelueschen 1976) may not degrade speech intelligibility in background noise. Thus, a hearing aid that reduces low frequencies by high-pass filtering and/or multiple-band compression might act to reduce background noise *and* preserve speech intelligibility. Furthermore, it frequently has been hypothesized that upward spread of masking effects is reduced by attenuating low-frequency sounds, resulting in improved speech intelligibility. However, upward spread of masking effects is nonlinear (Carter and Kryter 1962), affecting primarily high amplitude band-limited signals. Therefore, the rationale has been established for activating the high-pass filter circuit when input SPL exceeds a certain level, like the processing with BILL (adaptive high-pass filter or multi-band compression) hearing aids. However, most BILL hearing aids are activated when *input* signals reach 60 to 70 dB SPL; based upon the nonlinear growth of masking, it makes sense to activate the circuit when hearing aid output at the eardrum reaches a certain level. Then, the filter circuit compensates for the amount of gain applied for different persons, rather than always activating the circuit at the same level for all patients.

The TILL (K-amp) hearing aid reduces low amplitude, low frequency signals in an attempt to deliver high fidelity. This is somewhat at odds with the nonlinear growth of masking data (Carter and Kryter 1962), which indicate that upward spread of masking occurs for high amplitude signals. Furthermore, Skinner and Miller (1983) showed that under different conditions, broad-band amplification provided the highest speech intelligibility. Finally, Punch and Beck's (1980) data indicate that reduction of low frequencies degraded speech quality.

Assumption 3 Nonlinear Amplification Should Be Used To Prevent Hearing Aid Distortion

Hearing aid distortion has typically been expressed by using measures of harmonic distortion (ANSI 1987). Recently, it has been proposed that measures of intermodulation distortion be used for hearing aid measurements. Dyrlund (1989) reported that measurements of signal coherence are superior to traditional measures of distortion because a realistic (broad-band) test signal is used and because coherence measures the combined effects of harmonic *and* intermodulation distortion. *Coherence* is a spectral analysis method used to assess the overall linear performance of a system within its operating bandwidth. Coherence at a certain frequency is a measure of the proportion of all output power that depends linearly on the input signal at that frequency. *Noncoherence*, on the other hand, is caused by nonlinearities and additive noise.

The results of several recent studies (Preves and Newton 1989; Dyrlund 1989) show that the action of high-pass filtering or compression reduces intermodulation distortion compared to conventional, peak-clipping hearing aids. So, in that sense,

hearing aids that use this technology *will* result in lower distortion and provide more "headroom" (Preves 1990) than conventional, peak-clipping hearing aids.

Assumption 4 Speech Intelligibility in Noise Will Increase with BILL, PILL, and TILL Hearing Aids

The key factor uniting the other three assumptions is whether these strategies will result in improved speech recognition. First of all, recall that speech and noise are mixed at the input of a single microphone for all of these hearing aids. Therefore, regardless of the changes in frequency response, the signal-to-noise ratio will be the same because speech and noise are attenuated equally. This statement is supported by data from Fabry and Van Tasell (1990), using the Articulation Index (AI). The AI, developed in the 1940s by researchers at Bell Laboratories (French and Steinberg 1947), uses an individual's auditory thresholds plus long-term spectral measures of speech and background noise to calculate speech audibility for a specific listening situation. AI calculations result in an index that may vary from 0.0 to 1.0. The AI has previously been shown to be related monotonically to speech recognition scores under laboratory conditions (for example, see Skinner and Miller 1983; Pavlovic 1988). Fabry and Van Tasell (1990) evaluated this assumption for subjects wearing a master hearing aid in speech noise background. The master hearing aid was equipped with an adaptive high-pass filter circuit that could be enabled or disabled without affecting other hearing aid characteristics. Aided AI scores were calculated for a group of hearing-impaired subjects who wore the hearing aid under "filter-on" (BILL) and "filter-off" (FFR) conditions and rated the intelligibility of connected discourse in noise. No improvements were predicted by the AI (figure 6) and no differences were observed in rated speech intelligibility between BILL and FFR conditions (figure 7). In fact, for one subject, the AI actually predicted poorer speech intelligibility for the BILL condition than for the FFR condition (circled point in figure 6). The reason for this *poorer* predicted performance is shown in figure 8. Note that when the filter was activated, less speech was audible than for the filter-off (FFR) condition, resulting in a lower AI score (0.104 versus 0.132) and therefore lower predicted speech intelligibility.

Fabry and Van Tasell's (1990) results support the data from earlier studies (Klein 1989; Tyler and Kuk 1989; Van Tasell, Larsen, and Fabry 1988) that showed no significant differences in speech intel-

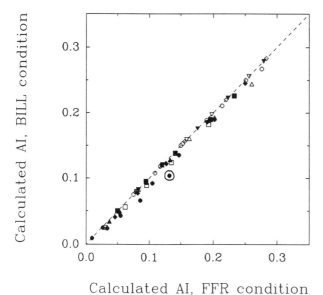

Figure 6. Calculated AI values for twelve hearing-impaired subjects wearing a master hearing aid in BILL-mode versus FFR mode. Dashed line indicates no difference between BILL and FFR AI values. Circled point indicates data from subject depicted in figure 8.

ligibility by subjects wearing BILL and FFR hearing aids for most realistic listening environments. However, the occasional listener still shows some improvements in nearly every study of commercially available "noise-reduction" devices (Dempsey 1987; Ono, Kanzaki, and Mizoi 1983; Stein and Dempesy-Hart 1984; Van Tasell, Larsen, and Fabry 1988). Lest

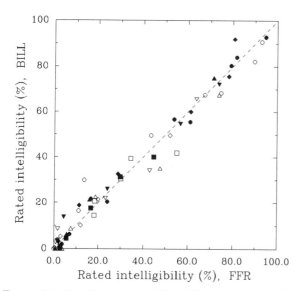

Figure 7. Rated speech intelligibility, in percent, by twelve hearing-impaired subjects wearing a master hearing aid in BILL-mode versus FFR-mode. Dashed line indicates no difference in rated intelligibility between the two conditions.

the laws of physics be denied, there are several explanations for these improvements.

When Hearing Aid Gain is Re-adjusted   In at least two published studies that compared "noise-reduction" devices to conventional hearing aids (Stein and Dempesy-Hart 1984; Wolinsky 1986) subjects were permitted to re-adjust the volume-control wheel after the adaptive-filter circuit was activated. When hearing aid gain is changed, slight improvements in speech intelligibility are possible for some subjects. Figure 9 illustrates, in terms of the Articulation Index, why this may occur. For the subject shown in this figure, increasing the volume when the filter circuit is activated improves the AI from 0.15 to 0.18, which predicts slightly higher speech intelligibility than for the filter-off condition.

When volume-control wheel changes are required after filter activation, the "automatic" nature of automatic signal processing loses its appeal, but slight improvements in signal-to-noise ratios are possible. Ono, Kanzaki, and Mazoi (1983) proposed that an adaptive high-pass filter circuit should be followed by automatic volume control (AVC) output compression. Thus, if the "target" gain in the high frequencies for a given person is different in quiet (filter-off) and noisy (filter-on) listening situations, AVC could be used to optimize gain—and AI values—in that frequency region *automatically*.

When Upward Spread of Masking Is Reduced   The results of several recent experiments have shown improvements in speech intelligibility by some (but not all) subjects wearing BILL hearing aids when certain band-limited, low-frequency noises are used (Van Tasell, Larsen, and Fabry 1988; Stein and Dempesy-Hart 1984). Presumably, these effects were either due to auditory effects, such as reduction in the upward spread of masking, or nonauditory factors, such as hearing aid distortion (Crain, Van Tasell, and Fabry 1989). Fabry, Leek, and Walden (1990) conducted an experiment that attempted to minimize the effects of *nonauditory* effects by using a laboratory model of a BILL hearing aid that added very little distortion or noise. In that study, they reported that upward spread of masking was present for normal and hearing-impaired subjects in the presence of a low-pass 1000-Hz noise with steep filter slopes (in excess of 100 dB/octave). Speech recognition was measured in the presence of this noise under two simulated hearing aid conditions: one in which a broad-band, fixed frequency response (FFR) was used, and another where speech and noise were high-pass filtered similar to BILL hearing aids. Speech recognition was greater

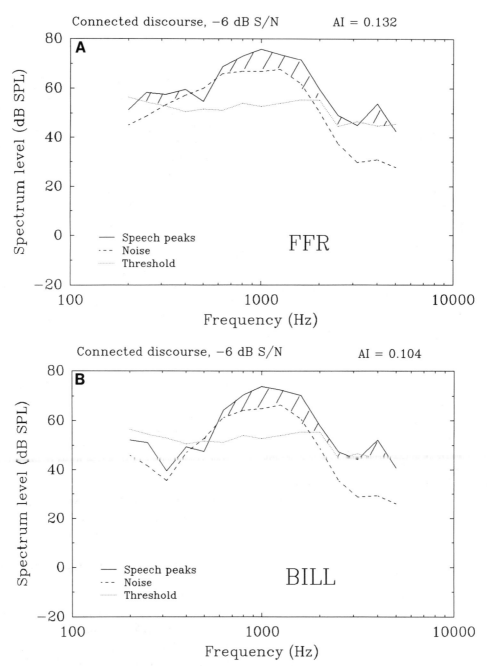

Figure 8.   Speech (solid line), noise (dashed line), and threshold (dotted line) levels for a hearing-impaired subject in aided FFR (top panel) and BILL (bottom panel) conditions. AI values for FFR and BILL conditions were 0.132 and 0.104, respectively.

under BILL than FFR conditions for nearly all subjects (figure 10); this improvement was related in a somewhat predictable sense to reduced upward spread of masking under the BILL condition. Normal and hearing-impaired subjects' masked thresholds were measured at 1500 Hz in the presence of the 1000 Hz low-pass noise for both FFR and BILL

conditions. Because there was no noise actually present at 1500 Hz, large differences between BILL and FFR masked thresholds were assumed to be related to a reduction in upward spread of masking under the BILL condition. Figure 11 shows this difference in masked threshold plotted as a function of the change in speech recognition for the two condi-

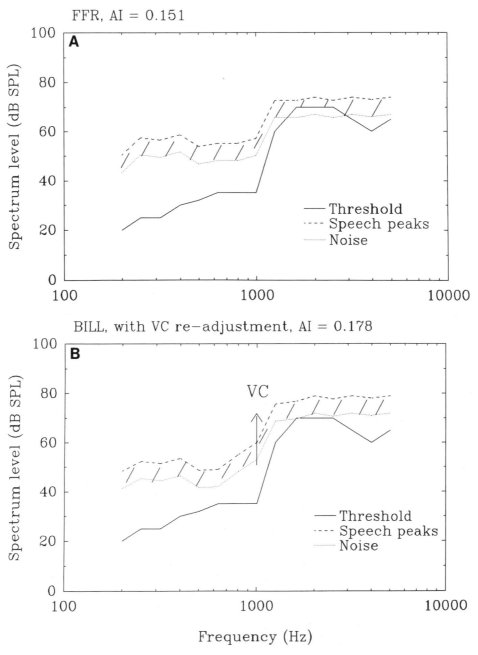

Figure 9. Data from hypothetical subject for FFR (top panel) and BILL (bottom panel) conditions when volume control was adjusted independently for the two conditions, resulting in higher AI value for BILL (0.178) than FFR (0.151) condition.

tions (BILL minus FFR). Calculation of the Pearson r correlation coefficient revealed a moderately high correlation of 0.61. This suggests that high-pass filtering similar to that used in BILL hearing aids were related in a somewhat predictable sense to upward spread of masking. However, there were sizeable differences across subjects, supporting previous findings that not all may benefit from such a device. Also, the benefits provided by this type of fil-

ter are restricted to certain types of low-frequency, band-pass noises that are rarely found outside the laboratory.

When Hearing Aid Distortion Is Reduced **Recall** that both Dyrlund (1989) and Preves and Newton (1989) reported that when compression and/or high-pass filtering was used, intermodulation distortion was reduced compared to peak-clipping

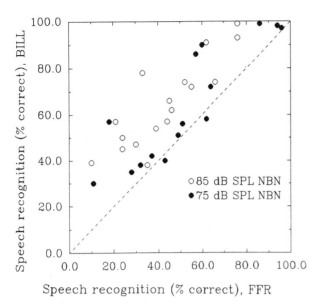

Figure 10. Speech recognition scores, in percent word recognition, for normal and hearing-impaired subjects for NU-6 words presented at 72 dB SPL in the presence of 75 dB SPL (filled circles) and 85 dB SPL (open circles) low-pass noise for BILL versus FFR conditions.

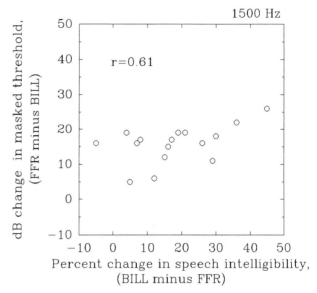

Figure 11. Data compare the change in masked threshold at 1500 Hz for a low-pass 1000 Hz noise versus the percent change in speech intelligibility under FFR and BILL conditions. Data on the ordinate are FFR masked thresholds *minus* BILL masked thresholds for the same subject; data on the abscissa are the difference in speech recognition for BILL *minus* FFR conditions for the same subject.

hearing aids. What remains to be seen is whether this lower distortion results in improved speech intelligibility. The debate has raged for years over whether compression hearing aids lead to higher speech recognition than peak-clipping hearing aids. Anyone who has ever listened to a compression hearing aid knows that the sound *quality* is much better than a peak clipping device, but several laboratory reports show no significant differences between peak-clipping and multiple-band compression when they are tested under laboratory conditions (Barfod 1976; Lippmann, Braida, and Durlach 1980). Villchur (1982) contends that the controlled conditions are part of the problem, claiming that speech stimuli used in the lab are frequently peak-equated to limit the dynamic fluctuations present in natural speech. This "pre"-compression of speech is not representative of realistic use conditions, and may bias the results against multiple-band compression. Although the recent trend has been toward the development of hearing aids with "full dynamic range compression" (Johnson, Pluvinage, and Benson 1989) more data are needed to determine the actual benefit in terms of speech intelligibility.

When Experiments Use the Listener's Own Hearing Aid This has been the default technique for conducting hearing aid experiments for many years.

Traditionally, the logic has been that if a person is willing to relinquish his or her own hearing aid for another device, it signifies some improvement that is not measurable with statistics. However, there are many problems with this experimental design, including a rather sizeable Hawthorne effect (Campbell and Stanley 1966). In addition, when patients' hearing aids are used, there may be no way to control for substantial differences in gain, frequency response, and output limitation level or type.

In the author's opinion, these are the only circumstances under which improvements in speech intelligibility are possible. Of these, preventing output distortion may be the most promising, because the circumstances under which upward spread of masking may occur are rather limited (perhaps only to psychoacoustics laboratories). Further research needs to be directed toward the relationship between distortion and speech intelligibility in realistic listening conditions. Additionally, more research is needed to determine the relationship between speech *quality* and level-dependent amplification. Also, other human factors such as increased wearing time, listening effort, or response time to speech stimuli should continue to be explored as potential metrics for use.

Conclusions

Resolved Issue

For commercially available "noise-reduction" hearing aids that use a single microphone, changes in speech intelligibility are not possible except under constrained conditions. This is true for those devices presently available for sale, but not for "true" digital hearing aids or those that use multiple microphones.

Unresolved Issues

1. Despite the fact that improved speech intelligibility in noise is not achieved, some individuals still elect to wear hearing aids that use level-dependent amplification. This suggests that factors other than speech intelligibility contribute to user satisfaction; further research is needed to determine which metric(s) is (are) most appropriate for determining candidacy.

2. Is level-dependent amplification necessary? If so, should the changes be fast (updated every few milliseconds) or slow (updated with gross changes in the listening environment)? Should these changes be manual or automatic? How many changes (or frequency responses) are necessary? None of these questions has been answered satisfactorily in the literature.

3. There is a need for development of standard measurement and evaluation techniques for use with current noise-reduction hearing aids. This is a variation on several top priorities for research on hearing aid selection and instrument measurement identified by respondents to a survey conducted at the first Vanderbilt Hearing Aid Conference (Bess 1982). Obviously, some advances have been made since 1982, especially in the area of hearing aid measurement with broad-band signals (see Preves et al. 1989), but further research is necessary to validate hearing aid performance. This is a particularly relevant issue for hearing aids that employ level-dependent amplification, to determine exactly what "target" gain values should be, whether they should be achieved in quiet or noisy backgrounds, when the filter is activated or deactivated, and so forth. For those devices offering multiple frequency responses, new target values will be required for optimizing hearing aid parameters to different background settings, and new strategies that are based upon a listener's personal listening environments

are likely to be developed. The research that promises to be the most valuable will use wearable, programmable hearing aids that are worn outside the laboratory in carefully controlled field studies.

References

American National Standards Institute 1987. Specifications for hearing aid characteristics. *ANSI S3.22–R1987.* New York.

Barfod, J. 1976. Multichannel compression hearing aids: Effects of recruitment on speech intelligibility. *Report Number 11.* The Acoustics Laboratory, Technical University of Denmark.

Bess, F.H. 1982. Amplification for the hearing impaired: Research priorities. In *The Vanderbilt Hearing Aid Report* eds. G.A. Studebaker and F.H. Bess. Upper Darby, PA: Monographs in Contemporary Audiology.

Campbell, D.T., and Stanley, J.C. 1966. *Experimental and Quasi-Experimental Designs for Research.* Chicago: Rand-McNally.

Carter, N.L., and Kryter, K.D. 1962. Masking of pure tones and speech. *Journal of Auditory Research* 2:66–98.

Crain, T.C., Van Tasell, D.V., and Fabry, D.A. 1989. Aided masking patterns with an adaptive frequency response hearing aid. Paper presented at the meeting of the American Speech-Language-Hearing Association, November 1989, St. Louis, MO.

Dempsey, J.J. 1987. Effect of automatic signal-processing amplification on speech recognition in noise for persons with sensorineural hearing loss. *Annals of Otology, Rhinology, and Laryngology* 96:251–53.

Dyrlund, O. 1989. Characterization of non-linear distortion in hearing aids using coherence analysis. A pilot study. *Scandinavian Audiology* 18(3):143–48.

Fabry, D.A., and Van Tasell, D.J. 1990. Evaluation of an articulation-index based model for predicting the effects of adaptive frequency response hearing aids. *Journal of Speech and Hearing Research* 33(4):676–89.

Fabry, D.A., Leek, M.R., and Walden, B.E. 1990. Do "adaptive frequency response" (AFR) hearing aids reduce upward spread of masking? *Journal of the Acoustical Society of America* 87(Supp. 1):S87.

French, N.R., and Steinberg, J.C. 1947. Factors governing the intelligibility of speech sounds. *Journal of the Acoustical Society of America* 19:90–119.

Gittles, T., and Wilson, F. 1987. Compression amplification with environment controlled release time. *Hearing Instruments* 38(8):39–41.

Goldberg, H. 1972. The utopian hearing aid: Current state of the art. *Journal of Auditory Research* 12:331–35.

Graupe, D., Grosspietch, J., and Basseas, S. 1987. A single-microphone-based self-adaptive filter of noise from speech and its performance evaluation. *Journal of Rehabilitation Research and Development* 24:119–26.

Johnson, J., Pluvinage, V., and Benson, D. 1989. Digitally programmable full dynamic range compression technology. *Hearing Instruments* 40(10):26–30.

Killion, M.C. 1990. A high fidelity hearing aid. *Hearing Instruments* 41(8):38–39.

Killion, M.C., Staab, W.J., and Preves, D.A. 1990. Classifying automatic signal processors. *Hearing Instruments* 41(8):24–26.

Klein, A. 1989. Assessing speech recognition in noise for listeners with a signal processor hearing aid. *Ear and Hearing* 10:50–57.

Klumpp, R.G., and Webster, J.C. 1963. Physical measurements of equally speech-interfering navy noises. *Journal of the Acoustical Society of America* 35:1328–1338.

Lippmann, R.P., Braida, L.D., and Durlach, N.I. 1980. Study of multichannel amplitude compression and linear amplification for persons with sensorineural hearing loss. *Journal of the Acoustical Society of America* 69(2):524–34.

Lybarger, S. 1947. Development of a new hearing aid with magnetic microphone. *Electrical Manufacturing* 1–13.

Mahon, W. (ed.). 1987. 1987 Buyer's guide to ASP hearing aids. *The Hearing Journal* 38(3):30–48.

Mangold, S., and Leijon, A. 1979. Programmable hearing aid with multi-channel compression. *Scandinavian Audiology* 8(2):121–26.

Moore, B.C. 1987. Design and evaluation of a two-channel compression hearing aid. *Journal Rehabilitation Research Development* 24(4):181–92.

Moore, B.C., and Glasberg, B.R. 1988. A comparison of four methods of implementing automatic gain control (AGC) in hearing aids. *British Journal of Audiology* 22(2):93–104.

Niederjohn, R.J., and Grotelueschen, J.H. 1976. The enhancement of speech intelligibility in high noise levels by high-pass filtering followed by rapid amplitude compression. *IEEE Transactions of Acoustics, Speech, and Signal Processing ASSP* 24:277–82.

Ono, H., Kanzaki, J., and Mizoi, K. 1983. Clinical results of hearing aid with noise-level-controlled selective amplification. *Audiology* 22:494–515.

Pavlovic, C.V. 1988. Articulation Index predictions of speech intelligibility in hearing aid selection. *Asha* 30(6/7):63–65.

Preves, D.A. 1990. Approaches to noise reduction in analog, digital, and hybrid hearing aids. *Seminars in Hearing* 11(1):39–67.

Preves, D.A., and Newton, J.R. 1989. The headroom problem and hearing aid performance. *The Hearing Journal* 42(10):19–26.

Preves, D.A., Beck, L. Burnett, E., and Teder, H. 1989. Input stimuli for obtaining frequency responses of automatic gain control hearing aids. *Journal of Speech and Hearing Research* 32(1):189–94.

Punch, J., and Beck, L.B. 1980. Low-frequency response of hearing and judgments of aided speech quality. *Journal of Speech and Hearing Disorders* 45:325–35.

Sammeth, C.A. 1990. Current availability of digital and hybrid hearing aids. *Seminars in Hearing* 11(1):91–100.

Sigelman, J., and Preves, D.A. 1987. Field trails of a new adaptive signal processor hearing aid circuit. *Hearing Journal* 40(4):24–27.

Skinner, M.W. 1980. Speech intelligibility in noise-induced hearing loss: Effects of high-frequency compensation. *Journal of the Acoustical Society of America* 67:306–317.

Skinner, M.W. 1991. Effects of frequency response, bandwidth and overall gain of linear amplification systems on performance of adults with sensorineural hearing loss. In *Acoustical Factors Affecting Hearing Aid Performance* (2nd edition), eds. G.A. Studebaker and I. Hochberg. Austin, TX: Pro-Ed.

Skinner, M.W., and Miller, J.D. 1983. Amplification bandwidth and speech intelligibility for two listeners with sensorineural hearing loss. *Audiology* 22:253-79.

Stein, L., and Dempesy-Hart, D. 1984. Listener-assessed intelligibility of a hearing aid self-adaptive noise filter. *Ear and Hearing* 5:199–204.

Thomas, I.B., and Niederjohn, R.J. 1970. The intelligibility of filtered-clipped speech in noise. *Journal of the Audio Engineering Society* 3:299–303.

Tyler, R.S., and Kuk, F.K. 1989. The effects of "noise suppression" hearing aids on consonant recognition in speech-babble and low-frequency noise. *Ear and Hearing* 10(4):243-49.

van Dijkhuizen, J.N., Festen, J.M., and Plomp, R. 1989. The effect of varying the amplitude-frequency response on the masked speech-reception threshold of sentences for hearing-impaired listeners. *Journal of the Acoustical Society of America* 86(2):621–28.

Van Tasell, D.J., Larsen, S.Y., and Fabry, D.A. 1988. Effects of an adaptive filter hearing aid on speech recognition in noise by hearing-impaired subjects. *Ear and Hearing* 9:15–21.

Villchur, E. 1973. Signal processing to improve speech intelligibility in perceptive deafness. *Journal of the Acoustical Society of America* 53:1646–1657.

Villchur, E. 1982. The evaluation of amplitude-compression processing for hearing aids. In *The Vanderbilt Hearing Aid Report* eds. G.A. Studebaker and F.H. Bess. Upper Darby, PA: Monographs in Contemporary Audiology.

Widex 1989. *Quattro Programming Manual*. Widex Corporation.

Wolinsky, S. 1986. Clinical assessment of a self-adaptive noise filtering system. *The Hearing Journal* 4(10):29–32.

Yund, E.W., Simon, H.J., and Efron, R. 1987. Speech discrimination with an 8-channel compression hearing aid and conventional aids in background of speech-band noise. *Journal of Rehabilitation Research and Development* 24(4):161–80.

CHAPTER 7

Clinical Implications and Limitations of Current Noise Reduction Circuitry

Ruth A. Bentler

In the last three to four years clinical audiologists have been inundated with "new" technology in analogue hearing aids. While many of these circuits may not qualify as "noise reduction" by our scientific standards, marketers tout a number of different designs as being capable of "reducing background/ environmental noise levels" or "improving ability to understand speech in noise." These designs include the *automatic* level dependent, *manual* multiple memory "choose your response," and, recently, the wide band "high quality reproduction of sound/ noise" designs. Several attempts have been made to classify this broad range of signal processing circuitry. *Adaptive frequency response* (AFR) has been suggested for those hearing aids that incorporate circuitry that automatically adapts the frequency response in response to level or spectral content of the environment (Fabry and Walden 1990). The same authors have suggested the term *programmable multifrequency response* (PMR) to refer to hearing aids (digitally controlled programmable hearing aids) incorporating several different frequency responses that are stored in memory and selectively activated by the user, as needed. These classifications do not account for some of the most recent developments in hearing aids such as the single memory programmable hearing aid or the adaptive compression™[1] circuit, to name a few. As a result, Killion, Staab, and Preves (1990) have proposed another classification system: (1) FFR (Fixed Frequency Response) hearing aids, or those utilizing compression limiting, wide range dynamic compression or (my addition) adaptive compression™; and (2) LDFR (Level Dependent Frequency Response) hearing aids or those circuits that (a) (Type 1) reduce low-frequency gain in response to high-intensity input, (b) (Type 2) reduce high-frequency response in response to high-level input, or (c) (Type 3) can be

programmed to do either. It becomes apparent that the direction in hearing aid design is toward the development of the ideal hearing aid from any environment—one that can provide *the* optimal frequency response in both quiet and noise. In attempting to determine what is optimal for which hearing-impaired listener, a wide variety of designs and innovations has been put forward. With multitudinous new "spec" sheets to filter through and decipher, many clinicians find wading through resultant marketing propaganda as disconcerting as attempting to revamp evaluation procedures to meet these innovations. As a result, decision making within the context of the hearing aid evaluation has become less scientific and more "seat of the pants." For a clinical audiologist seeking direction and/or guiding reassurance there remains a dearth of clinical evidence of circuit superiority rankings or appropriate protocol for evaluation. Until some empirical evidence surfaces relative to these issues, many clinicians will base decisions relative to appropriateness of circuitry on availability and experience with particular brands and models.

Over the last two years an attempt has been made at the University of Iowa to quantify advantages of several recent automatic "noise reduction" circuits for hearing-impaired individuals of varying degrees, configurations, and experience levels (Bentler 1989; Bentler et al. 1989). Three groups of subjects are being followed for one year: an *experimental group*, comprised of approximately 60 subjects fitted with one of four circuits marketed as "noise reduction" and followed closely; and two control groups: *control A*, a group of 43 subjects who followed standard clinic protocol for hearing evaluation, hearing aid evaluation and fitting, and follow-up, and *control B*, a group of 16 additional subjects who were followed closely (identical protocol to the experimental group) but without a "noise reduction" circuit. The circuits randomly assigned to the experimental group included the adaptive compres-

---

[1]Adaptive compression is now a trademark of Telex Corporation.

sion™, (high pass) adaptive frequency response, Zeta™, and frequency selective input compression designs. Three configurations of hearing loss were investigated: *flat* (less than 15 dB difference from 500 to 2000 Hz) *gently sloping* (less than 25 dB/octave slope from 1000 to 2000 Hz), and *steeply sloping* (greater than 25 dB/octave slope from 1000 to 2000 Hz). Two degrees of hearing loss were considered: *mild* (less than 40 dB average of 1000 and 2000 Hz, except for the steeply sloping category, then less than 30 dB loss at 250, 500, and 1000 Hz) and *moderately severe* (greater than 50 dB average at 1000 and 2000 Hz, except for the steeply sloping group, then greater than 30 dB loss at 250, 500, and 1000 Hz). All subjects within the experimental and control B groups were fitted according to NAL-R (Byrne and Dillon 1986). The purpose of the investigation essentially was to determine if any quantifiable differences could be shown to exist among the groups studied. Some of the preliminary results obtained in our study will be presented here.

Quantifying Advantage

Objective Measures

Clinical decision making in hearing aid selection historically has been based on "advantage." Whether the chosen hearing aid provided the closest match to some target values, the most improvement in speech recognition (or smallest size, longest battery life, and so on), it showed some advantage over those to which it was compared. With these current "noise reduction" designs, there is increasing evidence that speech recognition scores do not improve (Bentler et al. 1989; Fabry and Walden 1990; Klein 1989; Van Tasell, Larsen, and Fabry 1988) nor can they be expected to improve (without alterations in the volume control and/or use of band limited noise). Similarly, it becomes difficult to measure the insertion gain advantage provided by one circuit compared to any other due to the nonlinear nature and input dependent response characteristics of many adaptive response/multiple memory designs (Preves and Sigelman 1989). As a result, the protocol for quantifying advantage remains elusive within most clinical settings. To use unrealistic noise spectra as the background for speech recognition tasks provides no predictive information relative to speech recognition ability (Van Tasell, Larsen, and Fabry 1988), and to obtain insertion gain utilizing a swept pure tone provides no good pre-

diction of user gain. Other possibilities for determining benefits have been suggested, including the Articulation Index (AI) and SRT in noise.

Use of the Articulation Index theory (French and Steinberg 1947) has been advocated to predict the effects of various frequency responses on speech intelligibility. Its use with adaptive frequency response circuitry, however, requires a clear understanding and measurement of both electroacoustic characteristics of the hearing aid and background noise levels. The problem of accurately measuring the gain derived from any nonlinear (dependent upon input signal characteristics) amplification system makes AI calculations provisional. Fabry and Van Tasell (1990) found that for hearing-impaired subjects using a master hearing aid with an adaptive (low frequency) filtering circuit, the Articulation Index did not predict improvement in speech intelligibility in the AFR-on versus AFR-off condition, suggesting that use of AI as a part of a clinical protocol may not prove fruitful. Even if clinicians choose to use AI in predicting ("monotonically") relative performance between several hearing aids, it may be beyond the technical capabilities provided in their work setting. Calculation of the Articulation Index requires a fairly precise measurement of the gain provided to the listener during presentation of a particular speech stimulus. Because gain may vary with every change in input for current automatic circuits, it is difficult to get even an approximate estimate of user gain in even the best of circumstances. Many clinical settings do not have the hardware *or* the software (for calculations of AI with appropriate band weighting, etc.) to obtain such calculations.

Use of an adaptive procedure to obain the 50% performance in both quiet and noise (essentially SRT) is another potential tool. Using a protocol identical to that presented by Van Tasell, Larsen, and Fabry (1988), sound field SRTs were obtained in a background noise for 48 subjects. Figure 1 shows the long-term average speech spectrum of the 11 spondees used; this set of spondees has been shown to be highly homogeneous in intelligibility (Dubno, Dirks, and Morgan 1984). At the bottom of figure 1 the spectrum of the speech noise that was used is shown. Speech recognition threshold was obtained using a simple up–down method to track the 50% performance (Levitt 1971). Stimulus items were presented in random order. Each subject was familiarized with the entire list at a relatively high level—typically 72 dB SPL at the input to the hearing aid microphone—after which the presentation level was decreased in 5 dB steps until an incorrect re-

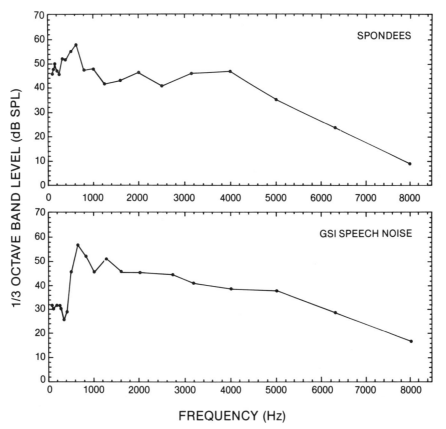

Figure 1. Average (rms) sound pressure level in one-third octave bands for speech stimuli (Van Tasell, Larsen, and Fabry 1988) and speech weighted noise.

sponse was made. After two reversals were made, the step size was reduced to 1 dB and testing continued until SRT was stabilized (a minimum of 16 reversals). The mean and standard deviation of the final 12 reversals were calculated; the mean was taken as SRT for that condition. The procedure was repeated with a 70 dB SPL noise level and again in quiet for reliability measures. Initial findings indicated that S/N ratio for 50% performance is indeed a reliable measure, but did not change significantly across subjects with the noise reduction circuit activated ("filter in") compared to measures taken with the noise reduction circuit inactivated ("filter out"). These findings are in agreement with those reported by Van Tasell, Larsen, and Fabry (1988). Consequently, additional data analyses were initiated in an attempt to glean further usefulness for the SRT findings. For each of the subjects, measures of satisfaction ratings, using a scale of 1 to 5 (1 = not satisfied, 2 = a little satisfied, 3 = moderately satisfied, 4 = very satisfied, 5 = totally satisfied), and the low predictability scores on the Speech Perception in Noise Test (Kalikow, Stevens, and Elliot 1977; Bilger

et al. 1984) were also obtained. It seemed possible that while the SRT in noise might not significantly change with the activation of the nonlinear circuit, there may be some relationship between S/N ratio necessary for 50% performance in a background of noise and performance on a speech recognition task (of low predictability words) and/or the subject's satisfaction with a given circuit. Results indicated no significant correlation between S/N required for 50% performance and SPIN (LP) scores or satisfaction ratings ($p = .05$). Further analysis indicated no significant correlation between "filter in"/"filter out" low predictability score change (as reported by Stein, McGee, and Lewis 1989) and the SRTs in noise ($p = .05$). Hawkins et al. (1988) suggest that a good speechreader can tolerate 10 dB more noise when viewing *and* hearing the talker and still achieve the same self-estimated percent achieved intelligibility. While that variable is considered or measured too infrequently in hearing aid evaluation procedures, it may account for the hearing aid success of some listeners and not others who exhibit similar SRTs in noise (without visual cues).

While the potential for SRT in noise may be promising, the logistics of obtaining those measures must be understood clearly. The typical speech spectrum noise currently available on commercial audiometers is a common choice of noise for many protocols; yet, there is evidence that moderate levels of noise may drive hearing aids into their saturation range (Crain, Van Tasell, and Fabry 1989; Frye 1987) because of a higher crest factor (peak to rms). As a result, the hearing aid may be saturating in the "filter out" condition but not during the "filter in" condition because in the latter case a considerable portion of the noise is filtered. The assumption may be made erroneously that the activation of the noise reduction circuit has accounted for the improved speech reception, when in fact the level of the noise may have created distortion at the output (reduced coherence) that did not exist in the "filter in" condition or in most real life situations. Conversely, in clinical setting, using a noise signal whose rms level is too low may not activate the noise reduction circuit, and thus the advantage that may have been gleaned from an improved signal-to-noise ratio would not be evident. In addition, the 5 dB step size currently utilized for SRT measurements is typically too large for measuring any subtle differences between circuits. While many commercial audiometers have a 1 dB step size available, the addition of this 40-minute protocol may not be practical. And finally, choice of stimuli for obtaining SRT is critical to the outcome. Use of a subset of highly homogeneous spondees (such as described by Dubno, Dirks, and Morgan 1984) is required to ensure reliable enough measures in "filter in"/"filter out" conditions to make comparisons.

Subjective Measures

More subjective methods of quantifying advantage are possible in the form of self-report inventories and/or satisfaction questionnaires. Although these subjective measures have not been shown to correlate well with objective measures (e.g., Bentler 1989; Bentler et al. 1989), their intended uses, namely description of the handicapping effects of a hearing loss for an individual and planning for rehabilitative follow-up, cannot be overlooked. (Yet audiologists utilizing this type of evaluative measure may well be in the minority according to McCarthy, Montgomery, and Mueller 1990.) If the ultimate goal is the user's perception of increased benefit, then satisfaction questionnaires or self-report inventories (including an expectation checklist such as was de-

veloped by Seyfried and Anderson 1989) must be considered in any fitting protocol.

To date, there is no evidence that those persons fitted and counseled appropriately with (automatic) noise reduction circuitry actually are served better. Long-term satisfaction ratings were obtained from new hearing aid wearers after six months and after one year of hearing aid use. Recall that both the experimental group and one control group (B) were followed closely (a minimum of six two-hour appointments over a year), while the subjects in the other control group (A) were clients sampled randomly from clinic files (and typically "checked in on" at the end of a trial, only). Using the same scale of 1 to 5 (1 = not satisfied, 2 = a little satisfied, 3 = moderately satisfied, 4 = very satisfied, 5 = totally satisfied), mean satisfaction rating at six months and one year (shown in figure 2) indicate similar mean ratings of satisfaction. It is apparent that the experimental group did not differ in mean rating of satisfaction from either group utilizing non-noise reduction hearing aids. Analyzing the same information for degree of satisfaction, table I shows that similar proportions of subjects from each group had ratings of not satisfied, slightly satisfied, etc. In fact, as shown in table II, 82.6% of the experimental group rated moderate or above satisfaction with their "noise reduction" design at six months and 85.8% of the same group rated moderate or above satisfaction at one year. For control group A (no noise reduction circuit, no close follow-up), 81.4% acknowledged moderate or better satisfaction at six months and 75.8% at one year. For control group B (no noise reduction circuit, closely followed) six month data indicate similar degrees of satisfaction. Although these "satisfaction" levels for all groups are somewhat higher than previously reported (Hossford-Dunn and Baxter 1985; Kochkin 1990; Oja and Schow 1984), there is no statistical evidence of greater satisfaction among those subjects using the noise reduction designs.

Other subjective measures that were obtained on the same group of subjects included a subsection of the Hearing Performance Inventory (HPI) (Giolas et al. 1979; Lamb, Owens, and Schubert 1983). This subsection, dubbed the HPI$_{38}$, consists of 38 questions assessing an individual's ability to understand speech in a variety of background sounds. The experimental group, as a whole, indicated significant improvement (reduction in HPI score) at both the 6 month and the 12 month administration for the fairly quiet, music, and people talking nearby subtests (figure 3). In fact, the cor-

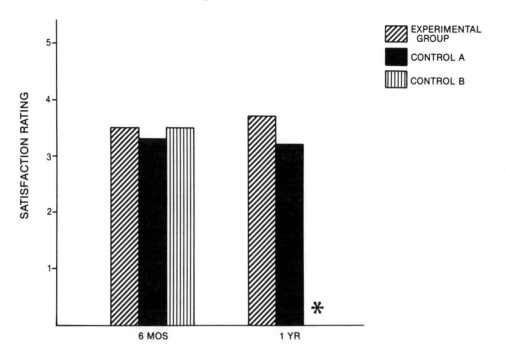

* CONTROL B data incomplete for 1 year

Figure 2.   Mean satisfaction ratings obtained at six months and one year for experimental and control groups (see text).

relation coefficient for satisfaction ratings to each subtest were moderate (see table III). In an effort to determine if experienced hearing aid users are better contenders for the automatic designs, as has been suggested by several manufacturers, the data were analyzed separately for the two subgroups (figure 4). It is evident that no difference exists between experienced and nonexperienced subgroups (ANOVA, $p = .05$). The data were re-sorted to determine if the mildly hearing-impaired (less than 40 dB PTA) groups might be deriving more benefit than the moderately severely hearing-impaired

Table 1.   Satisfaction Ratings of Three Groups by Degree

	Not Satisfied	A Little Satisfied	Moderately Satisfied	Very Satisfied	Totally Satisfied
Experimental Group			6 Months		
	8.5%	8.5%	34.8%	36.9%	10.8%
			1 Year		
	5%	10.2%	25.6%	46.2%	12.8%
Control A Group			6 Months		
	4.6%	13.8%	39.5%	28%	13.8%
			1 Year		
	13.8%	10.3%	27.6%	34.4%	13.8%
Control B Group			6 Months		
	6.3%	6.3%	43.7%	37.5%	6.3%
			1 Year		
	*	*	*	*	*

*Data not yet complete.

Table II. Percentage of Each Group Rating Moderate or Above Satisfaction

	6 Months	1 Year
Experimental Group	82.6%	85.8%
Control A Group	81.4%	75.8%
Control B Group	82.2%	*

*Data not yet complete.

(greater than 50 dB PTA) group. Using a Two-Way ANOVA, the mildly impaired group was noted to have significantly greater change in their HPI scores (for all three subsets) than the more severely impaired group (Newman Keuls, $p = .05$) from the initial scores (figure 5). The only configuration that showed significant change in the HPI over the year was the gently sloping subgroup, and no circuit type was shown superior to any other (figure 6). The conclusion that the more mildly hearing-impaired individual with a gently sloping configuration (experienced or not) appears to derive/ report the most benefit from *any* hearing aid should come as no surprise to the clinical audiologist!

The one advantage that repeatedly surfaces and cannot be overlooked in clinical interactions (Bentler et al. 1989) is that of perceptually improved listening conditions. Whether the circuit is adjusted manually or automatically reduces background noise, the result may be less annoyance, or "easier listening" (Preves and Sigelman 1989), an

Table III. Correlation Coefficient for HPI versus Satisfaction (Three Subtests) for Experimental Group

Initial		
Quiet	Music	People
−.38 (.02)	−.30 (.07)	−.32 (.05)
6 Months		
Quiet	Music	People
−.40 (.01)	−.36 (.02)	−.29 (.08)
1 Year		
Quiet	Music	People
−.44 (.007)	−.42 (.01)	−.46 (.005)

advantage that is difficult to quantify. Another advantage, however unintentional, surfaced during our data collection: that of allowing the client to change the response characteristics from linear to nonlinear (essentially "filter out" to "filter in"), a feature unavailable or underutilized in the past. In order to meet guidelines from our Human Subjects Committee, manufacturers were requested to provide user switches to activate the nonlinear circuit in two automatic noise reduction designs (specifically the Zeta™ and high pass adaptive filtering circuits). Virtually every subject acknowledged the usefulness of the switch, frequently noting that the

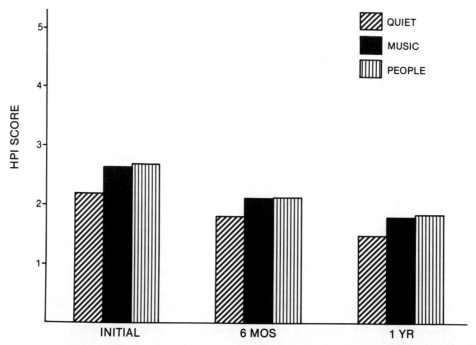

Figure 3. HPI₃₈ scores (3 subtests) for experimental group obtained initially, and at 6 months and 1 year postfitting.

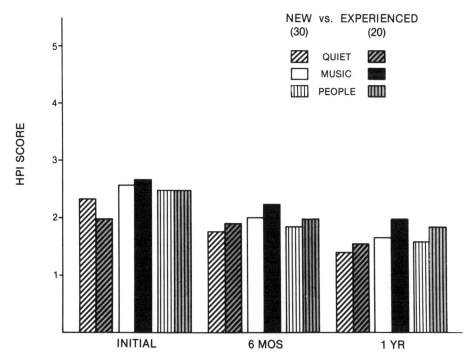

Figure 4. HPI$_{38}$ scores (3 subtests) for experienced versus new user subgroups obtained initially, and at 6 months and 1 year postfitting.

quality of "filter out" was more pleasing. Speech Reception Thresholds obtained in both switch positions indicated lower SRTs with the switch "off" ("filter out") in many cases, suggesting that "filter in" may have changed the frequency response, even in a quiet background, a speculation easily confirmed by probe microphone measurements utilizing a composite noise signal.

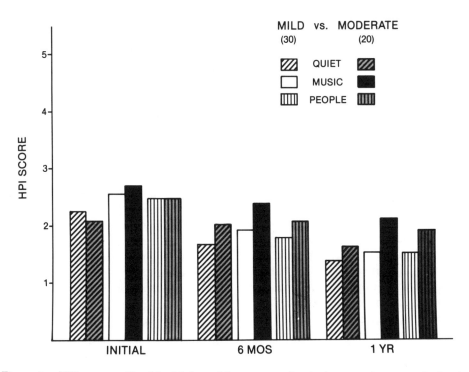

Figure 5. HPI$_{38}$ scores (3 subtests) for mild versus moderate degree subgroups obtained initially, and at 6 months and 1 year postfitting.

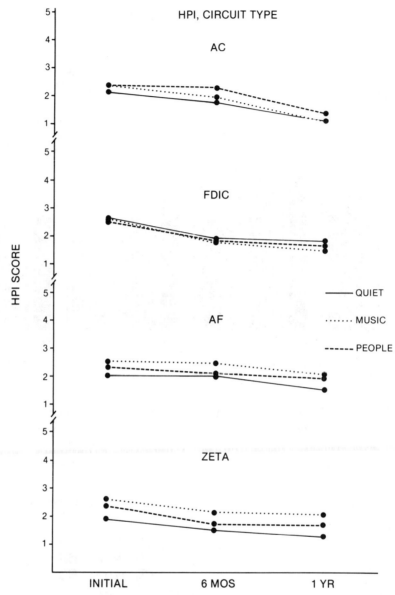

Figure 6.   HPI$_{38}$ scores (3 subtests) for four different circuit types obtained initially, and at 6 months and 1 year postfitting.

Implications/Limitations

The implications and limitations of many recent automatic and manually adjustable hearing aid designs are portentous. Once the clinician has sorted through the barrage of marketing "news," he or she must be cognizant of a number of unresolved (or perhaps unresolvable) fitting issues:

1. *How to measure gain with the noise reduction aids.* With the automatic design, "target" gain/output established with the (standard) swept pure tone often will not approximate that measured with

speech weighted or other environmental stimuli; that is, with each input, different output characteristics may be obtained (Stelmachowitz et al. 1990). Electroacoustic measurements require a complex input to realize the nonlinearity of the automatic circuit. What complex is optimal? What crest factor is representative of real life events?

2. *When to measure or match the target gain.* With multiple memory designs, it is very difficult for the audiologist to attempt logic in setting some target gain values. Should one memory be labelled "baseline" from which all other adjustments for multiple environments be made?

3. *Who is a candidate?* Clinical decision-making has evolved from "Which aid provides the most gain (or best target match)?" to "What are the limitations for a particular client relative to the available choices?" Handedness, manual dexterity, better/worse ear, social/occupational demands, expectations, and so on, are considerations used to provide some direction relative to the appropriateness of any aid. More complex considerations must be made for current designs such as cognitive skills, cost/benefit of analog versus some digitally programmable option, and so forth. The following cases are presented to emphasize the difficulty of obtaining a profile of the "totally satisfied" or "totally dissatisfied" client:

Example 1 Subjects EW and HvW were both fitted with the same (high pass) adaptive filtering circuit (figure 7). Both are employed females and experienced hearing aid users; both exhibit flat, moderately severe hearing losses, and both have nearly identical NST, SPIN, and HPI scores. Both report wearing their hearing aid for 16 hours per day, EW with "Total Dissatisfaction" and HvW with "Total Satisfaction." An interesting aside here is that HvW reports using her "filter in" condition approximately 5% of the time, whereas EW reports the noise reduction circuit is on 100% of the time. Expectation scores indicated that EW had higher positive expectations (for example, relative to comfort, need, and effectiveness) whereas HvW had

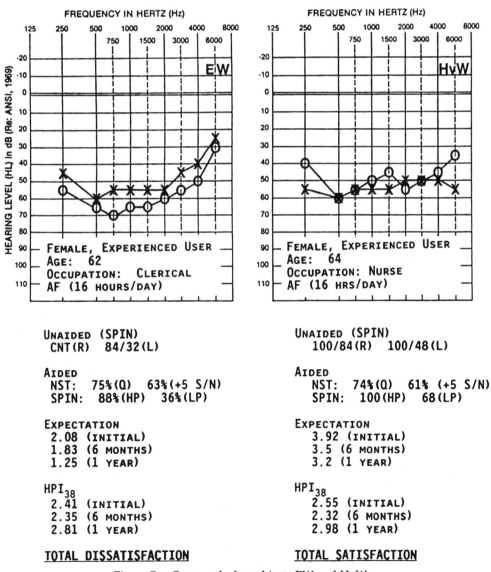

Figure 7.   Case study for subjects EW and HvW.

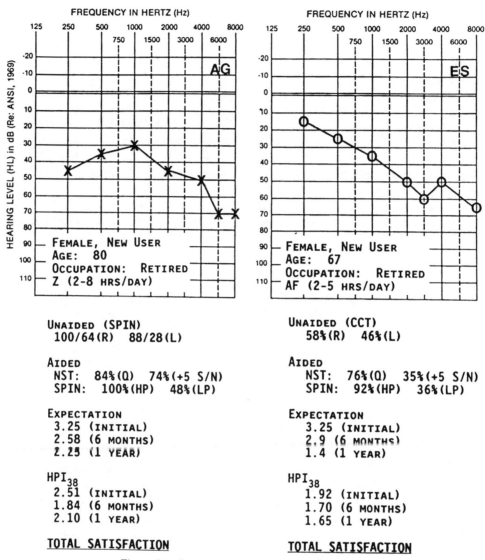

FREQUENCY IN HERTZ (Hz)

UNAIDED (SPIN)
100/64(R) 88/28(L)

AIDED
NST: 84%(Q) 74%(+5 S/N)
SPIN: 100%(HP) 48%(LP)

EXPECTATION
3.25 (INITIAL)
2.58 (6 MONTHS)
2.25 (1 YEAR)

HPI₃₈
2.51 (INITIAL)
1.84 (6 MONTHS)
2.10 (1 YEAR)

TOTAL SATISFACTION

UNAIDED (CCT)
58%(R) 46%(L)

AIDED
NST: 76%(Q) 35%(+5 S/N)
SPIN: 92%(HP) 36%(LP)

EXPECTATION
3.25 (INITIAL)
2.9 (6 MONTHS)
1.4 (1 YEAR)

HPI₃₈
1.92 (INITIAL)
1.70 (6 MONTHS)
1.65 (1 YEAR)

TOTAL SATISFACTION

Figure 8.   Case study for subjects AG and ES.

lower expectations, but more apparent benefit. Additionally, note that the HPI scores did not change for either subject over the year.

Example 2   Subjects AG and ES are both retired females, new users of amplification, with mild degree of hearing impairment (figure 8). Note identical expectation scores, and similar (initial) HPI scores. Each indicates "Total Satisfaction" with her new hearing aid, both at 6 months and 1 year of use. AG was fitted with the Zeta™; ES was fitted with a (high pass) adaptive filtering hearing aid. Either circuit proved ideal, although the cost differential (greater than $250) was significant.

Example 3   Subjects DY and PC are two retired males (both 72 years old), with very similar degrees and configurations of hearing loss (figure 9). DY,

however, is a new hearing aid user (10 hrs/day), whereas PC is an experienced hearing aid user of approximately five years (2 hrs/day). Unaided CCT scores are the same, as are NST and SPIN (HP) scores, although the SPIN (LP) scores indicate better performance without contextual cues for DY, who likewise rates "Total Satisfaction" with his noise reduction circuit compared to PC's "Total Dissatisfaction." Additionally, final HPI scores suggest that DY may be having less difficulty communicating in noisy environments than PC.

Example 4   Subjects JW and WR are retired farmers of similar age and fairly similar degree and configuration of hearing loss (figure 10). Unaided CCT, aided NST, and SPIN scores are nearly identical, again with the exception of LP SPIN. Expectation scores and (initial) HPI scores are nearly identi-

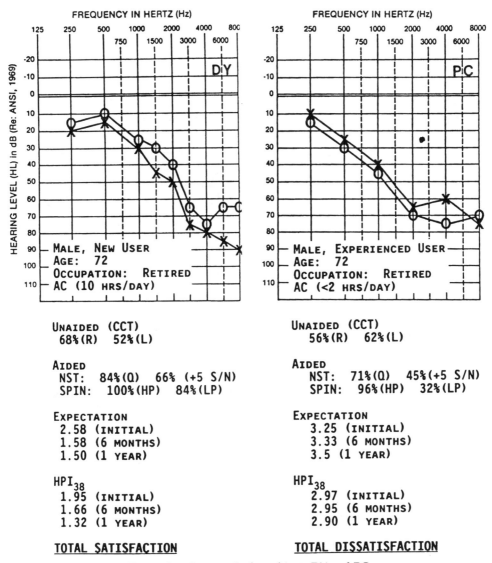

Figure 9. Case study for subjects DY and PC.

cal. In this example, however, JW (whose LP scores were higher throughout the year) reported "Total Dissatisfaction" with his frequency selective input compression circuit, whereas WR was "Totally Satisfied" with the same circuit. Note the very significant change in HPI for WR as well, which is consistent with his satisfaction rating.

It is obvious that individuals who are very similar on a number of measures may have very dissimilar outcomes.

Summary

The resultant "wait and see" attitude of many clinics is justified. With no apparent direction as to who benefits from what the most, coupled with the uncertainty of clinicians and researchers alike about appropriate fitting protocol, many clinical settings have not yet invested time or money in the newer designs. Added to this are preliminary suggestions that "noise reduction" circuits do not provide better objective or subjective measures of performance than more traditional analog circuits. In the event we might overlook those hearing aid users who do acknowledge significant benefit, however, protocols for evaluation of current noise reduction design should include the following:

1. For automatic circuits (specifically adaptive—or level dependent—frequency response circuits), a user switch should be requested from the manufacturer. Such a switch will allow the individ-

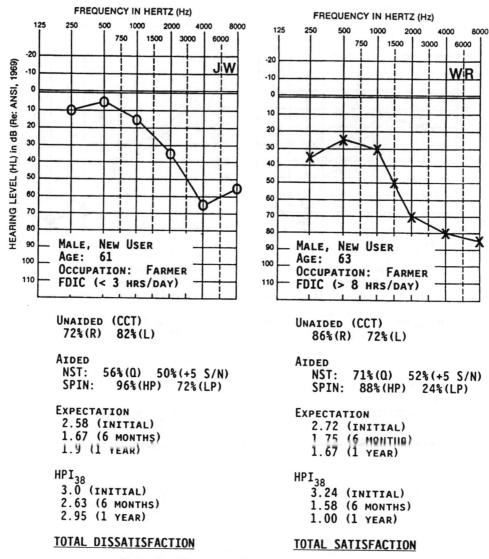

Figure 10.   Case study for subjects JW and WR.

ual to ascertain the benefits to be gained from "filter in" versus "filter out" in many different environments. Such an option would also allow for a single subject/client comparison of speech intelligibility, coherence, and some of the scaling procedures currently in use.

2.   For manual (multiple memory) designs, a trial/experience period should be provided. It has been my experience that many (new and experienced) hearing aid users cannot differentiate (as far as speech recognition or quality are concerned) between the available programs in various environments. The cost difference between a traditional analog hearing aid and a multiple memory design may be enough, however, that clinicians need to be accountable for such a recommendation.

3.   For both the automatic as well as the manual designs, use of subjective scales of benefit and/or performance should become a routine part of any fitting protocol. An understanding of a particular client's expectations and communication demands and breakdowns, as well as his or her perceived success, can provide specifics that group data will continue to overlook.

References

Bentler, R.A. 1989. Factors related to hearing aid user satisfaction. Poster at Annual Meeting of the American Speech-Language-Hearing Association, November 1989, St. Louis.

Bentler, R.A., Niebuhr, D.P., Getta, J.P., and Anderson, C.V. 1989. A study of the effectiveness of "noise reduction" circuitry. Poster at Annual Meeting of the American Speech-Language-Hearing Association, November 1989, St. Louis.

Bilger, R.C., Neutzel, J.M., Rabinowitz, W.M., and Rzeczowski, C. 1984. Standardization of a test of speech perception in noise. *Journal of Speech and Hearing Research* 27:32–48.

Byrne, D., and Dillon, H. 1986. The National Acoustics Laboratories' (NAL) new procedure for selecting the gain and frequency response of a hearing aid. *Ear and Hearing* 7:257–65.

Crain, T.R., Van Tasell, D.J., and Fabry, D.A. 1989. Aided masking patterns with an adaptive frequency response hearing aid. Paper read at the Annual Meeting of the American Speech-Language-Hearing Association, November 1989, St. Louis.

Dubno, J.R., Dirks, D.D., and Morgan, D.E. 1984. Effects of age and mild hearing loss on speech recognition in noise. *Journal of Acoustical Society of America* 76:87–96.

Fabry, D., and Van Tasell, D.J. 1990. Evaluation of an Articulation Index based model for predicting the effects of adaptive frequency response hearing aids. *Journal of Speech and Hearing Research* 33(4):676–89.

Fabry, D.A., and Walden, B.E. 1990. Noise reduction hearing aids: What is the fate of ART (adaptive response technology)? *ASHA; Journal of the American Speech and Hearing Association* 32:23–26.

French, N.R., and Steinberg, J.C. 1947. Factors governing the intelligibility of speech sounds. *Journal of the Acoustical Society of America* 19:90–119.

Frye, G.J. 1987. Crest factor and composite signals for hearing aid testing. *The Hearing Journal* 40:15–18.

Giolas, T., Owens, E., Lambs, H., and Schubert, E. 1979. Hearing performance inventory. *Journal of Speech and Hearing Disorders* 44:169–95.

Hawkins, D.B., Montgomery, A.A., Mueller, H.G., and Sedge, R.K. 1988. Assessment of speech intelligibility by hearing-impaired listeners. In *Noise as a Public Health Problem, Vol. 2* eds. B. Berglund, U. Berglund, J. Karlsson, and T. Lindvall. Stockholm, Sweden: Swedish Council for Building Research.

Hossford-Dunn, H. and Baxter, J.H. 1985. Prediction and validation of hearing aid wearer benefit: Preliminary findings. *Hearing Instruments* 36:34–41.

Kalikow, D., Stevens, K., and Elliot, L. 1977. Development of a test of speech intelligibility in noise using sentence materials with controlled word predictability. *Journal of the Acoustical Society of America* 61:1337–1351.

Killion, M.C., Staab, W.J., and Preves, D.A. 1990. Classifying automatic signal processors. *Hearing Instruments* 41(8):24–26.

Klein, A. 1989. Assessing speech recognition in noise for listeners with a signal processor hearing aid. *Ear and Hearing* 10:50–57.

Kochkin, S. 1990. Introducing MarkeTrak: A consumer tracking survey of the hearing instrument market. *Hearing Journal* 43:17–27.

Lamb, S.H., Owens, E., and Schubert, E.D. 1983. The revised form of the hearing performance inventory. *Ear and Hearing* 4:152–57.

Levitt, H. 1971. Transformed up-down methods in psychoacoustics. *Journal of the Acoustical Society of America* 49:467–77.

McCarthy, P.A. Montgomery, A.A., and Mueller, H.G. 1990. Decision making in rehabilitative audiology. *Journal of the American Academy of Audiology* 1(1):23–30.

Oja, G.L., and Schow, R.L. 1984. Hearing aid evaluation based on measures of benefit, use and satisfaction. *Ear and Hearing* 5:77–86.

Preves, D.A., and Sigelman, J.A. 1989. A questionnaire to evaluate signal processing hearing aids. *Hearing Instruments* 40(11):20–21, 24.

Seyfried, D.N., and Anderson, C.V. 1989. Use of a communication self report inventory to measure hearing aid counseling effects. Ph.D. diss., University of Iowa, Iowa City, IA.

Stein, L., McGee, T., and Lewis, P. 1989. Speech recognition measures with noise suppression hearing aids using a single subject experimental design. *Ear and Hearing* 10(6):375–81.

Stelmachowicz, P.G., Lewis, D.E., Seewald, R.C., and Hawkins, D.B. 1990. Complex and pure-tone signals in the evaluation of hearing aid characteristics. *Journal of Speech and Hearing Research* 33(2):380–85.

Van Tasell, D.J., Larsen, S., and Fabry, D.A. 1988. Effects of an adaptive filter hearing aid on speech recognition in noise by hearing impaired subjects. *Ear and Hearing* 9(11):15–21.

CHAPTER 8
Advanced Signal Processing Techniques for Hearing Aids

Harry Levitt

The development of microminiature electronics has had a profound impact on hearing aid development. The invention of the transistor was a particularly important advance in that it allowed for substantial reductions in the size of hearing aids. The subsequent development of integrated circuits led to even greater reductions in size and, as a consequence, it has been possible to develop hearing aids small enough to fit in the ear canal. Current technological advances in very large-scale integrated (VLSI) circuits now offer new possibilities for further advances in hearing aid design. Whereas there is still considerable emphasis on making hearing aids smaller and cosmetically more attractive, there is also an ongoing effort in developing advanced signal processing techniques for reducing background noise, increasing speech intelligibility and improving overall sound quality that can be implemented in modern hearing aids.

A particularly important recent advance has been the development of digital, or partially digital, hearing aids. Advanced signal processing hearing aids using analog techniques also have been developed. It is the purpose of this chapter to describe these new hearing aids, review their relative advantages, and discuss the audiological implications of these new technologies.

Modern signal processing hearing aids can be subdivided into three groups: (1) analog hearing aids in which conventional analog circuits (filters, amplifiers, limiters) are used to process the audio signal, (2) digital hearing aids in which the audio signal is processed by digital means, and (3) hybrid analog/digital hearing aids that combine analog and digital techniques. A common form of the hybrid analog/digital hearing aid is that in which analog circuits process the audio signal, the analog circuits being controlled by digital means.

Preparation of this paper was supported by Grant #H133E80019 from the National Institute on Disability and Rehabilitation Research.

In a conventional analog hearing aid, the acoustic signal is converted first to an electrical wave form that is a direct analog of the instantaneous pressure variations picked up by the microphone. This electrical analog of the acoustic signal is then filtered, amplified, and processed. In all of these operations the electrical signals are processed as continuous wave forms. In a digital hearing aid, the acoustic signal picked up by the microphone is first converted to an electrical analog signal and then converted to a digital signal. The digital signal takes the form of a series of binary numbers, i.e., numbers consisting of only two types of digit (0 and 1) are used. The binary numbers representing the audio signal then are processed using digital circuits of the type commonly used in computers. After the digital signal has been processed it is converted back to an analog electrical signal, which, in turn, is converted to an acoustic signal by the hearing aid receiver.

The process of converting an analog signal to digital form, known as *analog-to-digital conversion*, is illustrated in figure 1. The uppermost section of the diagram shows the wave form of a continuous signal. This wave form is then sampled at discrete intervals in time. The solid points show the value of the wave form at each sampling instant. The middle section of the diagram shows the sampled-data version of the analog signal. Note that this sampled-data signal is not a continuous wave form but exists only at discreet instants in time; the value of each sample is equal to the value of the wave form at each sampling instant.

The second stage of the digitization process converts the sampled data to numerical form. A binary code is commonly used in specifying the numerical value of each sample. The coding process requires that a series of comparisons be made. The sample is first compared to the midvalue of its range. If it exceeds the midvalue, the first digit in the code is 1, and if not, then it is 0. This first digit identifies,

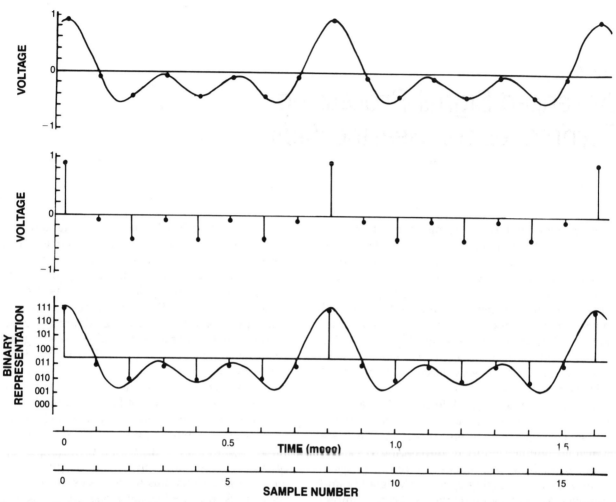

Figure 1. Converting a signal from analog to digital form. The uppermost section of the diagram shows the wave form of a continuous signal. The solid points show the value of the wave form at each sampling instant. The middle section of the diagram shows the sampled-data version of the analog signal. The lowest section of the diagram shows the sample values after 3-bit quantization. (The original wave form is also shown here in order to illustrate the accuracy of quantization.) Diagram reproduced from Levitt (1987).

very crudely, the region within which the sample lies. A second comparison then is performed to determine whether, within this region, the sample lies above or below the midvalue. As before, a 1 is assigned to the binary code if the sample lies above this midvalue, a 0 is assigned if it lies below. At this stage, the binary code consists of two digits having four possible values (00, 01, 10, 11). This binary code specifies the quartile within which the sample lies. The accuracy of the digitization process can be increased by increasing the number of binary comparisons and hence the number of binary digits used in specifying the binary code. A code consisting of three binary digits (abbreviated as *bits*) places the sample within one of eight (2^3) possible regions; a four bit code divides the range into sixteen (2^4) regions, and so on.

The lowest section of figure 1 shows a 3-bit binary representation of the sample values. The original analog waveform also is shown. The plotted points lie fairly close to the continuous curve indicating that, visually, a 3-bit approximation appears to provide a good approximation to the original sample values. The difference between the approximate binary representation of a sample and its true value is known as the *quantization error*.

An important practical question in the design of digital hearing aids is the precision of quantization that is necessary. The larger the number of bits used in representing the digitized samples, the smaller the quantization error and the greater the fidelity of the processed audio signals. The price paid for this increased fidelity is a larger analog-to-digital converter and greater power consumption. This is an important consideration if the hearing aid is to be small enough to fit on or in the ear.

It has been shown empirically that a quantization accuracy of 11 or 12 bits is needed in order for the quantization error to be inaudible in digital audio. When digital signals are processed, rounding errors are introduced in the numerical calculations. In order to prevent these rounding errors from being audible (as processing noise) many high quality digital audio systems use 16-bit quantization. For hearing-aid applications, the use of high precision quantization is prohibitively expensive in terms of size and power consumption of the required analog-to-digital converter.

It is possible to reduce the accuracy of quantization by several bits without introducing perceptible quantization errors by using quantization intervals that are not spaced linearly, e.g., smaller quantization intervals for low-level signals. Even with the use of optimized quantization strategies for hearing-aid applications, the number of bits needed to quantize speech signals adequately is still relatively high (on the order of 6 or 7 bits).

A second important issue in the design of digital hearing aids is the choice of sampling rate. It can be shown mathematically that the minimum sampling rate for an error-free digital representation of an analog signal should be at least twice the highest frequency contained in the analog signal. In order to ensure that this requirement is met, it is common practice to include a low-pass filter at the input to an analog-to-digital converter. This filter, known as an *anti-aliasing* filter, typically has a sharp rate of cut-off with substantial attenuation in the stop band. A similar filter, known as an *anti-imaging* filter, is commonly employed at the output of the digital-to-analog converter in order to eliminate any spurious frequency components that may have been introduced by the digital processing or conversion processes.

Once the audio signal has been converted to digital form it can be processed by means of numerical operations. See Levitt (1987) for an introductory tutorial on digital signal processing and its application to hearing aids.

There are advantages and disadvantages to both analog and digital techniques. Analog circuits have the advantage of being highly developed. Many years of effort have gone into the development of analog circuit chips for hearing aid applications. As a consequence, this technology is highly advanced, and sophisticated microminiature analog circuits of high quality are available for use in modern hearing aids. Furthermore, a substantial body

of expertise exists for the development of even more advanced analog circuit chips. In contrast, microminiature digital circuit chips for hearing aid applications are still in the early stages of development and there is limited expertise, at present, in the development of practical microminiature digital chips of extremely low power consumption. Digital circuits, on the other hand, have an important advantage in that highly advanced signal processing algorithms have been developed and can be implemented in digital form with relative ease.

Two broad classes of digital hearing aids have been developed as a result of these problems. One class of such instruments has been developed for research and clinical use (Levitt 1982; Levitt et al. 1986). These instruments are relatively large in size (e.g., desk mounted units) and are capable of implementing powerful methods of signal processing. An instrument of this type is often referred to as a digital master hearing aid (DMHA). The second type of digital hearing aid is small enough to be wearable, but has significantly reduced signal processing capabilities in comparison with a desk mounted DMHA (Nunley et al. 1983).

The relatively large DMHA can be used clinically for the prescriptive fitting of wearable programmable hearing aids and as a general purpose instrument for rehabilitation training. As a research tool, the DMHA has been found to be invaluable. DMHAs with powerful, programmable signal processing capabilities have been used effectively in evaluating the potential benefits of advanced signal processing algorithms in acoustic amplification (Levitt, Neuman, and Sullivan 1990).

The smaller, wearable digital hearing aids have not enjoyed the same degree of success. At present, the state of the art in microminiature digital circuitry is such that both the size and power consumption of the chips required for a wearable digital hearing aid are still relatively large. As a consequence, the first commercial digital hearing aid was a body worn unit (The Nicolet Phoenix hearing aid). Similarly, virtually all of the experimental wearable digital hearing aids developed thus far have been body worn units (Engebretsen, Morley, and Popelka 1987; Cummins and Hecox 1987). Microminiaturization of digital chips is continuing and it is likely that digital hearing aids small enought to fit behind the ear will be developed in the not too distant future. Several research laboratories are actively pursuing this goal and an experimental prototype has already been developed.

Major engineering compromises are necessary in order to produce substantial reductions in the size of digital hearing aids and, as a consequence, the first generation of behind-the-ear digital hearing aids is likely to embody only moderately sophisticated signal processing algorithms. The unanswered question is whether the signal processing capability that can be incorporated in a practical, personal digital hearing aid will be superior to that which can be achieved using a partially digital approach.

A substantial reduction in power can be obtained by eliminating the second stage of the analog-to-digital converter, i.e., the electrical analog signal is sampled at discrete intervals. These samples are not converted to numerical form but remain as sampled voltages. The hearing aid, under these conditions, operates as a sampled-data system and not as a fully digital system. Sampled-data and fully digital systems are very similar, as shown in figure 2. Both types of system require anti-aliasing and anti-imaging filters, a means for sampling the incoming analog signal, and a means for reconstructing a continuous analog signal after processing.

Although sampled-data systems are not as flexible as fully digital systems, they can be used to implement many of the signal processing algorithms developed for digital systems. In particular, filters with extremely fine frequency resolution and flexible control of both amplitude and phase characteristics can be implemented relatively easily using a sampled-data system.

An example of a hearing aid requiring precise control of both the amplitude and phase characteristics of a filter is shown in figure 3. This diagram shows the major components of a hearing aid designed to cancel acoustic feedback (Levitt, Dugot, and Kopper 1988). The input from the microphone is amplified and filtered in the usual way by means of a pre-amplifier, filter (F1), and power amplifier. The hearing aid also has an electrical feedback path running from the output of the power amplifier via the filter F2 back to the input stage (it is added to the incoming signal immediately after the pre-amplifier).

The amplitude and phase characteristics of F2 are adjusted adaptively by the microprocessor to make the electrical feedback signal equal in amplitude and opposite in phase to the acoustic feedback signal. When added together the electrical and acoustic feedback signals cancel. In order to facilitate the adaptive adjustment process, a switch is used to insert a probe-tube signal for scanning the frequency range while the microphone is momentarily disconnected. The monitor signal provides information to the microprocessor about whether the adaptive adjustments to filter F2 are resulting in cancellation of

the acoustic feedback and, if not, the direction of future adjustments to achieve cancellation.

Another way in which the size and power consumption of a modern signal processing hearing aid can be reduced is to combine analog and digital components in a hybrid instrument. A block diagram of a typical hearing aid of this type is shown in figure 4. In this hearing aid, the audio signal is processed by analog components (e.g., amplifiers, filters, limiters). These components are relatively small in size and draw very little power in comparison with digital signal processing chips in their current state of development. The analog components of the hearing aid, however, are controlled by digital means. Because the control signals used by the digital controller vary relatively slowly (compared to an audio signal) the sampling rate of the system is low and, in addition, the number of bits required to specify the control signals is much less than that required for an audio signal. As a consequence, both the size and the power consumption of the digital controller is quite small and can be incorporated in an instrument small enough to fit in the ear.

Although the use of an analog signal path reduces the possibilities for implementing advanced signal processing techniques, the digital controller allows for several important advantages of a digital system. These include programmability, memory, and adaptive filtering (Graupe, Grosspietsch, and Basseas 1987; Johnson et al. 1988; Pluvinage and Benson 1988). Most of the programmable hearing aids currently on the market are hybrid analog/digital units.

The reaction and degree of acceptance by hearing aid users with respect to the new generation of digital and hybrid analog/digital hearing aids have yet to be determined. It is already clear, however, that current methods of prescribing and fitting hearing aids need to be reconsidered.

Contrary to expectation, experimental evaluations of advanced signal processing techniques for amplitude compression, noise reduction, and reverberation reduction have not yet produced evidence of substantial improvements in intelligibility for the majority of subjects (Bustamante and Braida 1987; Levitt, Neuman, and Sullivan 1990). On the other hand, a few subjects seem to show benefit for selected forms of signal processing and, in many cases, improvements in overall sound quality have been reported (Neuman and Schwander 1987; Neuman, Levitt, Weiss, and Schwander 1987). At present, it is too early to judge whether a consistent pattern exists with respect to the benefits observed and the audiological characteristics of the subjects.

SAMPLED-DATA SYSTEM

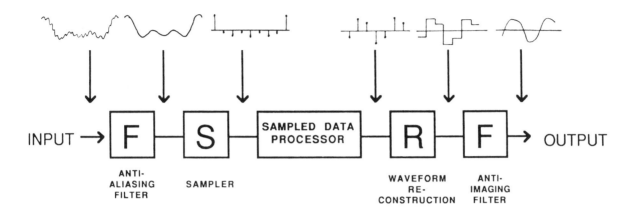

ALL DIGITAL SYSTEM

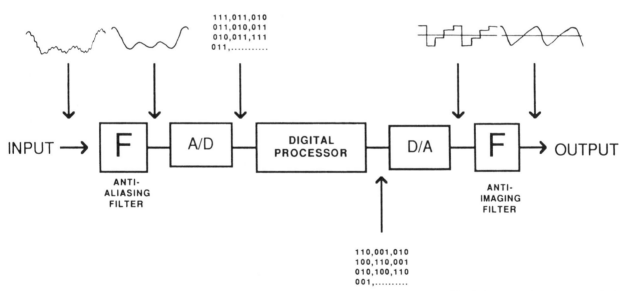

Figure 2.   Comparison between a sampled-data and an all digital system. The upper block diagram shows a sampled-data system. It consists of an anti-aliasing filter, a sampling circuit, a signal processor for operating on sampled-data sequences, a circuit for wave form reconstruction, and an anti-imaging filter. The lower block diagram shows the corresponding all-digital system. It consists of an anti-aliasing filter, an analog-to-digital converter (this unit contains both a sampler and a circuit for converting the samples to binary form), a digital signal processor (this could be a general-purpose digital computer), a digital-to-analog converter, and an anti-imaging filter. Diagram reproduced from Levitt (1987).

A common trend that has been observed in most of these studies is that large individual differences exist with respect to the effect of advanced signal processing on intelligibility and sound quality. Consequently, as hearing aids become more sophisticated, and as the range of different signal processing strategies increases, hearing aid dispensers will need to de-velop techniques for identifying which is the best signal processing strategy for each client. A digital master hearing aid with the capability of implementing the various signal processing strategies used in modern hearing aids appears to be a promising tool for this purpose.

A useful feature of both digital and hybrid ana-

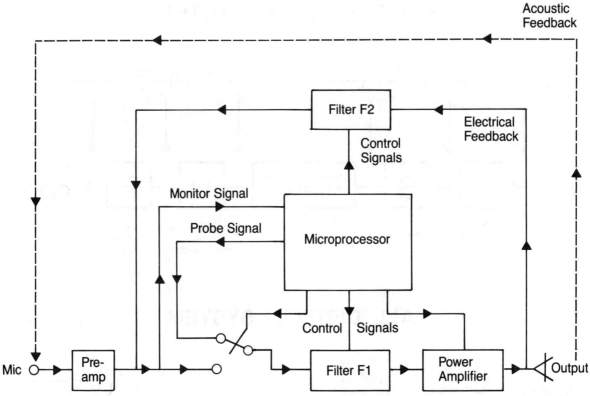

Figure 3. Digital hearing aid with feedback cancellation. The forward signal path consists of a microphone, preamplifier, filter F1, power amplifier, and output transducer. Cancellation of acoustic feedback is achieved by means of an electrical feedback signal taken from the output of the power amplifier passed through filter F2 and added to the input signal at the output of the pre-amplifier. Filter F2 is adjusted so that the electrical feedback signal is equal in amplitude but opposite in phase to the acoustic feedback signal. Diagram reproduced from Levitt (to appear).

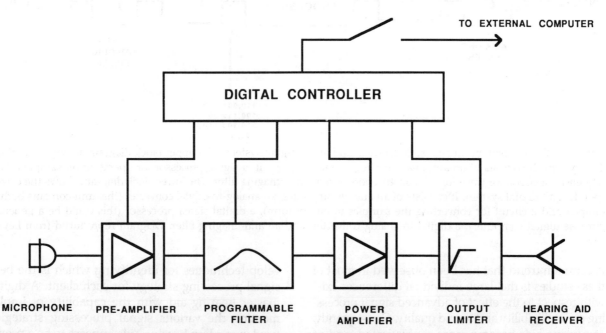

Figure 4. Hybrid analog/digital hearing aid. The audio signal is processed by conventional analog components: amplifiers, filters, limiters. These analog components, however, are controlled by digital means. The digital controller, in turn, can be programmed by an external computer. Diagram reproduced from Levitt (1987).

log/digital hearing aids is that they can be programmed by an external computer. As hearing aids become more sophisticated, there is a greater need for more efficient methods of prescribing these instruments. A modern two-channel compression hearing aid, for example, has many more variables than a conventional linear hearing aid. The problem of finding the optimum settings for a multivariable hearing aid is a very difficult problem and computerized adjustment procedures are essential for this task. Research is currently in progress on the development of computerized fitting strategies for modern programmable hearing aids (Engebretsen et al. 1986; Neuman, Levitt, Mills, and Schwander 1987). These developments are likely to result in a much greater dependence on computer-based techniques for hearing aid prescription.

An unexpected development with important clinical implications is that certain simple features associated with digital or hybrid analog/digital hearing aids, such as memory, are having a profound effect on the fitting and evaluation of hearing aids. The idea of a push-button memory that will allow the hearing aid user to switch from one type of hearing aid to another does not require the use of advanced signal processing techniques, yet this feature is reaping rich rewards in terms of providing users with more effective amplification for different acoustic environments (e.g., quiet versus noisy room). It is also a very effective tool for fitting and evaluating hearing aids under real life conditions. Given the growing difficulty of prescribing hearing aids of increasing sophistication, greater attention should be paid to the use of these simple features.

References

Bustamante, D.K., and Braida, L.D. 1987. Principle-component amplitude compression for the hearing impaired. *Journal of the Acoustical Society of America* 82:1227–1242.

Cummins, K.L., and Hecox, K.E. 1987. Ambulatory testing of digital hearing aid algorithms. In *Proceedings of the 10th Annual Conference on Rehabilitation Technology* eds. R.D. Steel and W. Gerrey. Washington, DC: RESNA-Association for the Advancement of Rehabilitation Technology.

Engebretsen, A.M., Morley, R.E., and Popelka, G.R. 1987. Development of an ear-level digital aid and computer-assisted fitting procedure: An interim-report. *Journal of Rehabilitation Research and Development* 24(4):55–64.

Engebretsen, A.M., Popelka, G.R., Morley, R.E., Niemoller, A.F., and Heidbreder, A.F. 1986. A digital hearing aid and computer-based fitting procedure. *Hearing Instruments* 37(2):8–14.

Graupe, D., Grosspietsch, J.K., and Basseas, S.P. 1987. A single-microphone-based self-adaptive filter of noise from speech and its performance evaluation. *Journal of Rehabilitation Research and Development* 24(4):119–26.

Johnson, J.S., Kirby, V.M., Hodgson, W.A., and Johnson, L.J. 1988. Clinical study of a programmable, multiple memory hearing instrument. *Hearing Instruments* 39(11):44–46.

Levitt, H. 1982. An array-processor, computer hearing aid. *ASHA* 24:805, (abstract).

Levitt, H. 1987. Digital hearing aids: A tutorial review. *Journal of Rehabilitation Research and Development* 24(4):7–19.

Levitt, H., Dugot, R. and Kopper, K.W. 1988. Programmable digital hearing aid system. U.S. Patent #4,731,850.

Levitt, H., Neuman, A., and Sullivan, J. 1990. Studies with digital hearing aids. *Acta-Oto-Laryngology* Suppl. 469:57–69.

Levitt, H., Neuman, A., Mills, R., and Schwander, T. 1986. A digital master hearing aid. *Journal of Rehabilitation Research and Development* 23(1):79–87.

Neuman, A.C., and Schwander, T.J. 1987. The effect of filtering on the intelligibility and quality of speech in noise. *Journal of Rehabilitation Research and Development* 24(4):127–34.

Neuman, A.C., Levitt, H., Weiss, M., and Schwander, T. 1987. Evaluation of noise reduction techniques for hearing aids. In *Proceedings of the Tenth Annual Conference on Rehabilitation Technology,* eds. R.D. Steele and W. Gerrey. Washington, DC: RESNA-Association for the Advancement of Rehabilitation Technology.

Neuman, A., Levitt, H., Mills, R., and Schwander, T. 1987. An evaluation of three adaptive hearing aid selection strategies. *Journal of the Acoustical Society of America* 82:1967–1976.

Nunley, J., Staab, W., Steadman, J., Wechsler, P., and Spencer, B. 1983. A wearable digital hearing aid. *The Hearing Journal* October:29–31, 34–35.

Pluvinage, V., and Benson, D. 1988. New dimensions in diagnostics and fitting. *Hearing Instruments* 39(8):28–29, 39.

CHAPTER 9

Implantable Auditory Systems

Thomas H. Fay

Suzuki (1988), Goode (1989), Abramson (1989), and Maniglia (1989) have each provided excellent and comprehensive reviews of the literature of implantable hearing devices from the earliest to the most recent efforts. A brief summary of developments is given here with emphasis on the three major categories of approach: (1) electromagnetic induction drivers, (2) piezoelectric crystal drivers, and (3) temporal bone vibrators. Following this is a discussion of our clinical experience at Columbia-Presbyterian Medical Center in New York with the partially implantable Swedish bone conduction (BC) device known presently as the Nobelpharma Auditory System or NAS and formerly as the Bone Anchored Hearing Aid or BAHA (Abramson et al. 1989).

Even though impressive advances in technological development of conventional hearing aids have been made in recent years, there remain serious objections to them by a large segment of those who are candidates for their use. High on any list of objections would be distress due to feedback or to the aid's poor performance in suppressing background noise. Other objections are unnatural sound reproducing quality for speech, music, and environmental sounds, difficulty of operation and manipulation, battery size and cost, and wearability problems that cause discomfort—such as tight-fitting occluding ear molds or bone conduction headbands. The most prevalent and perhaps the most important objection, however, is their conspicuousness. Major efforts by the hearing aid industry have been devoted to removing these objections, with differing degrees of success. Despite miniaturization and the use of microprocessors, there remain objections that are not fully addressed by such advances. The psychological barriers to acceptance of disability in any form are potent whether they apply to oneself or to others. Our culture has always had difficulty accepting hearing disability, and personal denial of its presence is widespread. Refusal to admit and accept the need for amplification is a problem that we all encounter regularly in our roles as hearing specialists, and not too infrequently within ourselves, despite our considerable knowledge.

It behooves us, therefore, to concentrate on removal of as many barriers to acceptance of wearable amplification as possible. Some of the objections already are being addressed through the developmental and clinical experimentation with implantable auditory devices.

Goode (1989), who has made important and creative contributions to this field, views an implantable hearing aid as an extension of conventional hearing aid technology wherein one or more of the four basic components are surgically implanted in the ear. He states that indications for an implantable hearing aid for a sensorineural loss are the same as those for a conventional aid, and that implantable aids also can be used for conductive losses that cannot be surgically corrected. Clearly, these indications are markedly different from those for the cochlear implant, which is designed for use only by profoundly deaf persons who cannot profit from acoustic amplification. Goode points out that the theoretical acoustic advantage of an implantable aid stems chiefly from eliminating the receiver and from driving the ossicles directly, thereby improving the sound fidelity. He further observes that only the output stage need be implanted, given the current significant technical problems involved in total implantation.

A number of important advances have been made recently in the development of several types of output transducers. Further refinements in the effectiveness of these devices will make it possible to sidestep some of the most troublesome stumbling blocks encountered with conventional hearing aids. Most important will be the replacement of the air conduction (AC) receiver as output transducer with vibrators of various types placed in different locations. Such devices can stimulate the inner ear without introducing a distorting column of vibrating air into the transmission linkage between microphone and movement of perilymph. In those partially implantable auditory systems currently in use, employment of vibrators as transducers has not only improved sound quality and speech intelligibility markedly, but has eliminated auditory feedback as well as the need for tight-fitting earmolds.

Important advances also are being made in the development of partially implantable bone conduction devices, chiefly through the development of new ways to couple the vibrator to the skull that reduce the need for massive driving power. Direct attachment to the skull can obviate the obnoxious pressure-exerting headband or the spring-loaded eyeglass temple pieces conventionally required to force the vibratory signal through the intervening skin and tissues to the temporal bone.

Improved sound quality and ease of wear notwithstanding, visibility is still a problem with most existing partially implantable systems because the external parts are contained in conventional hearing aid cases that are worn either behind or in the ear, in the usual manner. Hence, totally implantable devices remain a goal for the future. Some of the last major barriers to total implantation will fall when rechargable miniaturized power supplies and easily operated remote controls are developed. Then, with problems of visibility and conspicuousness under control, the possibility of overcoming some of the more inaccessible psychological reasons for objection to wearable amplification may well be at hand.

Electromagnetic Induction Drivers

As early as 1935, Wilska (1935, 1959) apparently achieved the first stimulation of the human middle ear by way of electromagnetic induction. He first placed bits of iron on the tympanic membrane and, in later trials, attached a small coil to it. The output of a variable frequency oscillator drove a primary induction coil placed over the ear canal that enabled the subject to hear pure tones. Regrettably, these tones were perceived as being double the pitch of the induced frequency. This problem was solved by superimposition of a strong constant magnetic field that unfortunately caused pain and discomfort to the subject. In another effort, a different coil was used, but it generated enough heat to cause sensations of burning and pain. Wilska soon terminated his efforts, but not before demonstrating that vibrations produced at the tympanic membrane by electrical methods are received in the inner ear in the same manner as an acoustical vibration (Goode 1989).

Rutschmann, Page, and Fowler, Jr. (1958) and Rutschmann (1959) reported that one of their subjects claimed satisfactory reproduction of radio programs monitored by an externally worn induction coil driving a 10 mg magnet glued to the umbo. When the magnetic field was driven by an oscillator, their normal hearing subjects achieved normal thresholds at 1 kHz.

Since 1969, Goode and his associates at Stanford University Medical School have concentrated their efforts on a partially implanted electromagnetic induction device. Using a single subject with exceptional hearing, he first glued a magnet to the umbo and drove it by a coil 3 mm away placed deep in the ear canal. Figure 1 is a schematic diagram of the concept in which sound entering the microphone of the amplifier A is transduced into a magnetic field by the coil B that induces analogous movement of the magnet C attached to the tympanic membrane or the ossicles. The subject achieved −10 dB HL equivalent thresholds at 500, 1000, and 2000 Hz with the device (Goode 1970). Unable to repeat the findings in subsequent subjects with normal hearing, Goode suspects that the original subject actually had thresholds of −20 dB HL or better (Goode 1989).

Glorig et al. (1972) used an external amplifier and coil to stimulate a magnet glued to the umbo of one subject who reported that speech clarity

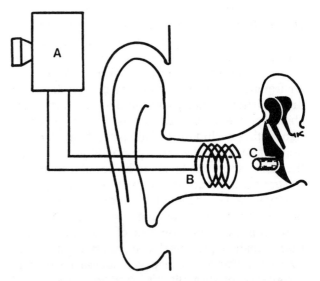

Figure 1. The principle of the electromagnetic implant hearing aid. (See text for details.) (Reprinted with permission from Goode, R. L. 1988. Electromagnetic implantable hearing aids. In *Middle Ear Implant: Implantable Hearing Aids, Advances in Audiology*, Vol. 4:24, ed. J.-I. Suzuki. Basel: S. Karger AG.)

was comparable to that achieved when wearing earphones.

Different magnet placements, weights, and coil locations have been explored by Goode and Glattke (1973) with the results favoring an intracanal coil location because of its proximity to the magnet, and magnet weights of 50 mg or less because of the adverse effect of increased mass on frequencies above 4000 Hz. Still later studies with increasingly powerful magnets eventually resulted in a system capable of use by patients with mild hearing loss. Clinical development of this system was not undertaken at the time (Goode et al. 1986).

One difficulty with an electromagnetic induction hearing system is that inductive reactance increases with frequency. Each doubling of frequency causes a 6 dB drop in current through the coil for the same voltage input. This requires increased amplifier output at higher frequencies (Goode 1988). Because energy transfer between coil and magnet is inversely proportional to the cube of the distance between them, Goode recommends placement of the coil deep in the ear canal as close as possible to the magnet for optimal location. The coil should not occlude the canal or cause pain or trauma to it or to the tympanic membrane. The magnet should be as strong as possible, but low in mass to avoid loading the middle ear, which would result in reduction of high-frequency transmission. He also suggests implanting the magnet within the middle ear space in contact with one of the ossicles in order to eliminate problems with water, cerumen, or desquamated skin in the ear canal causing irritation and infection around the magnet (1988).

Kartush and his associates (as reported by Bojrab, Clemis, and McGee 1988), as well as Heide et al. (1988) have produced results with the implantable electromagnetic induction device under development by the Richards Medical Company. This system utilizes a samarium cobalt magnet glued to the tympanic membrane and driven by a single unit containing all of the other components (i.e., microphone, amplifier, battery, and electromagnetic coil). Worn completely within the external auditory canal, this system represents a contemporary version of the approach of Wilska and of Rutschmann. Six conventional hearing aid users with sensorineural losses who were experimentally fitted with the device by Heide and his group achieved significant functional gain and reported superior subjective experiences as compared to their own aids. The unit produced no feedback, its sound quality was judged to be better than their own aids and performance in noise was found to be superior (Heide et al. 1988).

Fredricksson et al. (1973) glued a magnet to the stapes of monkeys and placed the electromagnetic coil entirely within the mastoid cavity. Cochlear microphonic responses remained stable over a 14-month period, and histologic preparations revealed no hair cell damage. Hough, Vernon, Dormer, Johnson, and Himelick (1986) and Hough et al. (1987) have described a three-coil system driving a magnet attached to an ossicle. The primary external coil transcutaneously energizes the subcutaneous secondary coil, which in turn drives the tertiary coil located in the mastoid cavity and by which the magnet on the ossicle is driven. As might be expected, there are power loss problems resulting from the several energy transduction points. Whenever energy is transduced or transmitted across one pathway link to another, signal strength and fidelity are altered. This simple fact can be of great importance in determining success or failure of an implantable system in general, as well as in an individual fitting. Power loss and frequency distortion are the chief considerations in this context.

Wilson and his colleagues (1990) at Washington University School of Medicine in St. Louis have shown the importance of minimizing the load placed on the ossicles by a vibrating electromagnetic transducer. Using monkeys as subjects, they demonstrated a decrease in auditory evoked potentials equivalent to a drop of about 20 dB in stimulus sound pressure level as the transducer, when attached to the long process of the incus, was progressively advanced in small increments toward the stapes. Apparently, the most efficient energy transfer to the inner ear results from minimal contact pressure between transducer and ossicle. Any increase in pressure, beyond that just sufficient to ensure stable placement of the transducer, appears to restrict the range of stapes footplate movement, thus diminishing its capacity for response. It is, therefore, essential to maintain accurate control over the ossicular loading of the transducer through its exact placement and stabilization. This applies equally to any form of ossicular replacement prosthesis.

Maniglia (1989) and his colleagues at Case Western Reserve University School of Medicine have reported extensive laboratory and animal research on several designs of partially implantable middle ear devices since 1985. Electromagnetic and piezoelectric circuits were compared in both cat and human temporal bones. Based on its broader and flatter frequency response, they selected the electromagnetic minicoil to drive a samarium-cobalt stapes magnet assembly for use in their short-term live animal experiments.

Amplitude-modulated radio signals were transmitted from an externally powered conduction coil to an internal induction coil functioning as an antenna. The received signals were either conducted by direct wiring or were further transmitted by radio to the electromagnetic driving coil, which was mounted approximately 2 mm from the samarium-cobalt stapes-magnet assembly without making direct contact with it. Auditory brainstem potentials showed an average of 35 dB gain for click stimuli transmitted by the implant in an anesthetized cat that had been conductively impaired by incus removal. The system consumed low current with radio transmission, and appears to compare favorably with a medium power hearing aid in acoustic gain and power requirements. Several variations of the basic components and magnet location have been proposed for ongoing animal research in further preparation for human implantation (Maniglia et al. 1988). Figure 2 shows a typical proposal from Man-

iglia et al. (1988) of a totally concealed partially implantable unit for human use. The magnet is located on the external surface of the tympanic membrane and anchored with titanium screws passing through the membrane that are fixed to the malleus. All other components are contained in the single unit located deep within the external canal. This proposal is one of several approaches that are currently under development for human experimentation by Maniglia and his group.

Piezoelectric Crystal Drivers

In response to applied pressure, a piezoelectric crystal will reverse its electrical charge, and is therefore capable of generating an electrical voltage. Also, when an electrical voltage is applied to the crystal, it will change its length, and is therefore capable of generating vibratory movement. Several investigators have applied this principle to the design of vibrating output transducers to drive various

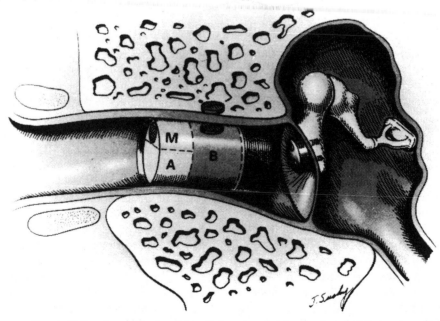

Figure 2. A design for an electromagnetic hearing device that is partially implanted, but totally concealed. The magnet is screwed to the malleus, and the external unit which contains the microphone M, the amplifier A, and the battery B, is located in the ear canal. (Reprinted with permission from Maniglia, A.J. 1989. Implantable hearing devices: State of the art. *Otolaryngologic Clinics of North America* 22(1):187.)

parts of the ossicular chain. The high impedance of the piezoelectric crystal matches the high impedance of the ossicular chain far more closely than other output transducers, such as the low impedance electromagnetic drivers. When connected directly to the ossicle, the vibrating crystal transmits the signal with greatly improved efficiency and fidelity, particularly in the high frequencies, thus ensuring the crystal an important role in future implant design.

In 1970, Vernon and colleagues first described using an ossicular driving piezoelectric ceramic crystal, the Denniston Probe, named for its developer. They reported successful stimulation of the cochlea by placing the probe at various tympanic membrane and ossicular chain locations in guinea pigs, and also in one human subject during a routine tympanotomy flap procedure (1970). The AC cochlear potential was measured in the animals in response to pure tone stimuli by both air conduction and vibratory modalities. Acceptable sensitivity and harmonic distortion results were achieved by both modes. The human subject reported extremely clear pure tone reception that was free of distortion and gave speech discrimination responses that were perfect. Five years later, Nunley et al. (1975, 1976) implanted a piezoelectric disc-shaped driver connected to the stapes of chinchillas that had been surgically deafened monaurally, leaving a normal experimental ear. When the driver was unpowered, its damping effect on the stapes caused a threshold shift that disappeared when power was applied. They reported conditioned hearing test results that showed significant amplified threshold improvement compared to the unamplified tests. They concluded that the device could be used to drive the stapes sufficiently to provide a level equivalent to normal hearing without overdriving and damaging the ossicular chain.

Japanese researchers—under the auspices of the Ministry of International Trade and Industry of Japan—began formal discussions in 1973 that led ultimately to the establishment in 1978 of a major five-year research and development project for an implantable artificial middle ear. This project, in which a piezoelectric ceramic crystal ossicular driver of bimorphic design was the crucial element, was initiated and sustained through the developmental research of Suzuki et al. (1983) and the clinical investigations of Yanagihara et al. (1983). Their combined efforts resulted in an important technical advance in ossicular driver design. For the vibrator, they used a ceramic crystal bimorph consisting of two piezoelectric crystals of reversed polarity joined together into a single unit. When one end of this device is fixed, the free end will vibrate up and down in an arc around the fixed end in response to applied electrical voltage changes (figure 3). When implanted (figure 4), the fixed end is firmly attached to the bony wall of the surgically enlarged mastoid cavity and the free end is attached directly to the head of the stapes or to its footplate by a columella. The arcing motion delivered to the stapes by this bimorph closely resembles that delivered by a normal functioning incus. The driver receives energy either directly by wire from the electrical output of the am-

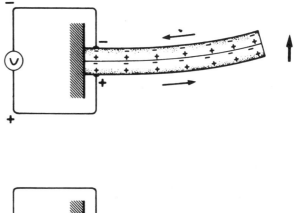

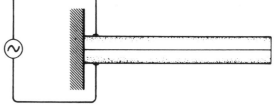

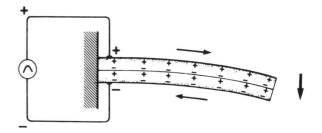

Figure 3. Functional principle of the piezoelectric ceramic crystal bimorph. A periodically alternating electric field applied to a crystal bimorph will cause it to vibrate. If one end is fixed, its free end will vibrate up and down. (Reprinted with permission from Yanagihara, N., Suzuki, J., Gyo, K., Syono, H., and Ikeda, H. 1984. Development of an implantable hearing aid using a piezoelectric vibrator of bimorph design: State of the art. *Otolaryngology— Head and Neck Surgery* 92(6):708.)

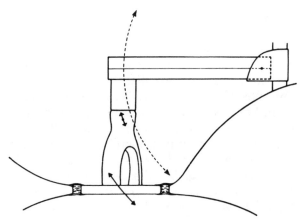

Figure 4. Vibration mode of the stapes. The stapes vibrates in an arc-like fashion around the same axis as the ceramic bimorph vibrator. (Reprinted with permission from Gyo, K., and Goode, R.L. 1988. Measurement of stapes vibration driven by the ceramic vibrator of a middle ear implant—Human temporal bone experiments. In *Middle Ear Implant: Implantable Hearing Aids, Advances in Audiology*, Vol. 4:111, ed. J.-I. Suzuki. Basel: S. Karger AG.)

plifier or from an implanted induction coil powered by the amplifier. Theoretically, any or all of these elements along with the microphone may be implanted. Practically, only the driver mechanism needs to be implanted. Suzuki, Kodera, and Yanagihara (1983) first implanted this device in six cats, and the units were kept functioning for six months with no loss of signal energy or deterioration of the vibrator, although there was a decrease in threshold sensitivity in two of the animals. Yanagihara and his colleagues temporarily attached this device directly to the stapes during tympanoplasty in human subjects who had suffered extensive damage to the middle ear. They could hear well with the vibrator and achieved speech discrimination scores superior to those with conventional hearing aids (Yanagihara et al. 1983). These observations may be explained on the basis of the measurable differences in sound transmission of a middle ear implant vibrator compared to a conventional hearing aid receiver that were reported by Suzuki, Kodera, and Yanagihara (1983). Using a probe microphone, they measured the vibration of the air column produced in the external canal by the air conduction aid and compared it to the vibration at the tip of the vibrator measured by a capacitive probe. Distortion in the air column was considerable and unavoidable due to the tight occlusion needed to prevent feedback. The vibrator, in contrast, followed the electri-

cal input signals faithfully. Additional explanation for these results may lie in the vastly improved impedance matching achieved by coupling the high impedance piezoelectric vibrator directly to the high impedance stapes and the resultant marked improvement in the fidelity of high frequency transmission (Khanna and Corliss 1986).

Gyo, Goode, and Miller (1987), working with fresh human temporal bones, found that either excessive tightness or looseness of the vibrator-stapes connection causes a loss in high frequency transduction efficiency, indicating the necessity to maintain optimal connection. When the connection was optimal, the sharp resonance peak at 5.5 kHz seen in the vibrator response when measured alone, was gently smoothed without significantly altering the high-frequency emphasis of its curve. This is an important consideration when permanently fixing a driver to an ossicle during implantation, and the effect achieved should be tested prior to final closure.

Although development of both total and partial middle ear implants was pursued in the government-sponsored project completed in 1983, both Suzuki and Yanagihara have since concentrated on the clinical application of the partially implantable middle ear implant (P-MEI). This is chiefly because of the problems in development of a small implantable battery that is rechargeable or that has sufficient power to avoid frequent surgical replacement. There are no such problems with external power supplies, and the investigators, concentrating on the P-MEI manufactured by Rion Company Limited jointly produced a total of 40 implants as of 1989 (Suzuki et al. 1989). Figure 5 shows the components of their system. The microphone, amplifier, battery, and primary induction coil are contained in a conventional postauricular hearing aid case. The signal is transmitted by electromagnetic induction to the secondary coil implanted under the retroauricular skin. The piezoelectric vibrator element is supported by a rigid column firmly attached at both ends to the temporal bone. This column permits a three-dimensional adjustment of the vibrator tip, which is coupled to the head of the stapes or to a columella standing on the stapes footplate. The vibrator is energized directly by a connecting wire from the internal coil.

Although the P-MEI could be applicable to patients with moderate sensorineural hearing loss, these investigators have limited them to patients with middle ear disease where the advantages are more definite. Their clinical results have been largely successful in terms of good sound quality

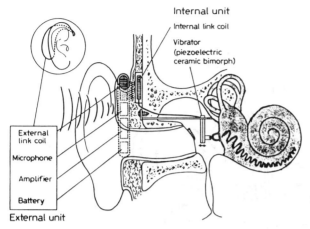

Figure 5. Functional principle of the partially implantable middle ear implant (P-MEI) using the piezoelectric ceramic bimorph vibrator. (Reprinted with permission from Yanagihara, N., Aritomo, H., Yamanaka, E., and Gyo, K. 1988. Intraoperative assessment of vibrator-induced hearing. In *Middle Ear Implant: Implantable Hearing Aids, Advances in Audiology*, Vol. 4:130, ed. J.-I. Suzuki. Basel: S. Karger AG.)

for speech, music, or environmental sound, and with few exceptions their patients generally have been quite satisfied. Their present best indications for the P-MEI are for patients with:

1. Bilateral hearing impairment;
2. Mixed type hearing impairment with bone conduction thresholds between 20 and 40 dB HL;
3. Middle ear anomalies and/or microtia with atresia of the auditory canal;
4. Chronic otitis media; or
5. Cholesteatoma.

Their best reasons for using the P-MEI are: the excellent sound quality achieved through direct stapes vibration and the resultant avoidance of conventional receivers with their requisite distorting air link; the extended high frequency range up through 8 kHz without distortion at levels affording 50 dB gain above air conduction thresholds; and as an alternative for use by those who are not satisfied with conventional air conduction aids following tympanoplasty (Suzuki et al. 1989).

Ironically, while the chief advantage of this type of implant stems from the direct connection between crystal driver and ossicle, its chief disadvantage may be the difficulty in maintaining this fragile connection on a permanent basis. Long-term follow-up is clearly warranted.

Tjellstrom (1988) has proposed the use of the Japanese piezoelectric bimorph stapes vibrator in conjuction with a percutaneous connector attached to an osseointegrated titanium implant in the temporal bone (figure 6). Mounting the hearing aid microphone, battery, and controls on the external abutment of the implant would eliminate the space-occupying internal coils and would make the battery and controls easy to reach by the patient. Using the same temporal bone-mounted connector, he also proposed mounting a direct-wired piezoelectric transducer onto an osseointegrated titanium fixture that is screwed directly into the bony otic capsule (figure 7). This would deliver the signal by bone conduction directly into the bony labyrinth with considerably more power than via the stapes, and would avoid the possibility of damage to the inner ear that is always inherent in direct vibratory contact with the ossicles. This is a fine example of creative combination of the best elements of differing approaches to cochlear stimulation. The high internal impedance of the ceramic bimorph can be made to match that of the skull, and piezoelectric drivers have been described with impedance characteristics that vary with frequency in a manner similar to that of the skull (Abramson 1989). Direct connection of such a device to the skull would improve the efficiency of energy transfer considerably. Furthermore, the resonant frequencies of piezoelectric crystals can be set well above audible frequencies, thus providing a flat response over a wide frequency range (Khanna and Corliss 1986). These characteristics, coupled with the availability of external signal controls, power source, and microphone, all mounted on the easily accessible percutaneous titanium abutment, render this a highly desirable proposal worthy of development. Tjellstrom (1988) points out that a primary task is the study of optimal modes of vibration for these proposals.

Temporal Bone Vibrators

Some people who need hearing aids cannot use air conduction instruments because of medical or anatomical contraindications such as draining ears or atresia. Medical and surgical treatments for these conditions have improved steadily, but there are still many for whom hearing impairment remains, forcing them to depend on bone conduction aids or to risk continual exacerbation of infection and otitis by using air conduction aids that inhibit the free cir-

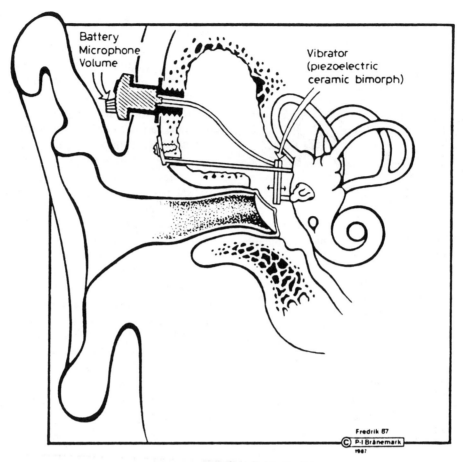

Figure 6. Schematic drawing of a piezoelectric bimorph inducing vibrations in the stapes. The energy is provided through a percutaneous connector attached to an osseointegrated titanium implant. (Reprinted with permission from Tjellstrom, A. 1988. Vibratory stimulation of the cochlea through a percutaneous transducer. In *Middle Ear Implant: Implantable Hearing Aids, Advances in Audiology,* Vol. 4:48, ed. J.-I. Suzuki. Basel: S. Karger AG.)

culation of air in the external canal. Those who can benefit from a conventional bone conduction aid must contend with a variety of unfortunate concomitants such as:

1. Discomfort caused by pressure applied to the skull
2. Insecure position of the aid and shifting vibrator
3. Poor sound quality
4. Unfortunate cosmetic aspects
5. Problems with feedback
6. Off-the-head microphone location.

All of these problems can be eliminated by implanting some sort of device directly into the temporal bone to serve as an anchor for a skin-penetrating metallic abutment to which a bone vibrator can be connected. Hakansson et al. (1985) called this new principal *direct bone conduction,* and

this is the basic concept of the Swedish Nobelpharma Auditory System, or NAS, which was until recently called the Bone Anchored Hearing Aid, or BAHA.

The pioneering work of Branemark and his associates (1969) at the University of Gothenburg, Sweden, using osseointegrated titanium dental implants in the jawbones of edentulous patients, led to the development of the percutaneous titanium screw implant in the temporal bone by Tjellstrom, Hakansson, Liden, and others. The first implant was inserted at Gothenburg in 1977 (Hakansson et al. 1985). As of 1989, over 500 had been inserted worldwide: 300 in Sweden and 200 elsewhere (Hakansson, Tjellstrom, and Carlsson 1990). The device, approved for use in Canada, remains experimental in the United States where, as of 1990, it was still awaiting the Food and Drug Administration's approval. In cooperation with the Swedish group, in-

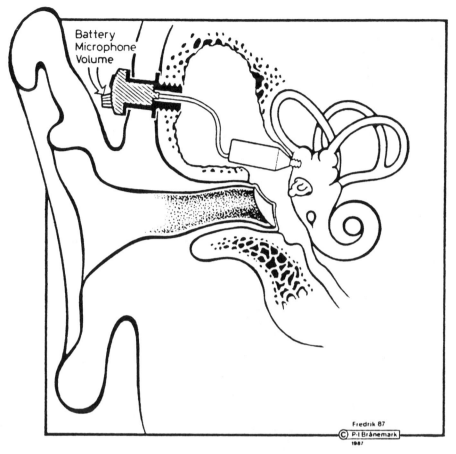

Figure 7.   Schematic drawing of a piezoelectric transducer, including a counterweight, anchored in or close to the otic capsule with an osseointegrated titanium screw. Battery, microphone, and volume control are mounted externally on a percutaneous connector attached to an osseointegrated titanium implant. (Reprinted with permission from Tjellstrom, A. 1988. Vibratory Stimulation of the cochlea through a percutaneous transducer. In *Middle Ear Implant: Implantable Hearing Aids, Advances in Audiology,* Vol. 4:49, ed. J.-I. Suzuki. Basel: S. Karger AG.)

vestigational trials have been undertaken at Columbia University (Fay, Abramson, and Russo 1986; Fay and Abramson 1988; Abramson et al. 1989), the University of Minnesota, the University of Texas at San Antonio, and the University of California at San Francisco.

Osseointegration of an implant may be defined as direct contact between the loaded implant surface and living bone tissue, without the development of intervening connective or fibrous tissue. Bone can bond directly to the titanium oxide layer on the surface of the metal without an intervening fibrous capsule. Figure 8 shows the absence of such tissue between the wedges of the titanium screw and bone tissue in a successful dental implant. When such tissue is present in a temporal bone implant, it can reduce the efficiency of energy transfer

from metal to bone, and it could ultimately lead to implant rejection.

The Swedish implantation process involves two separate surgical procedures performed under local anesthesia on an outpatient basis. In the first stage, the titanium screw is inserted into the temporal bone. A bony plug is removed and the fixture is gently screwed into place. The wound is completely closed over and allowed to heal for up to four months, during which the integration between bone and metal takes place. In stage two, the skin is re-opened and the titanium abutment screw that protrudes is attached to the osseointegrated fixture. Non-hair-bearing skin is placed over it and a central core of skin is removed to allow the fixture to protrude percutaneously (figure 9). The NAS may then be attached and worn freely as needed (figure 10).

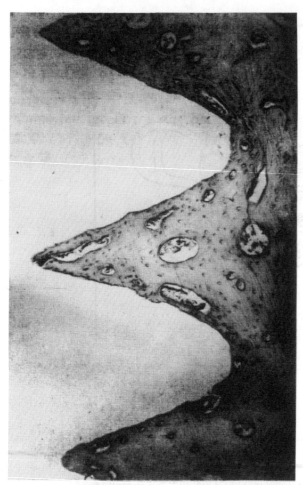

Figure 8. Photomicrograph of the osseointegrated wedges of a titanium screw in the bone tissue of a successful dental implant. Note the absence of an intervening fibrous capsule at the interface between bone and metal. (Reprinted with permission from Branemark, P.-I., Breine, U., Adell, R., Hansson, B.O., Lindstrom, J., and Ohlsson, A. 1969. Intra-osseous anchorage of dental prostheses. I. Experimental studies. *Scandinavian Journal of Plastic and Reconstructive Surgery* 3:91.)

Attachment is accomplished simply by inserting the instrument's T-shaped metal projection, called the bayonet, into the abutment slot and then turning the device 90 degrees, where it is held in firm contact by friction. This direct connection of the vibrator with the bone reduces by 10 to 15 dB the power output that is required to achieve perception levels equivalent to those obtained with conventional bone conduction transducers. It further obviates the headband, because pressure is no longer required to overcome the impedance of the skin and subcutaneous tissues. Figure 11 is a schematic diagram of the device showing its attachment to the implanted abutment. Note that the package is com-

pletely self-contained and head-borne, including the microphone, which is inauspiciously located behind the auricle. This can be a nuisance and sometimes confusing in terms of localization, but our subjects all seem to have adjusted to this minor drawback. Indications for the NAS are:

1. Patients using bone conduction hearing aids
2. Patients with congenital atresia
3. Patients using air conduction hearing aids but experiencing
   a. infection and chronic draining ears
   b. discomfort
   c. acoustic feedback due to a large meatus.

Contraindications for the NAS are:

1. Patients with mixed hearing loss in which the sensorineural component as indicated by the bone conduction pure tone average is greater than 45 dB HL and discrimination is less than 60%
2. Patients with pure sensorineural hearing loss
3. Patients who are emotionally unstable or developmentally delayed
4. Patients under the age of 16 years.

Those who are candidates for the NAS, as indicated by these criteria, are evaluated audiologically with a battery of tests while seated in the sound field of a sound-treated room at a distance of 1 meter in front of the loudspeaker at zero degrees azimuth. The ear with the better bone conduction is usually selected for the NAS, and the nonselected ear is occluded. The battery of four tests is presented under each of three conditions: unaided, patients wearing their own aid if it is worn on the selected ear, and patients wearing a standard Starkey bone conduction aid on the selected ear. The four sound field tests are: warble tone thresholds at all octave and semi-octave frequencies from 250 Hz through 8000 Hz, SRT, PB max, and the synthetic sentence inventory (SSI) of Speaks and Jerger (1965). Here the measure sought is the signal-to-noise ratio in dB at which 50% identification of the sentences occurs when they are presented at a constant level of 63 dB SPL and the speech spectrum background noise is varied.

These tests permit comparison of the patient's performance unaided, while wearing the accustomed aid if it is worn on the selected ear, and while wearing a conventional bone conduction aid that has adequate power and is known to be functioning properly. The assumption is that optimum performance by bone conduction of the selected ear has been sampled. If this performance is satisfactory,

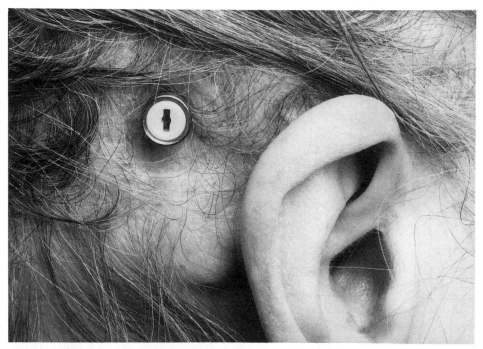

Figure 9.   Patient showing the skin penetrating titanium abutment with the coupling element in situ. (Photo by J.-O. Yxell. Reprinted with permission from Hakansson, B., Tjellstrom, A., Rosenhall, U., and Carlsson, P. 1985. The bone-anchored hearing aid. *Acta Otolaryngologica (Stockholm)* 100:233.)

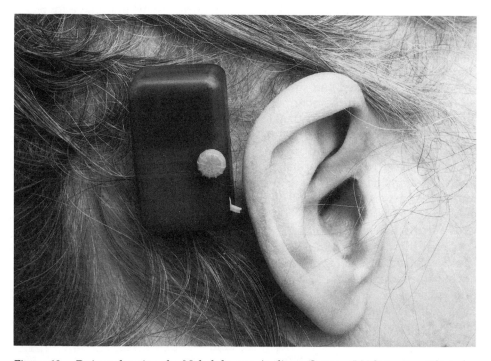

Figure 10.   Patient showing the Nobelpharma Auditory System (NAS) in situ. (Photo by J.-O. Yxell. Reprinted with permission from Hakansson, B., Tjellstrom, A., Rosenhall, U., and Carlsson, P. 1985. The bone-anchored hearing aid. *Acta Otolaryngologica (Stockholm)* 100:232.)

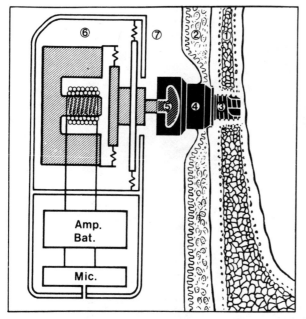

Figure 11. Schematic diagram of the bone anchored system (NAS): 1. skull bone, 2. soft tissue, 3. titanium screw, 4. titanium abutment, 5. coupling, 6. transducer, 7. housing. (Reprinted with permission from Hakansson, B., Tjellstrom, A., Rosenhall, U., and Carlsson, P. 1985. The bone-anchored hearing aid. *Acta Otolaryngologica (Stockholm)* 100:231.)

the patient is considered an audiologically suitable candidate for the surgical procedures.

Immediately prior to the first stage operation, a repeat audiogram is obtained to rule out the possibility of significant change in hearing status. After the second stage has been completed and suitable healing and tissue integration with the abutment has occurred, the NAS is attached and the patient is trained in its management and operation. When the patient is accustomed to the device and any fitting problems have been solved, the final evaluation is done. This final session includes a complete duplication of the preoperative test battery with the nonselected ear occluded as before, plus the addition of the NAS as a fourth listening condition.

Of the 16 patients that we have evaluated at Columbia-Presbyterian Medical Center to date, four of them were not suitable candidates because of insufficient sensorineural reserve. Their BC pure tone averages exceeded 45 dB HL, and the power output of the available instrument was either inadequate to reach them or would have forced the aid to be operated at maximum output for those patients whose BC average fell between 40 dB and 50 dB HL. This was unacceptable for an experimental surgical procedure, and we reduced the original experimental

upper limit for the BC average then used by the Swedes from 50 dB to 45 dB HL. A more recent generation instrument has slightly more power, and these patients may later become candidates for it or succeeding generations of instruments. Of the remaining 12 patients who were suitable audiologically, one was unsuitable because of questionable motivation due to normal hearing on one side in conjunction with complete atresia and absent auricle on the pure conductive side. His primary motivation was toward improved physical appearance through the use of a bone anchored auricular prosthesis rather than improved hearing. The other 11 suitable candidates received the first stage insertion of the titanium screw.

One patient was lost to the study when he moved out of the state and elected not to proceed to the second stage. The remaining ten completed the procedures and were fitted with their NAS over a three-year period from 1985 to 1988. The mean audiometric pure-tone averages for these ten patients are shown in table I with their ranges. The air conduction mean of 60 dB and the bone conduction mean of 20 dB indicate a mean air-bone gap for the group of about 40 dB. Table II presents the mean sound field postoperative measures for the unaided condition, the bone anchored system (NAS), and the standard bone conduction hearing aid. For warble tones, the mean average for 500, 1000 and 2000 Hz was reduced from 50 dB unaided to 23 dB by the bone anchored system and to 17 dB by the standard BC aid. Similarly, the mean speech reception thresholds (SRT) were reduced from the unaided 53 dB to 26 dB by the bone anchored system and to 19 dB by the standard BC aid. The excellent unaided mean discrimination score of 97% for the group was maintained at 98% for the bone anchored system and at 96% for the standard BC aid.

Figure 12 contains the synthetic sentence identification data for each of the ten subjects. The individual signal-to-noise ratios at which 50% identification occurred are shown by the asterisks for the bone anchored system (NAS) and by the open circles for the standard BC aid. All aids were set at the most comfortable listening level and the nontest ear was occluded. The subjects are arranged according to their ratios achieved with the NAS, starting with

Table I. Postoperative Hearing Measures. Mean Audiometric Pure Tone Averages. (N=10)

	Mean (dB HL)	Range
Air Conduction	60	50–78
Bone Conduction	20	10–38

Table II. Postoperative Hearing Measures. Mean
Sound Field Measures. (N = 10)

	Unaided		Bone Anchored System (NAS)		Standard BC Aid	
	Mean	Range	Mean	Range	Mean	Range
Warble tone average (dB HL)	50	42–60	23	15–35	17	5–37
SRT (dB HL)	53	45–60	26	20–30	19	5–30
PB %	97	72–100	98	80–100	96	76–100

the best ratio of −5 dB at the bottom and rising to
the worst ratio of +4 dB at the top, covering a range
of 9 dB. The standard BC aid ratios also encompass
a 9 dB range from −7 dB to +2 dB. It was better
than the NAS in six cases, both units were the same
in one, and the NAS was better in three cases.
When compared to the unaided condition in which
no one was able to hear anything at all, both bone
conducting devices performed well. When the advantages of comfort, appearance, and the head-
borne microphone are considered, the NAS, with
its lesser power, did *very* well.

The pre-implantation audiometric evaluation
for our most severe case (patient HA) is shown in

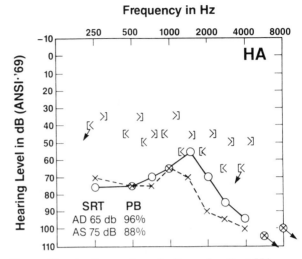

Figure 13. Audiometric evaluation of patient HA, pre-
implantation. (Reprinted with permission from Abramson, M., Fay, T.H., Kelly, J.P., Wazen, J.J., Liden, G., and
Tjellstrom, A. 1989. Clinical results with a percutaneous
bone-anchored hearing aid. *Laryngoscope* 99:709.)

figure 13. His bone conduction pure tone average
was just at the limit of 45 dB HL, but he was also
probably our most motivated patient—a 62-year-
old successful businessman with a long history of
bilateral middle ear effusion coupled with a failed
left stapes mobilization and a combination of right
mastoidectomy and fenestration. AC aids reverbe-
rate and feed back in the large cavity of his right ear
and they induce drainage in the left. He was wearing a BC aid on the left side, but was very eager to
try anything that would get rid of the headband and
its discomforts.

Figure 14 presents his post-implantation unaided sound field warble tone results shown as triangles, along with his standard BC aid shown as
open circles and NAS results shown as solid circles.
Also included for reference are his masked audiometric pure tone bone conduction thresholds for
the left ear. Both aided curves interweave nicely and
indicate serviceable functional gain.

Patient HA's aided SSI ratios, shown in figure
15, are of particular interest in that they suggest
what a more powerful bone anchored device could
do for him and others with less sensorineural reserve than our present limitations allow. Even
though he achieved the poorest ratio of all subjects
with the NAS, shown by the solid line, that +4 dB
ratio was improved to +1 dB when he wore his own
conventional BC aid, shown by the dashed line, in
the usual transcutaneous mode, that is, with the
headband pressing the vibrator against his mastoid. However, when an NAS attachment bayonet

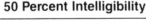
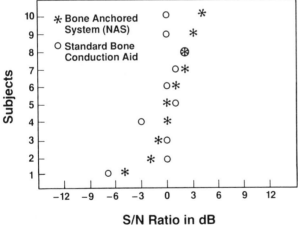

50 Percent Intelligibility

* Bone Anchored System (NAS)
O Standard Bone Conduction Aid

Subjects

S/N Ratio in dB

Signal Level = 63 dB SPL
Noise Level = Variable

Figure 12. Aided Synthetic Sentence Identification (SSI)
test in sound field. Signal level is constant at 63 dB SPL.
Noise is increased until 50% intelligibility occurs. (Reprinted with permission from Abramson, M., Fay, T.H.,
Kelly, J.P., Wazen, J.J., Liden, G., and Tjellstrom, A. 1989.
Clinical results with a percutaneous bone-anchored hearing aid. *Laryngoscope* 99:709.)

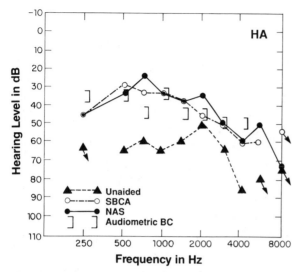

Figure 14. Post-implantation comparison of unaided and aided sound field warble tone results of patient HA. NAS—Nobelpharma Auditory System; SBCA—Standard Bone Conduction Hearing Aid;]-] Left mastoid audiometric masked bone conduction thresholds. (Reprinted with permission from Abramson, M., Fay, T.H., Kelly, J.P., Wazen, J.J., Liden, G., and Tjellstrom, A. 1989. Clinical results with a percutaneous bone-anchored hearing aid. *Laryngoscope* 99:709.)

was glued to the flat surface of his own BC vibrator and affixed directly to his NAS titanium abutment, he achieved a −2 dB ratio, shown by the dotted line, in this now percutaneous mode, with the hearing aid controls at the same settings as in the transcutaneous mode. This 6 dB improvement in ratio over the NAS clearly demonstrates his need for

a more powerful model, and the 3 dB ratio improvement over the transcutaneous mode indicates the greater efficiency of the percutaneous mode. As a result of this experiment, the patient was provided an extra back-up to his NAS that does not require a headband. Any body BC aid can be adapted to do this, but it will still have the disadvantages associated with locating the microphone and amplifier on the body and the cord connecting it to the vibrator.

Our last case (patient DV) is our best, and figure 16 shows her pre-implantation audiometric evaluation. This 52-year-old woman with long-standing bilateral chronic otitis media had bilateral mastoid surgery for cholesteatoma, but still had good bone conduction on both sides. She had been wearing binaural AC aids, but she suffered intermittent drainage in both ears. We fitted her left ear with the NAS and she continues to wear her AC aid in the right ear when she wants balanced hearing. Now, she can remove the AC aid when her ear begins to drain and still be able to hear without having to wear a headband.

Her post-implantation sound field warble tone results with her right ear occluded, shown in figure 17, indicate serviceable functional gain with the NAS, shown by the solid circles as well as with the standard BC aid shown by the open circles. Her masked audiometric pure tone bone conduction thresholds for the left ear are also included for reference.

Patient DV's performance with the SSI, for which she achieved the best results of all ten patients, is shown in figure 18. Unable to hear any of the sentences unaided in quiet, she achieved a −7

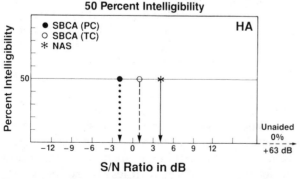

Figure 15. Aided Synthetic Sentence Identification (SSI) test in sound field of patient HA. SBCA (PC)—Standard Bone Conduction Hearing Aid (Percutaneous); SBCA (TC)—Standard Bone Conduction Hearing Aid (Transcutaneous); NAS—Nobelpharma Auditory System. (Reprinted with permission from Abramson, M., Fay, T.H., Kelly, J.P., Wazen, J.J., Liden, G., and Tjellstrom, A. 1989. Clinical results with a percutaneous bone-anchored hearing aid. *Laryngoscope* 99:710.)

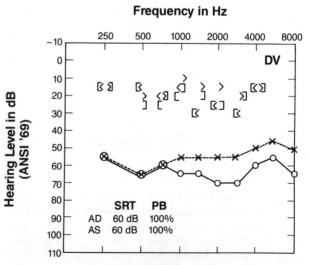

Figure 16. Audiometric evaluation of patient DV, pre-implantation.

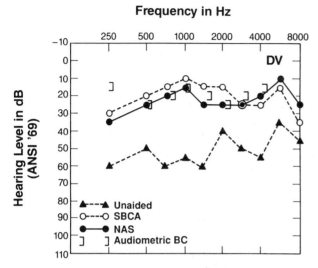

Frequency in Hz

Figure 17. Post-implantation comparison of unaided and aided sound field warble tone results of patient DV. NAS—Nobelpharma Auditory System; SBCA—Standard Bone Conduction Hearing Aid;]-] Left mastoid audiometric masked bone conduction thresholds.

dB ratio with the standard BC aid, shown by the solid circle, and a −5 dB ratio with the NAS shown by the asterisk. In contrast, her own AC aid only provided a +4 dB ratio. This is our best example of what can be done for many unhappy people who do not like wearing conventional BC aids.

Our ten patients were strongly positive in their responses to questionnaires after extensive periods of wear. The six patients who had previously worn aids rated the NAS significantly superior to them with respect to communicative effectiveness, comfort, convenience, and appearance (Abramson et al. 1989). Disadvantages include power limitations for BC losses worse than 45 dB average, location of the microphone behind the pinna emphasizing rear

sound sources, and insertion difficulties encountered by the wearer with the teflon inserts that hold the device in the abutment.

A transcutaneous partially implanted bone conduction system has been jointly developed by Hough and his associates in Oklahoma City and Vernon and his group in Portland, Oregon with the corporate support of Xomed-Treace of Jacksonville, Florida (Campos 1988). This device, the Audiant Bone Conductor™, is also based on the Branemark System, but it differs from the percutaneous Nobelpharma device in that a magnet attached to a titanium screw is inserted under the skin. Figure 19 shows a cross section of the concept and the signal delivery system. The original subcutaneous portion comprised a rare earth samarium cobalt magnet contained in a titanium disk that was sealed in silicone and attached to the temporal bone by a Herbert orthopedic titanium screw, in a single stage operation. The newer version of the implant, known as the XA2-II, contains a rare earth magnet (neodymium iron boron) that is completely enclosed within a titanium alloy case, thus rendering the entire surface of the implant magnetic.

The external portion of the Audiant™ is available in two processor configurations. The earlier and more powerful unit (figure 20) comprises a body-worn section that contains the microphone, battery, and amplifier, and is connected by a cord to a separate small head-borne section. This contains a second magnet to hold it in place over the implanted portion, and an induction coil to transmit the electromagnetic signal through the skin to the internal magnet that vibrates the temporal bone directly.

The more recent configuration is known as the Xomed Audiant "At the Ear" or ATE™ sound processor, shown in figure 21. All external parts are

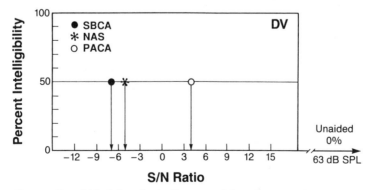

Figure 18. Aided Synthetic Sentence Identification (SSI) test in sound field of patient DV. SBCA—Standard Bone Conduction Hearing Aid; NAS—Nobelpharma Auditory System; PACA—Patient's Air Conduction Aid.

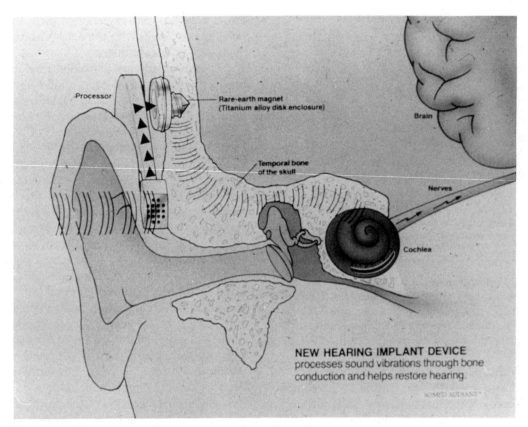

Figure 19.   Cross-section of the concept and signal delivery of the Audiant Bone Conductor™. (Reprinted with permission from Xomed-Treace.)

contained in its smaller postauricular case except for the microphone which projects forward on an extendable boom that rests on the pinna, thus affording forward-facing sound pick-up. The processor is designed to be held in place by its magnet, but is also equipped with a wire hook to be placed behind the pinna for additional support, if needed. Slippage caused by inadequate magnet strength, as well as discomfort and the possibility of tissue damage due to excessive pressure from long periods of wear were important problem areas with the original version. However, improved magnets for which five strengths are now available, and user compliance with schedules of wear that provide adequate tissue rest during periods of non-use, have largely brought these problems under control.

Hough introduced his first body-worn implanted device in 1985 and later reported the results from some of the first groups of patients. He recommended it for essentially the same group of candidates as for the percutaneous Swedish device, except that he limited the audiometric criteria to 80% or better speech discrimination, air conduction pure-tone average not less than 40 dB HL in the implanted ear, and a maximum bone conduction

pure-tone average of 25 dB HL (Hough, Himelick, and Johnson 1986; Hough, McGee, Himelick, and Vernon 1986). These constraints were imposed because of power limitations and loss of signal strength encountered in transcutaneous stimulation. The ATE™ version provides approximately 10 dB HL less output than the body-worn version, hence the maximum bone conduction average for that processor is actually reduced to 15 dB HL (Tollos 1990).

Hakansson and his colleagues (1990) attribute the substantial differences in performance between the percutaneous bone anchored system and the transcutaneous Audiant™ transducer to the great differences in length of gap in their magnetic circuits and to their differences in suspension properties. They define the gap as the length of the magnetic path that consists of nonmagnetic material. In the Swedish NAS system, the gap is small, consists entirely of air, and is completely contained in the external portion. In the Audiant™ transducer, where there is no metallic contact between the external and internal parts, the length of the relatively large gap is determined by the thickness of the intact soft tissue between them. Large gaps contribute to considerable loss of power and to second harmonic distortion (Hakansson et al. 1990; Hakansson, Tjellstrom, and Carlsson 1990).

Difficulties with power limitation, wearing discomfort, and skin irritation encountered with the original version of the Audiant™ have been verified by several investigators. Reporting from North America are Wade, Tollos, and Naiberg (1989), Weber (1989), Roush and Rauch (1990), and Browning (1990) in the United Kingdom. Careful evaluation of all other possible solutions are urged by these reporters before deciding to implant the Audiant™ in either mode. Counseling is important when reviewing options, and decisions to use the ATE™ should not be based on appearance alone.

Despite these difficulties, the Audiant™ is a viable alternative to conventional amplification in those cases that are essentially conductive, that have met the most stringent requirements for implantation, and in which the problems encountered with other alternatives are at least equal to or greater than those present in the Audiant™. All patients who are considered candidates for any of the available implantable systems should always understand clearly the disadvantages as well as the advantages prior to implantation.

With the development of adequate power supplies, sufficient signal strength at the cochlea, easily manipulable external controls, and the demonstration of long-term stability, a variety of approaches and pathways will be available for our creative ap-

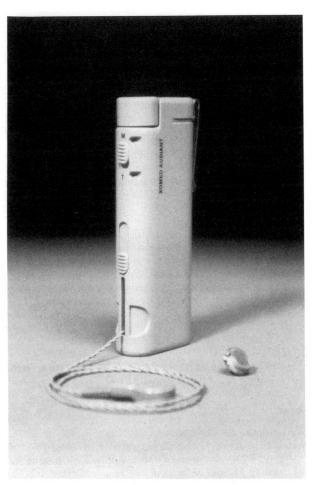

Figure 20. Audiant Bone Conductor™ body processor. (Reprinted with permission from Xomed-Treace.)

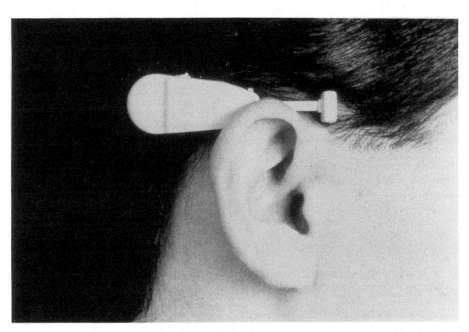

Figure 21. Audiant Bone Conductor™ At-the-Ear (ATE™) processor. (Reprinted with permission from Xomed-Treace.)

plication to our patients' needs. Implantable auditory devices will play a central role in future hearing aid developments, and it will be incumbent upon manufacturers to assure the availability of adequate supplies of compatible replacement instruments and parts throughout the lifetimes of wearers.

References

Abramson, M. 1989. Implanted hearing aids and sound-conducting devices. In *Otolaryngology—Head and Neck Surgery Update I*, eds. C.W. Cummings, J.M. Fredrickson, L.A. Harker, C.J. Krause, and D.E. Schuller. St. Louis: The C.V. Mosby Company.

Abramson, M., Fay, T.H., Kelly, J.P., Wazen, J.J., Liden, G., and Tjellstrom, A. 1989. Clinical results with a percutaneous bone-anchored hearing aid. *Laryngoscope* 99:707–710.

Bojrab, D., Clemis, J., and McGee, T. 1988. Semi-implantable hearing devices. Paper read at the Middle Section, Triological Society, January 1988, Ann Arbor, Michigan. Cited in Maniglia, A.J. 1989. Implantable hearing devices: State of the art. *Otolaryngologic Clinics of North America* 22:175–200.

Branemark, P.-I., Breine, U., Adell, R., Hansson, B.O., Lindstrom, J. and Ohlsson, A. 1969. Intra-osseous anchorage of dental prostheses. I. Experimental studies. *Scandinavian Journal of Plastic and Reconstructive Surgery* 3:81–100.

Browning, G.G. 1990. The British experience of an implantable, subcutaneous bone conduction hearing aid (Xomed Audiant). *The Journal of Laryngology and Otology* 104:534–38.

Campos, C.T. 1988. A chronology of an implantable bone conductor hearing device. *Hearing Instruments* 39:37–38.

Fay, T.H., and Abramson, M. 1988. Patient selection criteria for the bone anchored hearing aid (BAHA). Paper read at the annual convention of the American Speech-Language-Hearing Association, October 1988, Boston.

Fay, T.H., Abramson, M. and Russo, R.L. 1986. Patient selection criteria for the bone anchored hearing aid (BAHA). Paper read at the 27th Annual Convention of the New York State Speech-Language-Hearing Association, April 1986, Kiamesha Lake, New York.

Fredricksson, J.M., Tomlinson, D.R., Davis, E.R., and Odkvist, L.M. 1973. Evaluation of an electromagnetic implantable hearing aid. *Canadian Journal of Otolaryngology* 2:1, 53–62.

Glorig, A., Moushegian, G., Bringewald, P.R., Rupert, A.L., and Gerken, G.M. 1972. Magnetically coupled stimulation of the ossicular chain: Measures in kangaroo rat and man. *Journal of the Acoustical Society of America* 52:694–96.

Goode, R.L. 1970. An implantable hearing aid: State of the art. *Transactions of the American Academy of Ophthalmology and Otolaryngology* 74:128–39.

Goode, R. L. 1988. Electromagnetic implantable hearing aids. In *Middle Ear Implant: Implantable Hearing Aids, Advances in Audiology*, Vol. 4:22–31, ed. J.-I. Suzuki. Basel: S. Karger AG.

Goode, R.L. 1989. Current status of electromagnetic implantable hearing aids. *Otolaryngologic Clinics of North America* 22:201–209.

Goode, R.L., and Glattke, T. 1973. Audition via electromagnetic induction. *Archives of Otolaryngology* 98:23–26.

Goode, R.L., Aritome, H., Gonzales, J., and Gyo, K. 1986. The implantable hearing aid. In *Tissue Integration in Oral and Maxillofacial Reconstruction*, ed. D. van Steenberghe. Amsterdam: Excerpta Medica.

Gyo, K., and Goode, R.L. 1988. Measurement of stapes vibration driven by the ceramic vibrator of a middle ear implant—Human temporal bone experiments. In *Middle Ear Implant: Implantable Hearing Aids, Advances in Audiology*, Vol. 4:107–116, ed. J.-I. Suzuki. Basel: S. Karger AG.

Gyo, K., Goode, R.L., and Miller, C. 1987. Stapes vibration produced by the output transducer of an implantable hearing aid. *Archives of Otolaryngology Head and Neck Surgery* 113:1078–1081.

Hakansson, B., Liden, G., Tjellstrom, A., Ringdahl, A., Jacobsson, M., Carlsson, P., and Erlandson, B.-E. 1990. Ten years of experience with the Swedish bone-anchored hearing system. *Annals of Otology, Rhinology and Laryngology* Supp. 151, 99(10–2):1–16.

Hakansson, B., Tjellstrom, A., and Carlsson, P. 1990. Percutaneous versus transcutaneous transducers for hearing by direct bone conduction. *Otolaryngology—Head and Neck Surgery* 102:339–344.

Hakansson, B., Tjellstrom, A., Rosenhall, U., and Carlsson, P. 1985. The bone-anchored hearing aid. *Acta Otolaryngologica (Stockholm)* 100:229–39.

Heide, J., Tatge, G., Sander, T., Gooch, T., and Prescott, T. 1988. Development of a semi-implantable hearing device. In *Middle Ear Implant: Implantable Hearing Aids, Advances in Audiology*, Vol. 4:32–43, ed. J.-I. Suzuki. Basel: S. Karger AG.

Hough, J., Himelick, T., and Johnson, B. 1986. Implantable bone conduction hearing device: Audiant™ bone conductor. *Annals of Otology, Rhinology and Laryngology* 95:498–504.

Hough, J., McGee, M., Himelick, T., and Vernon, J. 1986. The surgical technique for implantation of the temporal bone stimulator (Audiant ABC). *The American Journal of Otology* 7:315–21.

Hough, J., Vernon, J., Dormer, K., Johnson, B., and Himelick, T. 1986. Experiences with implantable hearing devices and a presentation of a new device. *Annals of Otology, Rhinology and Laryngology* 95:60–65.

Hough, J., Vernon, J., Meikel, M., Himelick, T., Richard, G., and Dormer, K. 1987. A middle ear implantable hearing device for controlled amplification of sound in the human: A preliminary report. *Laryngoscope* 97:141–51.

Khanna, S.M., and Corliss, E.L.R. 1986. Consideration in stimulating the cochlea via a bone-anchored vibrator. In *Tissue Integration in Oral and Maxillofacial Reconstruction*, ed. D. van Steenberghe. Amsterdam: Excerpta Medica.

Maniglia, A.J. 1989. Implantable hearing devices: State of the art. *Otolaryngologic Clinics of North America* 22:175–200.

Maniglia, A.J., Ko, W.H., Zhang, R.X., Dolgin, S.R., Rosenbaum, M.L., and Montague, Jr., F.W. 1988. Electromagnetic implantable middle ear hearing devices of the ossicular-stimulating type: Principles, designs, and experiments. *Annals of Otology, Rhinology and Laryngology* Supplement 136:3–16.

Nunley, J.A., Agnew, J., and Smith, G.L. 1976. A new design for an implantable hearing aid. *ISA BM* 76313:69–72.

Nunley, J.A., Agnew, J., Smith, G.L., and Murphy, P. 1975. Stimulation of the chinchilla's ossicular chain with an implanted hearing device. *The Journal of Auditory Research* 15:258-61.

Roush, J., and Rauch, S.D. 1990. Clinical application of an implantable bone conduction hearing device. *Laryngoscope* 100:281–85.

Rutschmann, J. 1959. Magnetic audition–Auditory stimulation by means of alternating magnetic fields acting on a permanent magnet fixed to the eardrum. *IRE Transactions of Medical Electronics* 6:22–23.

Rutschmann, J., Page, H.J., and Fowler, Jr., E.P. 1958. Auditory stimulation: Alternating magnetic fields acting on a permanent magnet fixed to the eardrum. Paper read at the meeting of the American Physiological Society, 1958, Philadelphia. Cited in Goode, R.L. 1989. Current status of electromagnetic implantable hearing aids. *Otolaryngologic Clinics of North America* 22:201–209.

Speaks, C., and Jerger, J. 1965. Method of measurement of speech identification. *Journal of Speech and Hearing Research* 8:185–92.

Suzuki, J.-I. (ed.) 1988. *Middle Ear Implant: Implantable Hearing Aids, Advances in Audiology*, Vol. 4. Basel: S. Karger AG.

Suzuki, J.-I., Kodera, K., and Yanagihara, N. 1983. Evaluation of middle-ear implant: A six-month observation in cats. *Acta Otolaryngologica* 95:646–50.

Suzuki, J.-I., Kodera, K., Suzuki, M., and Ashikawa, H. 1989. Further clinical experiences with middle-ear implantable hearing aids: Indications and sound quality evaluation. *ORL Journal of Otorhinolaryngology and Related Specialties* 51:229–34.

Tjellstrom, A. 1988. Vibratory stimulation of the cochlea through a percutaneous transducer. In *Middle Ear Implant: Implantable Hearing Aids, Advances in Audiology*, Vol. 4, ed. J.-I. Suzuki. Basel: S. Karger AG.

Tollos, S.K. 1990. Personal communication.

Vernon, J., Brummett, B., Doyle, P., and Denniston, R. 1970. Cochlear potential evaluation of an implantable hearing aid. *Surgical Forum XXI Otorhinolaryngology* 21:491–93.

Wade, P.S., Tollos, S.K., and Naiberg, J. 1989. Clinical experience with the Xomed Audiant osseointegrated bone conducting hearing device: A preliminary report of seven cases. *The Journal of Otolaryngology* 18:79–84.

Weber, B. 1989. Implantable bone conduction hearing devices: Issues in patient selection and audiologic management. Paper read at the annual convention of the American Speech-Language-Hearing Association, October 1989, St. Louis.

Wilska, A. 1935. Eine methode zur bestimmung der horschwellenamplituden des trommelfells bei verschiedenen frequenzen. *Skandinavian Archives of Physiology* 72:161–65. Cited in Goode, R.L. 1989. Current status of electromagnetic implantable hearing aids. *Otolaryngologic Clinics of North America* 22:201–209.

Wilska, A. 1959. A direct method for determining threshold amplitudes of the eardrum at various frequencies. In *The Middle Ear*, ed. H.G. Kobrak. Chicago: University of Chicago Press.

Wilson, E.P., Deddens, A.E., Lesser, T.H.J., and Fredrickson, J.M. 1990. Implantable hearing aids: Changes in the auditory evoked potential of the monkey in response to increased loading of the stapes. *American Journal of Otolaryngology* 11:149–52.

Yanagihara, N., Aritomo, H., Yamanaka, E., and Gyo, K. 1988. Intraoperative assessment of vibrator-induced hearing. In *Middle Ear Implant: Implantable Hearing Aids, Advances in Audiology*, Vol. 4:124–133, ed. J.-I. Suzuki. Basel: S. Karger AG.

Yanagihara, N., Gyo, K., Suzuki, J., and Araki, H. 1983. Perception of sound through direct oscillation of the stapes using a piezoelectric ceramic bimorph. *Annals of Otology, Rhinology and Laryngology* 92:223–27.

Yanagihara, N., Suzuki, J., Gyo, K., Syono, H., and Ikeda, H. 1984. Development of an implantable hearing aid using a piezoelectric vibrator of bimorph design: State of the art. *Otolaryngology—Head and Neck Surgery* 92:706–712.

PART III
Electroacoustic Measurements

CHAPTER 10

Acoustic Measures of Hearing Aid Performance

David B. Hawkins

There has been a significant shift in recent years in the orientation to evaluation and selection of hearing aids. In the past, the emphasis was on the individual's ability to understand speech with a hearing aid, with little attention directed to the electroacoustic characteristics being evaluated or selected. In contrast, the most common approach today seems to rely almost exclusively on acoustic measures of hearing aid performance. If certain acoustic performance criteria are satisfied, the assumption is made that speech intelligibility has been optimized. In other words, a dramatic reversal of emphasis seems to have occurred. Decisions in the past were made with the assistance of behavioral responses from the hearing aid wearer to speech stimuli. Decisions now seem to be influenced heavily by the hearing aid's acoustic response in the ear canal of the hearing-impaired person.

Many believe that the current emphasis on real-ear performance of hearing aids is breaking new ground. However, literature in the 1940s stated clearly that the frequency response in a 2-cm³ coupler was not equivalent to that in a real ear canal. For instance, figure 1 shows a correction curve published in 1944 by LeBel to convert from the 2-cm³ coupler to the real ear. This curve will look familiar to those who are knowledgeable in the area of correction factors. LeBel stated in 1944 that "We have been using a curve of this general nature for some time, with uniformly improved results in fitting" (p. 66). LeBel also discussed the "fallacy" of using uncorrected 2-cm³ coupler responses.

There are two acoustic measurement procedures in use today that emphasize the response in the real ear. The first entails determination of the real-ear frequency response through assessment of unaided and aided sound-field thresholds, or functional gain. The second method of acoustic evaluation utilizes probe-tube microphone measurements (PTMs) to assess a variety of aspects of hearing aid performance.

Although the idea of the real-ear response may not be brand new, some of the techniques are, and

the purpose of this chapter is to discuss some advantages and disadvantages of these newer procedures and to describe some important variables in the implementation of an acoustic approach to the selection of hearing aids.

Terminology

As in any relatively new area, there has been some confusion in terminology related to measurements of hearing aid performance in ways other than the standard 2-cm³ coupler. If measurements are made on a Knowles Electronics Manikin for Acoustic Research (KEMAR), then the terminology is straightforward, as it is outlined in ANSI S3.35 (1985). When functional gain measurements are made, the terminology is simple and also clear. Functional gain is the difference between an unaided and aided sound-field threshold. The greatest confusion has been caused in the area of PTMs, as some of the analogous ANSI terms have been used (Preves 1987) and a number of others have been created. A recently formed ANSI working group (ANSI S3.80 Committee on Probe Microphone Measurements of Hearing Aid Performance) has generated some "consensus" terms for PTMs (Schweitzer et al. 1990). Use of these terms should be helpful in facilitating communication.

A comparison of the ANSI terms for manikin measurements and the consensus PTM terms is shown in table I. Also included are other terms that have appeared in the literature. For instance, the manikin unoccluded ear gain is analogous to the real-ear unaided response, or REUR, known to some as the free-field to eardrum transfer function or the ear canal resonance or external ear effect. This measurement shows the increase that occurs at the tympanic membrane as a result of head and body diffraction effects and concha and ear canal resonances.

The real ear aided response, REAR, represents

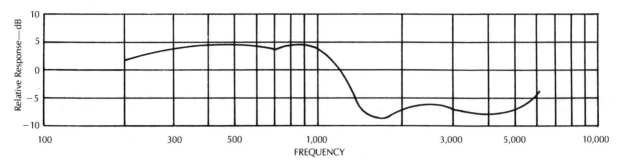

Figure 1.   Correction curve from the 2-cm³ coupler to real-ear performance. (From LeBel 1944.)

the SPL that is developed near the tympanic membrane while a hearing aid is worn. There is no analogous measurement in the ANSI manikin standard, as the reference SPL is subtracted, yielding a gain value.

Real ear insertion gain, REIG, is the difference in dB at a single frequency between the unaided response (REUR) and the aided response (REAR) and is analogous to functional gain. If insertion gain is measured across frequency, then the term is real-ear insertion response, REIR, with the manikin terminology being Simulated Insertion Gain Frequency Response, or SIGFR.

The maximum SPL that a hearing aid is capable of producing in a real ear has been called the real ear saturation response, RESR. The hearing aid is driven to saturation and the SPL is measured in the ear canal. The ANSI manikin standard calls this the Simulated In-Situ SSPL90 Frequency Response. A frequent term in the clinical literature has been real-ear SSPL90.

Examples of PTM data are shown in figures 2 through 4. A typical REUR is shown in figure 2. The peak in the unaided response of an average adult (and KEMAR) occurs around 2700 Hz and is between 15 to 20 dB. Figure 3 shows a REAR obtained on a person wearing a hearing aid. The actual SPL generated by the hearing aid in the ear canal is displayed as a function of frequency. The RESR is simply a REAR with a 90 dB SPL input in order to saturate the hearing aid.

Figure 4 shows an example of a REIR. The ordinate is now gain and the plot shows the insertion gain across frequency. If the hearing aid does not have a good high-frequency response, which is rather common, then the insertion response shows

Table I.   Terminology Comparisons

Measurement	ANSI S3.35 (In situ standard)	ANSI S3.80 (Probe-Tube Committee)	Other Terms
SPL near TM unaided	Manikin unoccluded ear gain (1 Freq.) Manikin frequency response (Curve)	Real ear unaided response (REUR)	FF eardrum TF Wearer unoccluded gain (1 Freq.) Wearer frequency response (Curve) Ear canal reson. Ext. ear reson. Ext. ear effects Open ear response Unaided response
SPL near TM aided		Real ear aided response (REAR)	In situ output response
Difference (dB) near TM between unaided and aided	Simulated insertion gain (1 freq.)	Real ear insertion gain (REIG) (1 freq.)	Insertion gain Real ear gain
	Simulated insertion gain freq. response (curve)	Real ear insertion response (REIR) (curve)	Insertion gain freq. response Real ear response
Maximum output of hearing aid near TM	Simulated in situ SSPL90 frequency response	Real ear saturation response (RESR)	Real Ear SSPL90

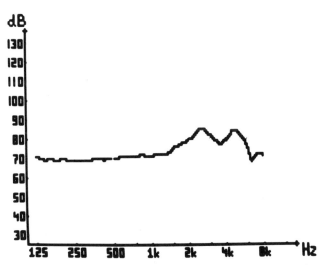

Figure 2. Real Ear Unaided Response (REUR) obtained on an adult with a 70 dB SPL input.

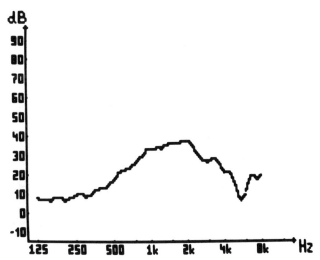

Figure 4. Real Ear Insertion Response (REIR) derived from the REUR and REAR shown in figures 1 and 2.

a negative slope in the high frequencies, as shown in this tracing.

Behavioral Measures of Unaided and Aided Performance: Functional Gain

The first recent clinical method devised to assess the real-ear frequency response directly was functional gain, where the aided sound-field threshold is subtracted from the unaided sound-threshold threshold. In the unaided condition, all head and body diffraction effects are present and the concha and ear canal are open and resonating. In the aided condition, head and body diffraction effects are

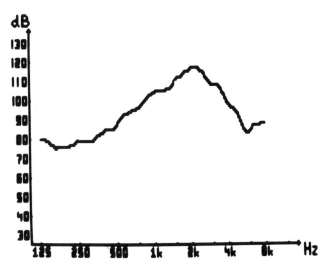

Figure 3. Real Ear Aided Response (REAR) obtained with a 70 dB SPL input.

again operative, the hearing aid microphone is located appropriately, and the actual acoustic load (the individual's residual air volume and middle ear impedance) is present. This measurement, popularized by Pascoe's work in 1975, represents the actual amplification provided by a hearing aid compared to the unaided listening condition. Assessing the real-ear frequency response through functional gain measurements was particularly popular during the late 1970s and early 1980s and is still used extensively, especially with young children.

Limitations of Functional Gain

There are some limitations associated with the functional gain approach. First, functional gain provides information only at octave, or at best half-octave, intervals. Significant peaks or dips in the real-ear frequency response can go unnoticed with this approach.

The accuracy of the sound-field threshold can be compromised in steeply sloping high-frequency hearing losses and/or cases where the unaided threshold is within normal limits. In the case of steeply sloping hearing losses, the client may respond to energy that is not at the center of the narrow-band signal. In other words, energy at a frequency lower than the center frequency of the signal may exceed threshold before the energy at the center frequency of the test signal. An invalid unaided and/or aided sound-field threshold can result, producing inaccurate functional gain.

There is also the potential for masking to occur in aided threshold measurements. Macrae and Frazer (1980) and Macrae (1982) have shown that masked aided thresholds can occur if the effective masking levels produced by the hearing aid circuit noise and/or amplified room noise exceed the real aided threshold. This is primarily a problem when the client has unaided thresholds in the near-normal or normal range. The result of masked aided sound-field thresholds is an underestimation of the actual amount of functional gain.

In some cases, the use of functional gain can provide an unrealistic estimate of real-ear gain of a hearing aid. For instance, if the client has less than a moderate-to-severe hearing loss and appropriate gain values would lead to aided thresholds in the range of less than 40 dB HL, then for the aided threshold measurements the input levels to the hearing aid will be quite low, (e.g., less than 45 to 50 dB sound pressure level [SPL]). If the hearing aid being evaluated has a linear input-output function up to 60 or 70 dB SPL inputs and then goes into some type of compression for higher input levels (a fairly typical input-output function in many compression hearing aids), the functional gain measured with the low-level inputs could be substantially greater than that measured for typical speech inputs of 60 to 70 dB SPL. This is not to say that the functional gain values will be inaccurate, but they will apply only to low-level inputs.

Another similar instance can occur when the hearing aid has a relatively low SSPL90 combined with a rather high amount of gain, such as might occur in a person with a moderate-to-severe hearing loss and low loudness discomfort levels. In the functional gain measurements, the low-level inputs probably will not saturate the hearing aid and thus the real-ear gain would be substantial. When typical speech inputs are applied, saturation could occur easily and as a result the gain would be reduced. This concept is shown in figure 5 from Stelmachowicz and Lewis (1988). The solid line represents the input-output function and is referenced to the left ordinate; the dashed line represents gain and applies to the right ordinate. This hearing aid, which has high gain and a low SSPL90, is saturated for inputs of 50 dB SPL and above. Notice that for low-level inputs the gain is between 65 and 70 dB, but for inputs typical of speech levels (60 to 70 dB SPL), the gain is 40 to 50 dB. Again, both measurements are assessing actual performance, but one must ask which is more representative of actual use conditions. With some "automatic signal processing" circuits in hearing aids today, or recently developed circuits like the one described by Killion (1988, 1990) in which the frequency response is level dependent, real-ear gain must be described with several

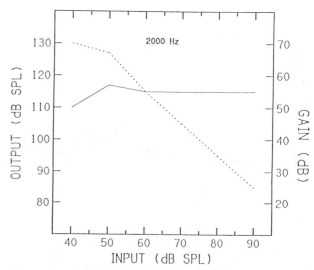

Figure 5.   Input/output function (solid line, left ordinate) and gain characteristics (dashed line, right ordinate) at 2000 Hz for a hearing aid with high gain and low SSPL90. (From Stelmachowicz and Lewis 1987.)

input levels. Functional gain would be a restrictive measurement in such cases, as it would be assessing real-ear gain with only one input level, that necessary to reach threshold for that individual person.

The variability associated with functional gain measurements can also prove to be a problem. Hawkins et al. (1987) measured the variability for repeated sets of aided sound-field thresholds with the volume control wheel being reset for comfortable listening after each measurement. This situation occurs when several hearing aids or several settings of one hearing aid are being compared. The resulting critical differences for several probability levels at different test frequencies are shown in table II. If a 0.05 level of confidence is chosen, the critical differences are approximately 15 dB. Recent data from Humes and Kirn (1990) support these rather large test-retest variations in functional gain. The variability would be expected to be less if the volume control wheel were fixed by the audiologist and larger when children are being evaluated.

Another limitation is that functional gain pro-

Table II.   Critical Differences (dB) for Aided Sound-Field Thresholds at Four Probability Levels (From Hawkins et al. 1987)

	Frequency (Hz)					
p	250	500	1000	2000	3000	4000
.05	11.9	15.7	15.1	15.1	16.1	16.5
.1	10.0	13.2	12.7	12.7	13.5	13.8
.2	7.8	10.2	9.9	9.9	10.7	10.8
.3	6.3	8.3	8.0	8.0	8.5	8.7

vides information only about the frequency response of the hearing aid. No information is provided about other aspects of hearing aid performance, such as distortion or SSPL90. Although this is not a criticism of the procedure per se, assessment of functional gain can be time-consuming; if information is generated about only one aspect of hearing aid performance, this can be viewed as a limitation if alternative measurement options yield additional performance data.

A final concern, conceptual and perhaps semantic in nature, relates to the plotting of aided sound-field thresholds on an audiogram. The implication of such a procedure is that the hearing aid improves the person's threshold. The approach becomes one of a static input signal with thresholds becoming better and thus allowing more of that input to be perceived. In reality, a hearing aid does not perform this function. The thresholds of a damaged cochlea and/or eighth nerve are not changed by a hearing aid. They are poor and will remain so. The hearing aid simply takes the input signal and amplifies it to some point above the constant elevated threshold. This concept is discussed further, later in this chapter.

In summary, functional gain measurements have proved useful in facilitating understanding of how hearing aid frequency responses are represented in a real ear. If care is taken in the measurement of functional gain, it can still prove useful in selection and evaluation of hearing aids. In some cases it can provide unique, important, and essential information that has more validity than other acoustic measurement alternatives. For instance, Stelmachowicz and Lewis (1988) reported a case of a child with probable vibro-tactile thresholds. Functional gain accurately indicated that aided thresholds showed minimal improvement with a power hearing aid as no auditory capabilities were present, whereas PTMs showed 50 to 60 dB of gain, suggesting that substantial aided benefit might be expected.

Measures of SPL in the Ear Canal: Probe-Tube Microphone Measurements (PTM)

In the last decade PTMs have provided an attractive alternative and/or addition to functional gain as a method of evaluating real-ear performance of hearing aids. The attractiveness of PTMs as an alternative to functional gain centers around seven advantages: (1) the measurements are more time efficient;

(2) information is obtained across the entire frequency range of interest rather than octave intervals; (3) less cooperation is required from the client in that behavioral responses are not necessary—the only requirements are the ability to tolerate the probe tube in the ear canal and to remain reasonably immobile; (4) off-frequency listening and masked aided thresholds are not problems; (5) a range of input levels can be used to define the real-ear response of the hearing aid if it operates in linear and nonlinear modes; (6) measurements other than frequency response are available, such as the real-ear saturation response (RESR) of the hearing aid; and (7) the ability to use a broad-band input signal, allowing more accurate assessment of compression and automatic signal processing hearing aids (Preves et al. 1989).

Variables Affecting PTMs

Although PTMs offer many advantages, they must be made with caution and with knowledge of a variety of factors that affect the measurements. The variables discussed here include the type of sound-field equalization, the loudspeaker azimuth, the reference microphone location, the probe-tube insertion depth, and the signal level.

Sound-Field Equalization There are two main approaches to sound-field equalization with PTMs: substitution and modified comparison (Preves 1987; Preves and Sullivan 1987). The selection is important because the method utilized to equalize the sound field for PTMs can affect the SPLs that are measured in the ear canal.

The substitution method is the most accurate approach in that all head and body diffraction effects will be evident in the measurements. The sound field is equalized with the client absent, then the person is seated at the precise calibration location. Errors will occur if the client moves from the calibrated position. It is, however, possible to assess accurately the effects of loudspeaker azimuth as long as the loudspeaker distance is held constant. The only disadvantage of the substitution method is the potential for client movement to cause errors. As a result, this method should be used primarily with individuals (typically adults) who can remain immobile during the measurements or when the use of a head holder is appropriate.

In the modified comparison method, a reference microphone is situated on the client's head at one of three typical locations: above the ear, on the cheek, or lateral to the concha. This microphone serves to maintain the loudspeaker output at a constant SPL or to make measurements from which corrections are applied to the probe-tube measured output to simulate a flat input at this point. By keeping the SPL constant at this reference microphone location, much of the head and body diffraction effects are subtracted out of the measurement. In this sense, the modified comparison method is technically less accurate than the substitution method. The loss of accuracy will be primarily for absolute measures of SPL in the ear canal (REAR) when the hearing aid is not saturated. Relative measures of gain, such as REIG, should be equivalent with the substitution and modified comparison methods.

The main advantage of the modified comparison method is that minor movements of the client during testing do not affect the results. This feature makes the modified comparison method attractive to many audiologists, especially when working with children. For a more detailed discussion of sound-field equalization the reader is referred to Preves (1987) and Preves and Sullivan (1987).

Loudspeaker Azimuth The location of the loudspeaker can be an important factor in PTMs. The most commonly recommended locations are 0° and plus or minus 45° (plus 45° if the hearing aid is on the right ear and minus 45° with the left ear aided). Killion and Revit (1987) evaluated several loudspeaker locations to determine which produced the most reliable measurements. The least variability was observed with a 45° azimuth and 45° elevation, closely followed by a 45° azimuth with 0° elevation. Assuming that most audiologists, for practical reasons, will select a 0° elevation, the 45° azimuth loudspeaker location would seem logical from a reliability perspective.

Regardless of which location is chosen, the audiologist should be aware that different SPLs will be measured in the ear canal with various loudspeaker locations. This is particularly true if the substitution method is employed. As a example, figure 6 shows REURs from Shaw (1974) with three loudspeaker orientations. The head diffraction effects are seen clearly as the signal source moves from 0° to 45° to 90°. If individual REURs are being used to correct prescription formulas (Mueller 1989) for deviations from the "average" reference REUR, it is important that this reference REUR be obtained with the same loudspeaker azimuth and same test equipment.

A related issue is the effect of loudspeaker location on relative measures such as the REIR. This is important if the audiologist is attempting to match REIG target values. Ickes, Hawkins, and Cooper

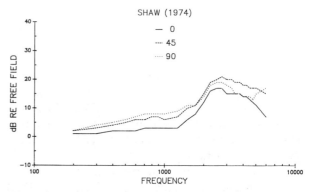

Figure 6.   Field to eardrum transfer function from three loudspeaker azimuths: 0°, 45°, and 90°. (Data from Shaw 1974.)

(1991) measured the REUR, REAR, and REIR with loudspeaker azimuths of 0°, 45°, and 90°. Figure 7 shows these results for a behind-the-ear (BTE) hearing aid on a KEMAR with an over-the-ear reference microphone. It is clear that some differences can occur for all three measurements, with the 90° azimuth producing the most deviant response, primarily in the higher frequencies.

Reference Microphone Location When the modified comparison method is employed, a reference microphone must be placed at some location on the head. As stated earlier, the most common locations have been over the ear, on the cheek, and lateral to the ear. A recent study by Feigin, Nelson Barlow, and Stelmachowicz (1990) measured the differences in SPLs from a cheek and over-the-ear reference microphone location to a BTE hearing aid microphone. Some notable differences were found, suggesting that if absolute SPL measurements in the ear canal were of interest, the location of the reference microphone could affect the result. In other words, although the reference microphone might be maintaining the SPL at that location, there can be frequency-dependent changes by the time the sound arrives at the hearing aid microphone.

Ickes, Hawkins, and Cooper (1991) examined the effects of three loudspeaker azimuths (0°, 45°, and 90°) and three reference microphone locations (over the ear, cheek, and lateral to the tragus) upon the REUR, REAR, and REIR for both a BTE and in-the-ear (ITE) hearing aid. The effects of changes in loudspeaker azimuth and reference microphone location were restricted in general to frequencies above 2000 Hz. Figure 8 shows these data for the REUR; also shown are Shaw's data with the substitution method. The largest variations are seen with the 90° azimuth and the at-the-ear reference

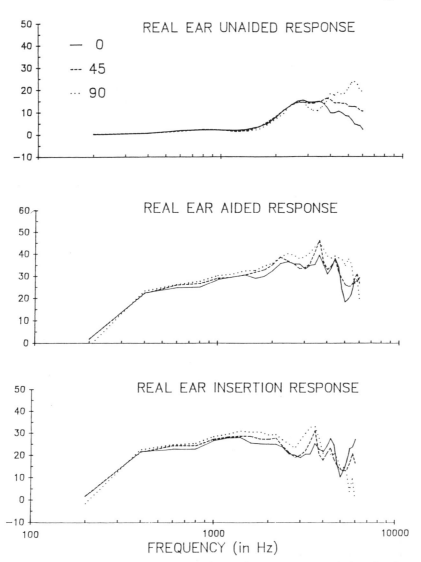

Figure 7.   REUR, REAR, and REIR obtained on a KEMAR with three loudspeaker azimuths (0°, 45°, and 90°) with an over-the-ear reference microphone location and a behind-the-ear hearing aid. (From Ickes, Hawkins,
and Cooper 1991.)

microphone location. Figure 9 shows the REIRs for
the same conditions with an ITE hearing aid. Although the differences among conditions are reduced due to the fact that the REIR is a difference
measurement, there are some substantial variations, again primarily with the 90° azimuth and the
at-the-ear reference microphone location.

These data, taken with the loudspeaker
azimuth results, would lead to a conclusion that a
45° azimuth with an over-the-ear or cheek reference
microphone placement would be preferable.

Probe Tube Placement   The most important procedural consideration in making accurate PTMs is
the placement of the probe tube in the ear canal. It is
especially important in measuring the REUR and
REAR, where the absolute SPL in the ear canal is of
interest.

The particular location of the probe tube in the
ear canal is important due to pressure maxima and
minima as a result of standing wave patterns. These
maxima and minima occur at different locations for
various frequencies. Locating the probe tube at a
pressure minima for a given frequency will result in
a measurement that can be significantly lower than
that actually occurring at the tympanic membrane.
An example of the error at 3000 Hz as a function of
probe tube location is shown in figure 10, taken
from Dirks and Kincaid (1987). The abscissa is the
distance from the tympanic membrane and the or-

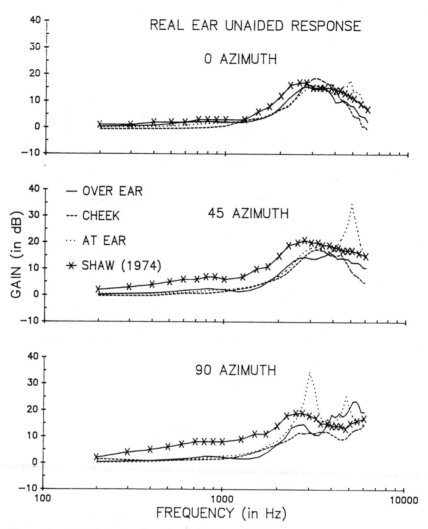

Figure 8.   REUR obtained at three different loudspeaker azimuths (0°, 45°, and 90°) with three different reference microphone locations (over the ear, cheek, and at the ear). Data from Shaw (1974) using a substitution method are shown for comparison. (From Ickes, Hawkins, and Cooper 1991.)

dinate is the difference between the probe and tympanic membrane SPL. The negative numbers indicate that the probe tube is underestimating the actual SPL at the tympanic membrane. As probe distance from the tympanic membrane increases, the error increases until it reaches a maximum at 25 mm, close to the quarter wave length for a 3000 Hz tone. Notice that the impedance of the middle ear has an effect on the magnitude of the error and the specific location of the minima.

Dirks and Kincaid (1987) developed a series of curves showing the error that will be present as the probe tube is positioned at differing locations in the ear canal for frequencies from 1000 to 8000 Hz. These data are shown in figure 11. If the probe tube is located 10 mm from the tympanic membrane, the error would be approximately 10 dB at 8000 Hz,

5 dB at 6000 Hz, 3 dB at 4000 Hz, 2 dB at 3000 Hz, 1 dB at 2000 Hz, and less than 1 dB at 1000 Hz. If the probe tube is located 5 mm from the tympanic membrane, the accuracy of the probe measurements would be within 2 dB through 8000 Hz. There is a direct relationship between distance of the probe tube from the tympanic membrane and accuracy of the measurement in the high frequencies. The closer to the tympanic membrane the probe tube is placed, the more accurate will be the measurement in the higher frequencies.

There are three basic considerations in placing the probe tube in the ear canal. First, it should be close enough to the tympanic membrane to achieve the accuracy the audiologist desires in high frequencies. A location of 5 mm or closer to the tympanic membrane would be ideal. Such a location

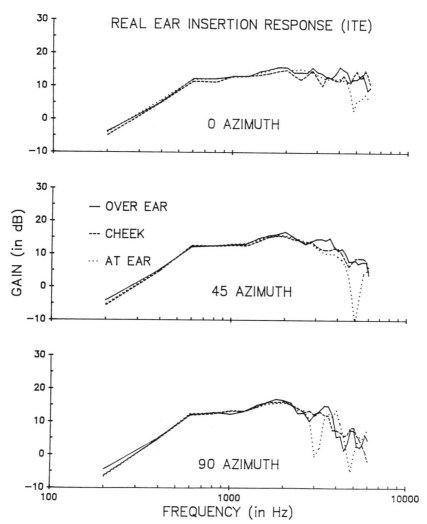

Figure 9. REIR for an in-the-ear hearing aid at three loudspeaker azimuths (0°, 45°, and 90°) and three reference microphone locations (over the ear, cheek, and at the ear). (From Ickes, Hawkins, and Cooper 1991.)

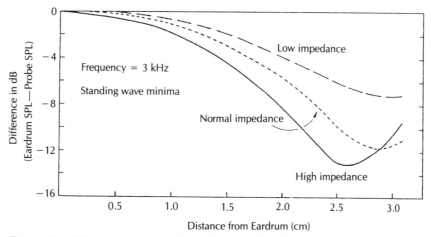

Figure 10. Difference between the eardrum and probe measured SPL at 3000 Hz for an average, low normal, and high normal impedance transmission line as a function of distance of the probe from the eardrum. (From Dirks and Kincaid 1987.)

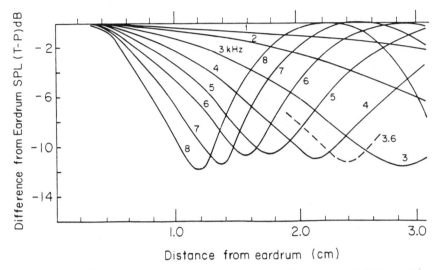

Figure 11. Difference between the eardrum and probe measured SPL at eight frequencies as a function of distance of the probe from the eardrum. (From Dirks and Kincaid 1987.)

should yield SPL measurements with an accuracy of within 2 dB through 6000 Hz. Second, it is important that the probe tube extend at least 5 mm past the tip of the canal portion of the earmold or ITE hearing aid. Burkhard and Sachs (1977) have shown that inaccuracies can occur in the higher frequencies if the probe tube is too close to the tip of the earmold. Third, the probe tube should be placed so that the client does not experience discomfort; this typically means not touching the tympanic membrane. Given these three considerations, there are a variety of methods for placement of the probe tube at an appropriate insertion depth in the ear canal. One method consists of several steps: (1) before inserting into the ear, place the probe tube next to the earmold or ITE and extend it at least 5 mm past the tip; (2) mark the probe tube (or place a collar) next to the outer edge of the earmold; (3) place the earmold and probe tube in the ear and determine an anatomical landmark where the mark or collar rests; (4) remove the hearing aid and earmold, replace the probe tube with the mark at the appropriate location, and measure the REUR; and (5) replace the earmold or ITE, being careful to keep the mark in the same location. Although this procedure works well, it can be time consuming and cumbersome.

An alternative method is to place the probe tube at a constant insertion depth past the ear canal opening, the tragus, or the intratragal notch. The length of the average adult ear canal is 25 mm (Zemplenyi, Gilman, and Dirks 1985). The typical distance from the ear canal opening to the tragus or intratragal notch is 10 mm, yielding a total distance

from this external location to the tympanic membrane of 35 mm. Hawkins, Alvarez, and Houlihan (1991) utilized an insertion depth of 30 mm past the tragus, resulting in a placement that should be 5 mm from the tympanic membrane in the average adult. This location produced a statement of discomfort in two of 25 subjects. A more conservative approach from the standpoint of avoiding touching the tympanic membrane would be to place the probe tube 25 to 27 mm past the tragus, resulting in a placement 8 to 10 mm from the tympanic membrane. Such a placement should yield absolute SPL measurements with an accuracy within 3 dB through 4000 Hz. This approach is appealing because it is quick, reproducible, and has been shown to yield reliable results (Hawkins, Alvarez, and Houlihan 1991).

A third alternative has been suggested by Sullivan (1988). Based upon the pressure maxima and minima principles described earlier and illustrated in figure 11, a 6000 Hz warble tone is introduced and the SPL is monitored as the probe tube is inserted slowly into the ear canal. When the lowest SPL reading is obtained, it is surmised that the distance from the tympanic membrane at that location should be between 13 and 16 mm, based upon the calculated pressure minima. The probe tube is marked at an external location for this insertion depth, 10 mm is added, and the probe tube is reinserted, thus yielding a predicted insertion depth of 23 to 26 mm, which according to Sullivan should be within 3 to 6 mm of the tympanic membrane.

Finally, several newer probe tube measurement

systems have incorporated procedures that make estimates of the probe tube distance from the tympanic membrane through acoustic measurements. Although the accuracy of such measurements has not been verified, this procedure represents a needed development, as it holds promise for a more accurate method of placement and replacement of the probe tube in the ear canal.

If the primary interest is measuring REIG and not absolute SPL in the ear canal, the exact location of the probe tube is not as important as the necessity for the probe tube to stay in the same location for both the REUR and REAR. Because the REIR is a difference value (REAR minus REUR), an error caused by probe tube placement can be tolerated if it is present in both measurements. Dirks and Kincaid (1987) have demonstrated this point by showing that although the REUR and the REAR are inaccurate at a 14 mm distance from the tympanic membrane location on a KEMAR, the REIR is identical to that measured at the eardrum location if the probe tube does not move.

In summary, for accurate SPL measurements in the higher frequencies, it is necessary to locate the probe tube at least 5 mm past the tip of the earmold or ITE and within 5 to 10 mm of the tympanic membrane. For accurate REIG measurements, the probe tube should stay in the same location for both the REUR and REAR. Because many applications of probe tube measurements may involve the assessment of both absolute SPLs and the REIR, the audiologist should try to satisfy both the depth and constant location criteria.

Signal Level Most commercial probe-tube microphone units are capable of delivering signals from the loudspeaker over a 50 to 90 dB SPL range. The appropriate signal level depends upon the purpose for the measurement. Making the easy assumption that SPL in the unaided ear canal increases linearly with intensity, the choice of signal level for the REUR is relatively unimportant. The level must, however, be high enough to be above the noise floor and low enough to prevent any loudness discomfort. Signal levels of 60 to 70 dB SPL are typically sufficient to meet both these criteria.

In contrast, the choice of signal level can be important for certain REAR and all REIR measurements. One important application of the REAR is assessment of the RESR. Because the purpose is to determine the maximum SPL that the hearing aid can deliver to the ear, it is important that the hearing aid be saturated during this measurement. In other words, the signal level must be sufficiently

high so that, when combined with the gain of the hearing aid, the maximum output is achieved. If the hearing aid volume control wheel is rotated to its maximum point before feedback, then an input level of 85 to 90 dB SPL typically will cause the hearing aid to saturate and an accurate measure of RESR can be obtained.

When measuring the REIR, a different situation exists. Ideally, typical input levels of 60 to 70 dB SPL would not saturate a well-fitted hearing aid. If saturation does occur, however, the gain of the hearing aid will be reduced. When making REIR measurements, the critical issue in the choice of level should probably be the selection of a typical input to the hearing aid. If this were the criterion, then a 65 to 70 dB SPL speech-weighted noise (which would have lower level per cycle values across frequency) or a 60 dB SPL swept warble tone would be most appropriate. The signal level, when combined with the gain of the hearing aid, should not saturate the hearing aid. As mentioned earlier, however, certain types of circuitry may need to be assessed at several different input levels to obtain an accurate picture of the overall functioning of the hearing aid.

An example of how the REIR can be affected by an inappropriately high signal level is shown in figure 12 from Hawkins and Mueller (1986). In this figure, the REIR is shown for a hearing aid with a relatively low SSPL90 when the input is both 60 and 80 dB SPL. Notice that the REIG is substantially greater with the 60 dB SPL input. If an attempt were being made to match certain target REIG values, the choice of input level in this case would be very im-

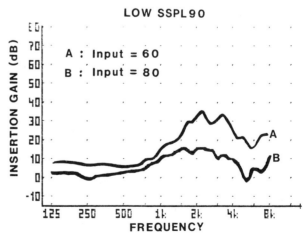

Figure 12. REIRs obtained with a hearing aid having a low SSPL90 for an input SPL that did not cause saturation (Curve A: 60 dB SPL) and an input SPL that did cause saturation (Curve B: 80 dB SPL). (From Hawkins and Mueller 1986.)

portant. The 80 dB SPL input would be too high and would result in an inappropriate conclusion. This problem of a high SPL input causing reduced and misleading REIG values will occur typically in a hearing aid with a lower SSPL90 combined with a moderate amount of gain. For several case studies on this issue, the reader is referred to Stelmacho-wicz and Lewis (1988).

One final aspect of the signal input level issue should be mentioned. If a complex signal is being employed, it is important to know the crest factor, which represents the number of decibels that the peak exceeds the rms level of the signal. If a high crest factor is present, as in a click, the peaks of the wave form can cause the hearing aid to saturate at a lower overall signal level (Frye 1987).

Clinical Applications of PTMs

Although numerous applications have been mentioned for PTMs, this discussion focuses on three major uses: adjusting or selecting hearing aids for (1) target RESR, (2) target REIR, and (3) target REAR for the long-term speech spectrum.

Adjusting for Target RESR   It is important that the maximum SPL the hearing aid can deliver to the person's ear does not exceed discomfort levels nor create additional hearing loss. SSPL90 values obtained in a 2-cm³ coupler typically underestimate the RESR, with the difference increasing in the higher frequencies. It is not uncommon for a hearing aid with a 2-cm³ coupler maximum SSPL90 of 120 dB SPL to generate over 130 dB SPL in a real ear canal. Given rather large variability in individual real ear 2-cm³ coupler differences, PTMs become an excellent means of setting the maximum output in the ear canal for a given person and hearing aid. In her chapter Stelmachowicz describes a method for determining the SPL present in the ear canal at the point of loudness discomfort and how the type of signal affects the measurement and its interpretation. If the SPL in the ear canal at LDL is known, then it is a rather simple and quick procedure to set the RESR of the hearing aid. The procedure is especially useful for children with whom accurate measures of loudness discomfort cannot be reliably obtained. The hearing aid can be adjusted to produce a RESR that is believed to be safe and comfortable.

Adjusting for Target REIR   Perhaps the most popular use of PTMs at this time is to assist in adjusting the hearing aid to match a target REIR. Under this approach, audiologists have typically decided to follow the recommendations of a published fre-

quency response selection procedure that prescribes a specific REIR for a given set of pure-tone thresholds. PTMs can be useful in two ways with this approach. First, a hearing aid must be selected that has a good chance of providing the desired REIR. Because hearing aid manufacturers can deal only in 2-cm³ coupler values, the desired REIR must be converted to a 2-cm³ coupler response. After the conversion, a BTE hearing aid can be selected from specification sheets or 2-cm³ coupler gain values can be communicated to the manufacturer for ordering an ITE. PTMs can be useful in deriving the 2-cm³ coupler response with the best likelihood of yielding the desired REIR. Although most prescription procedures provide average corrections to convert from the desired REIR to 2-cm³ coupler gain for the purposes of selecting a BTE or ordering an ITE, PTMs allow the audiologist to generate the correction factors for each individual, thus enhancing the chances that the selected or ordered coupler curve will produce the desired REIR. Mueller (1989) has described a procedure that corrects for the deviation of an individual's REUR from the average REUR assumed in selection procedures. This approach, although helpful, does not take into account the 2-cm³ coupler/real ear difference portion (Sachs and Burkhard 1972) of the correction factor. Punch, Chi, and Patterson (1990) described a more complete procedure in which a coupler response is determined through using the individual's REUR and calculating the 2-cm³ coupler/real ear difference by measuring the REAR and subtracting that from the coupler gain at the same volume control wheel setting. This procedure should assist the audiologist in determining a desired 2-cm³ coupler response that has a high probability of producing the REIR target. Such an approach should be particularly helpful with ITE hearing aid ordering.

A second use of PTMs is in the adjustment of the actual hearing aid to best match the target REIR. The volume control wheel, tone controls, and vent diameter can be altered to obtain an acceptable REIR. The measurements are not time consuming and the reliability can be good if care is taken in the measurements. Whether speech intelligibility is maximized once the targets have been achieved is a entirely different and speculative question.

Adjusting for a Target REAR for the Long-Term Speech Spectrum   The underlying assumption of several hearing aid prescription procedures is that the long-term speech spectrum should be amplified to a certain place within the residual auditory area (Cox 1983, 1985, 1988; Seewald and Ross 1988; Seewald, Ross, and Stelmachowicz 1987). If a speech spectrum input signal is available on the probe-tube instrument, it becomes a relatively easy procedure to adjust hearing aid parameters until target ear canal SPLs for the amplified speech spectrum are best achieved. Such a procedure has been described in the literature by Hawkins et al. (1989), Cox and Alexander (1990) and Stelmachowicz and Seewald (1991).

Test-Retest Reliability of PTMs

When consideration is given to the various procedural issues in PTMs, it is not surprising that some variability exists in the measurements. In discussing reliability, Tecca (1990) indicated that three types of test-retest variability should be considered when evaluating PTMs. The first is immediate test-retest variability. In this type, the probe tube is not removed from the ear, calibrations are not repeated, and the system is not turned off. Examples of measurements that would be evaluated in terms of immediate test-retest standards would be repetition of REIRs as the tone control is changed or repeated RESRs as the output control is altered. Although no data are presented, Tecca states that test-retest differences of greater than 2 dB should be considered significant.

A second type of variability is called short-term test-retest. In this case, the hearing aid is removed for some reason and the probe tube is reinserted. Several data sets are available that provide information on the variability of this type of measurement for REIG. Ringdahl and Leijon (1984) reported standard deviations of the test-retest differences that ranged from 1 dB at 250 Hz to 4.7 dB at 6000 Hz. Revit (1987) calculated similar values from Hawkins (1987) that ranged from 1.9 dB at 1000 Hz to 5.9 dB at 6000 Hz. Most recently, Hawkins, Alvarez, and Houlihan (1991) examined short-term test-retest variability for the REUR, REAR, and REIG. Their results indicated that the 95% confidence intervals for the REUR were ± 2 to 3 dB at 3000 Hz and below and ± 4 to 5 dB at 4000 and 5000 Hz. Confidence intervals for REAR and REIG were ± 2 to 3 dB below 1000 Hz, ± 3 dB in the 1000 to 2000 Hz region, and ± 4 to 6 dB at 3000 Hz and above.

The third type of variability mentioned by Tecca (1990) was long-term test-retest. One might predict that this type of variability might be slightly higher than those reported above for short term as a result of different calibration values, minor changes in middle ear pressure, and so forth.

There is no doubt that test-retest variability of probe-tube measurements can be quite good if care is taken. The major variable affecting the repeat-

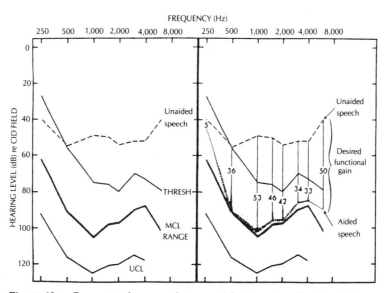

Figure 13. Conceptual approach to amplification described by Skinner et al. (1982). Left panel shows the unaided long-term speech spectrum, pure-tone thresholds, most comfortable loudness levels (MCL) and uncomfortable loudness levels (UCL). Right panel shows the desired result with amplification. The unaided long-term speech spectrum is amplified so that it is close the MCLs. The numbers represent the necessary real-ear gain to achieve this result. (From Skinner et al. 1982.)

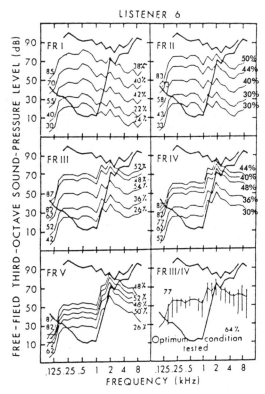

Figure 14. Results of different frequency response shaping on the word recognition ability of listener with a high-frequency sensorineural hearing loss. The solid lines represent thresholds and UCLs. The light lines indicate the 75th percentile levels of the words for the overall levels shown on the left. The word recognition scores associated with various input levels are shown on the right side of each light line. (From Skinner 1980.)

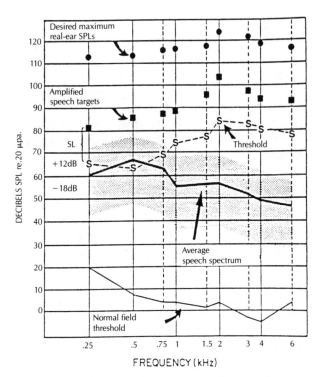

Figure 15. Schematic of the conceptual approach to amplification advocated by Seewald, Ross, and Stelmachowicz (1987). Targets values are adopted for the amplified long-term speech spectrum (solid boxes) and the desired RESR. All values are expressed in dB SPL. (From Seewald, Ross, and Stelmachowicz 1987.)

that are observed are probably a result of variability and not true differences between the measurements themselves.

Conceptual Approaches to Acoustic Performance Measures

Acoustic performance of a hearing aid can be expressed in several ways: output and/or gain in one of several types of couplers, functional gain or aided sound-field thresholds, and SPL and gain measured in the ear canal. Although 2-cm³ coupler measures are useful for communication purposes and ordering, they offer little in terms of selection, fitting, and evaluation of performance. The use of ear simulators and manikins represent a step in the right direction, but the mean simulation still requires corrections for the individual person.

Assessment of acoustic performance via aided sound-field thresholds or functional gain has attempted to bring a higher level of realism (Preves 1984) to the selection process. Although there are certain advantages to this approach, there are many

ability of these measurements is probably probe-tube location and the ability to retain it at that location. The audiologist should be most careful about this aspect of the procedure and attempt to develop a consistent and reliable method.

Relationship between Functional Gain and REIG

When probe-tube measurements first became popular, there was some skepticism expressed that insertion gain might not be the equivalent of functional gain. The argument was that the insertion gain measurement took place in the ear canal, whereas functional gain assessed the processed signal through to the central auditory system. Three studies, Mason and Popelka (1986), Dillon and Murray (1987) and Humes, Hipskind, and Block (1988) have addressed this issue by comparing insertion gain and functional gain on the same sets of subjects. The results are convincing that the two measurements are equivalent. The differences

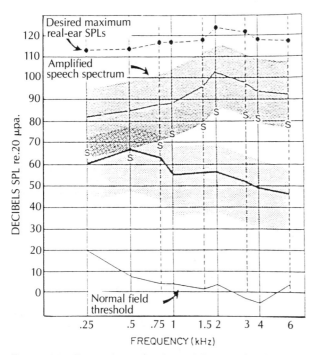

Figure 16. Desired result of amplification for the theoretical case shown in figure 15. The long-term speech spectrum has been amplified to the target values and placed within the person's residual auditory area. The hearing aid limits the real-ear output of the hearing aid at the line with solid dots. The peaks of the amplified speech spectrum do not saturate the hearing aid. (From Seewald, Ross, and Stelmachowicz 1987.)

potential disadvantages which were outlined earlier. Furthermore, if the aided thresholds are plotted on an audiogram, the implication is that the hearing aid has improved the hearing sensitivity of the individual. This common approach appears to be conceptually weak. The weakness was first made clear to me about 1980 by Gerald Popelka, and this understanding has helped enormously in thinking about what a hearing aid can do and perhaps should do. An alternative is to show the input speech spectrum amplified into the residual dynamic range above fixed auditory thresholds. This approach is most clearly seen now in the work of Skinner and colleagues (Skinner et al. 1982; Skinner 1988) and Seewald and colleagues (Seewald, Ross, and Stelmachowicz 1987; Seewald and Ross 1988). For instance, figure 13 shows an approach of Skinner et al. (1982) as described in the first *Vanderbilt Hearing-Aid Report*. The left panel shows the unaided situation. Speech spectrum information is audible only below 500 Hz. The right panel shows the desired result. The speech spectrum has been amplified by the amount of gain indicated by the numbers and placed near the most comfortable loudness

(MCL) curve. The thresholds have remained constant, but now the amplified speech spectrum is above threshold.

Skinner (1980) also has plotted such results in dB SPL, an approach that has even more appeal. Figure 14 shows how useful this approach can be in understanding the concept of the residual dynamic range and how performance changes as a result of the input level and the resulting audible information. The solid lines represent the thresholds and loudness discomfort levels. The six panels show results for different frequency response shapes, the lighter lines showing the amplified speech spectrum for various overall input levels. Notice that in this case the dynamic range above 3,000 Hz is so narrow as to be essentially nonfunctional.

Figure 15 shows a similar approach from Seewald, Ross, and Stelmachowicz (1987). Thresholds (S--S) are plotted in dB SPL and indicate that little speech spectrum information is audible without a hearing aid. The solid boxes represent target levels for the amplified speech spectrum, and the solid circles represent the desired RESR. Goals are thus established for the gain and SSPL90 and the entire residual auditory area is determined. Figure 16 shows the desired result according to Seewald, Ross, and Stelmachowicz. The amplified speech spectrum has been amplified above the impaired thresholds to prescribed levels and does not saturate the hearing aid.

Although approaches such as these do not tell us about speech intelligibility per se or sound quality, they are very informative and represent an enlightened approach to selecting and evaluating acoustic performance of hearing aids. Such an approach, in combination with PTMs, represents a step forward in assessing the acoustic performance of amplification.

References

American National Standards Institute. 1985. Methods of measurement of performance characteristics of hearing aids under simulated *in-situ* working conditions. ANSI S3.35–1985. New York: American National Standards Institute, Inc.

Burkhard, M., and Sachs, R. 1977. Sound pressure in insert earphone couplers and real ears. *Journal of Speech and Hearing Research* 20:799–807.

Cox, R. 1983. Using ULCL measures to find frequency-gain and SSPL90. *Hearing Instruments* 34:17–21, 39.

Cox, R. 1985. A structured approach to hearing aid selection. *Ear and Hearing* 6:226–39.

Cox, R. 1988. The MSU hearing instrument prescription procedure. *Hearing Instruments* 39:6–10.

Cox, R., and Alexander, G. 1990. Evaluation of an in-situ output probe-microphone method for hearing aid fitting verification. *Ear and Hearing* 11:31–39.

Dillon, H., and Murray, N. 1987. Accuracy of twelve methods for estimating the real ear gain of hearing aids. *Ear and Hearing* 8:2–11.

Dirks, D., and Kincaid, G. 1987. Basic acoustic considerations of ear canal probe measurements. *Ear and Hearing* 8(No. 5 Supplement):60S–67S.

Feigin, J., Nelson Barlow, N., and Stelmachowicz, P. 1990. The effect of reference microphone placement on sound-pressure levels at an ear-level hearing aid microphone. *Ear and Hearing* 11:321–26.

Frye, G. 1987. Crest factor and composite signals for hearing aid testing. *The Hearing Journal* 15–18.

Hawkins, D. 1987. Variability in clinical ear canal probe microphone measurements. *Hearing Instruments* 38:30–32.

Hawkins, D., and Mueller, H. 1986. Some variables affecting the accuracy of probe tube microphone measurements. *Hearing Instruments* 37:8–12, 49.

Hawkins, D., Alvarez, E., and Houlihan, J. 1991. Reliability of three types of probe tube microphone measurements. *Hearing Instruments* 42:14–16.

Hawkins, D., Montgomery, A., Prosek, R., and Walden, B. 1987. Examination of two issues concerning functional gain measurements. *Journal Speech and Hearing Disorders* 52:56–63.

Hawkins, D., Morrison, T., Halligan, P., and Cooper, W. 1989. Use of probe tube measurements in hearing aid selection for children: Some initial clinical experiences. *Ear and Hearing* 10:281–87.

Humes, L., and Kirn, E. 1990. The reliability of functional gain. *Journal Speech and Hearing Disorders* 55:193–97.

Humes, L., Hipskind, N., and Block, M. 1988. Insertion gain measured with three probe tube systems. *Ear and Hearing* 9:108–112.

Ickes, M., Hawkins, D., and Cooper, W. 1991. Reference microphone location and loudspeaker azimuth effects on probe tube microphone measurements. *Journal of the American Academy of Audiology.*

Killion, M. 1988. An "Acoustically invisible" hearing aid. *Hearing Instruments* 39(10):40–44.

Killion, M. 1990. A high fidelity hearing aid. *Hearing Instruments* 41(8):38–39.

Killion, M., and Revit, L. 1987. Insertion gain repeatability versus loudspeaker location: You want me to put my loudspeaker W H E R E? *Ear and Hearing* 8(No. 5 Supplement): 68S–73S.

LeBel, C. 1944. Pressure and field response of the ear in hearing aid performance determination. *Journal of Acoustical Society of America* 16(1):63–67.

Macrae, J. 1982. Invalid aided thresholds. *Hearing Instruments* 33:21–22.

Macrae, J., and Frazer, G. 1980. An investigation of variables affecting aided thresholds. *Australian Journal of Audiology* 2:56–62.

Mason, D., and Popelka, G. 1986. Comparison of hearing-aid gain using functional coupler, and probe-tube measurements. *Journal of Speech and Hearing Research* 29:218–26.

Mueller, H. 1989. Individualizing the ordering of custom hearing instruments. *Hearing Instruments* 40:18–22.

Pascoe, D. 1975. Frequency responses of hearing aids and their effects on the speech perception of hearing-impaired subjects. *Annals of Otology, Rhinology and Laryngology* 84(Supplement 23):1–40.

Preves, D. 1984. Levels of realism in hearing aid measurement techniques. *The Hearing Journal* 13–19.

Preves, D. 1987. Some issues in utilizing probe tube microphone systems. *Ear and Hearing* 8(No. 5 Supplement):82S–88S.

Preves, D., and Sullivan, R. 1987. Sound field equalization for real ear measurements with probe microphones. *Hearing Instruments* 38:20–26, 64.

Preves, D., Beck, L., Burnett, E., and Teder, H. 1989. Input stimuli for obtaining frequency responses of automatic gain control hearing aids. *Journal of Speech and Hearing Research* 32:189–94.

Punch, J., Chi, C., and Patterson, J. 1990. A recommended protocol for prescriptive use of target gain rules. *Hearing Instruments* 41(4):12–19.

Revit, L. 1987. New loudspeaker locations for improved reliability in clinical measures of the insertion gain of hearing aids. MA thesis, Northwestern University, Evanston, IL.

Ringdahl, A., and Leijon, A. 1984. The reliability of insertion gain measurements using probe microphones in the ear canal. *Scandinavian Audiology* 13:173–78.

Sachs, R., and Burkhard, M. 1972. Earphone pressure response in ear and couplers. *Journal of the Acoustical Society of America* 52:183(A).

Schweitzer, H., Sullivan, R., Beck, L., and Cole, W. 1990. Developing a consensus for "real ear" hearing instrument terms. *Hearing Journal* 41(2):28, 46.

Seewald, R., and Ross, M. 1988. Amplification for young hearing-impaired children. In *Amplification for the Hearing-Impaired*, ed. M. Pollack. Orlando, FL: Grune & Stratton.

Seewald, R., Ross, M., and Stelmachowicz, P. 1987. Selecting and verifying hearing aid performance characteristics for children. *Journal of the Academy of Rehabilitative Audiology* 20:25–37.

Shaw, E. 1974. Transformation of sound pressure from the free field to the eardrum in the horizontal plane. *Journal of the Acoustical Society of America* 56:1848–1861.

Skinner, M. 1980. Speech intelligibility in noise-induced hearing loss: Effects of high-frequency compensation. *Journal of the Acoustical Society of America* 67(1):306–317.

Skinner, M. 1988. *Hearing Aid Evaluation.* Englewood Cliffs, NJ: Prentice Hall.

Skinner, M., Pascoe, D., Miller, J., and Popelka, G. 1982. Measurements to determine the optimal placement of speech energy within the listener's auditory area: A basis for selecting amplification characteristics. In *The Vanderbilt Hearing-Aid Report: State of the Art-Research Needs*, eds. G. Studebaker and F. Bess. Upper Darby, PA: Monographs in Contemporary Audiology.

Stelmachowicz, P., and Lewis, D. 1988. Some theoretical considerations concerning the relation between functional gain and insertion gain. *Journal of Speech and Hearing Research* 31:491–96.

Stelmachowicz, P., and Seewald, R. 1991. Probe-tube microphone measures in children. *Seminars in Hearing.*

Sullivan, R. 1988. Probe tube microphone placement near the tympanic membrane. *Hearing Instruments* 39:43–44, 60.

Tecca, J. 1990. Clinical application of real-ear probe tube

measurement. In *Handbook of Hearing Aid Amplification, Volume II: Clinical Considerations & Fitting Practices*, ed. R. Sandlin. Boston, MA: College-Hill Press.

Zemplenyi, J., Gilman, S., and Dirks, D. 1985. Optical method for measurement of ear canal length. *Journal of Acoustical Society of America* 78(4):2146–2148.

CHAPTER 11

Clinical Issues Related to Hearing Aid Maximum Output

Patricia G. Stelmachowicz

In his chapter Hawkins provides an overview of both functional gain and probe-tube microphone measures of hearing aid performance. He reviews some of the variables that affect real-ear measures and discusses the clinical utility of these measures. The following discussion addresses two topics introduced briefly by Dr. Hawkins. Initially, this chapter focuses on the issue of stimulus type, particularly in the measurement of hearing aid maximum output. Then, the use of probe-tube microphone measures to estimate real-ear loudness discomfort levels (LDLs) will be discussed.

Stimulus Issues

As mentioned by Hawkins in his chapter, the currently available clinical probe-tube microphone systems employ a wide variety of signals including pure tones, warble tones, narrowband noise, clicks, broadband noise, speech-shaped noise, and multitonal complexes. Most systems offer more than one signal option and the rationale associated with each option differs considerably. Because pure-tone signals traditionally have been used to specify hearing aid performance both behaviorally and electroacoustically, they provide a link with both manufacturer's specifications and past clinical experience. Warble tones, narrow-band noise, and clicks have been used to minimize the effects of standing-wave patterns when signals are presented in the soundfield. Broadband noise, speech-shaped noise, and multitonal complexes have been used under the assumption that they provide an input that more closely approximates that encountered in daily life. In addition, the use of complex signals may be less time consuming, may be more appropriate than pure-tone signals for the measurement of certain

types of nonlinear hearing aids, and may be useful in the measurement of higher-order distortion products. While all of these rationales may be reasonable, it is important to understand that these signals may not always produce equivalent results when estimating hearing aid characteristics. Under certain circumstances one type of signal may be preferable to another. The following discussion addresses stimulus effects first in terms of hearing aid gain, measured with relatively low-level signals, and then in terms of maximum output, measured with high-level signals.

Frequency-Gain Characteristics

In general, the estimated frequency-gain characteristics of a hearing aid will be similar regardless of the signal used, provided the measurements are made within the linear operating range of the instrument (Frye 1987; Stelmachowicz et al. 1990). If the hearing aid is operating in saturation or if it is a nonlinear instrument, then differences will occur in the estimated frequency-gain characteristics with different signal types. Figure 1 illustrates the 2-cm³ coupler gain of a high-gain behind-the-ear hearing aid when the input was either a swept pure tone or a speech-shaped multitonal complex. In this example, only minor differences are apparent between the two responses. In clinical practice, this relatively close agreement appears to occur for a linear instrument as long as the input level of the complex signal is low. If the input level is higher or if impulsive signals with high-crest factors are used, the hearing aid may be driven into saturation by the complex signal but not by the pure tone. In this situation, the two signal types will produce different estimates of gain. An example of this is shown in figure 2. The dashed line, representing gain with a swept pure-tone input, is replotted from figure 1. The rms level of the complex signal has been increased to 70 dB SPL. Thus, the levels in figure 1 closely approximate

This work was supported in part by NIH.

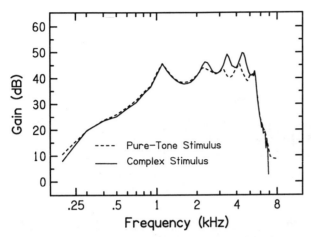

Figure 1.   Gain as a function of frequency for a high-gain hearing aid (Phonak Audinet C-D™; Tone = L; SSPL = 108; volume = 3½). The dashed line depicts gain measured with a 60 dB SPL pure-tone input and the solid shows the gain measured with a 60 dB SPL speech-shaped complex.

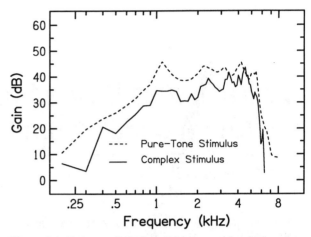

Figure 2.   Gain as a function of frequency for the hearing aid in figure 1. The dashed line shows gain with a 60 dB SPL pure-tone input. The rms level of the complex stimulus (solid line) has been raised to 70 dB SPL.

the ⅓-octave band levels of average speech. In the pure-tone case, the high-frequency average gain is 41 dB, whereas it is only 34 dB using the higher level complex input. This situation will occur most often for hearing aids adjusted to saturate at a relatively low level.

Under some circumstances, the use of complex signals may be more appropriate than pure-tone signals. A number of investigators have suggested that pure-tone signals will provide an erroneous estimate of low-frequency gain for instruments with automatic gain control (AGC) or other nonlinear signal processing capabilities (Kinghorn 1976; Preves et al. 1989; Studebaker 1979). This effect occurs because a swept pure-tone may activate the AGC circuit at some frequencies but not at others. The use of a broadband signal will minimize this measurement artifact. Thus, it appears that the choice of stimuli for measures of hearing aid gain may depend upon hearing aid characteristics, signal characteristics, and the question to be answered.

Maximum Output

Thus far, we have restricted the discussion to the case of relatively low-level input signals. For many reasons, it is important to consider how a hearing aid functions in response to high-level inputs. If the maximum output of a hearing aid is set too high, hearing aid rejection, and/or potential damage to the auditory system may occur. If the incoming signal level plus gain produce SPLs that are allowed to exceed the user's loudness discomfort levels

(LDLs), changes in the volume control setting will not alleviate the problem. For most instruments, reducing the gain by lowering the volume control setting will not reduce the maximum output. If the input signal is intense enough, the maximum output will be reached, even if the hearing aid gain is minimal. Even in hearing aid systems where the gain and maximum output co-vary with volume control changes, reducing the gain to avoid loudness discomfort is not the method of choice because it affects the audibility of lower-level signals adversely. Thus, careful selection of maximum output is imperative to a successful hearing aid fitting.

To illustrate the effect of signal type on the maximum output of a hearing aid, a broadband, high-gain hearing aid (Phonak Audinet PPC-L™) is used. In figure 3, the 2-cm³ coupler maximum output of this hearing aid is compared for two different signal types. The dashed line represents the SSPL90 curve using a swept pure tone as the input signal. The solid line represents the output when the input was a speech-shaped multitonal complex with components spaced at 100 Hz intervals. The rms level of this complex was 89 dB SPL and it was empirically verified that the hearing aid was in saturation. Note that there is a 15 to 20 dB difference in measured maximum output using these two stimulus types. The irregularities observed when using a complex signal are caused by higher order distortion products that only can be observed when the hearing aid is required to process more than one signal simultaneously, which is the typical situation for speech inputs and other common environmental signals. When swept pure tones are used, only one signal is processed by the hearing aid at

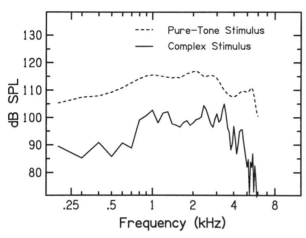

Figure 3. Maximum output (in dB SPL) as a function of frequency for a 90 dB SPL swept pure tone (dashed line) and a speech-shaped complex with an rms level of 89 dB SPL (solid line) for a high-gain hearing aid (Phonak Audinet PPC-L™: L1; 125; volume = 3).

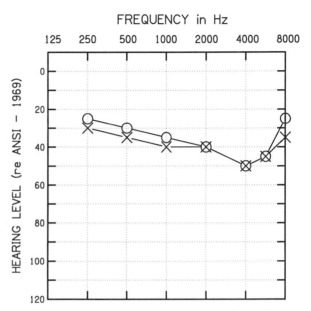

Figure 4. Pure-tone air conduction thresholds from a six-year-old boy with a mild-to-moderate sensorineural hearing loss. The Os and Xs represent the right and left ears, respectively.

any given point in time. It is worth noting that the differences seen here occur because output is being measured at each frequency individually. When using a complex signal, the maximum output at any one frequency will be lower than that obtained with a pure-tone stimulus, but the *overall rms output* should agree well with the high-frequency average SSPL90 defined with a pure-tone input. In this case, the rms level for the complex stimulus was 113.3 dB compared to a high-frequency average SSPL90 of 116.0 dB SPL with a pure-tone input. It should be obvious from this figure that the clinical decisions regarding desired maximum output would differ considerably if a complex signal rather than pure-tone signals were used to characterize output as a function of frequency.

An example from our clinical caseload may help to illustrate this point. Figure 4 depicts the pure-tone air conduction audiogram of a six-year-old boy with a mild-to-moderate sensorineural hearing loss. The child had an older sibling with a more severe hearing loss that may have been progressive in nature. The child was seen at our facility with concerns for possible progression of his hearing loss and reports of loudness discomfort. His parents reported that he has repeatedly complained of amplified sounds being too loud and recall at least one instance where he appeared to suffer increased hearing loss after a day's usage of the hearing aid coupled to his FM system. The child had been followed audiologically and was fitted with relatively high-gain binaural behind-the-ear (BTE) hearing aids. In the classroom, he utilizes an auditory trainer coupled to his personal hearing aid. In

our facility, probe-tube microphone measures (Fonix 6500™) of gain and output were obtained using a swept pure-tone input. The real-ear insertion response (REIR) and the real-ear saturation response (RESR) at the recommended use settings of the hearing aid fitted to his left ear are shown in the top and bottom panels of figure 5. Note that while the REIR is not excessive, the peak maximum output is 123 dB SPL at 2000 Hz. Recall that this child has a 40 dB HL auditory threshold at 2000 Hz. The corresponding 2-cm^3 coupler maximum output was 119 dB SPL; thus, this does not represent a case of unusually large real-ear-to-coupler differences. Given the degree of hearing loss and the complaints of loudness discomfort, we considered this output excessive. From the available audiological records, it appears that real-ear measures were performed at the center where the hearing aids were obtained. According to those records, the probe-tube microphone system used a speech-shaped complex signal with components spaced at 250 Hz intervals. As shown previously, this type of signal will underestimate maximum output for different signal types. On the basis of real-ear measures using this signal, the written report stated that "the hearing aid should cause him no discomfort." If a swept pure-tone input had been used, it is likely that a different conclusion would have been drawn from the real-ear measures. One could argue that we do not listen to pure-tone signals and thus, the use of a speech-shaped complex may be more indicative of real-life

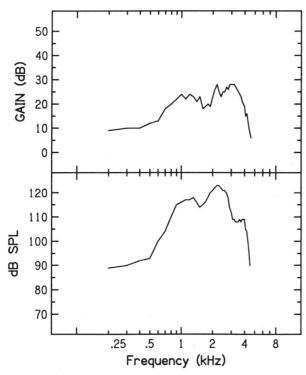

Figure 5. Top panel illustrates real-ear insertion response (REIR) as a function of frequency. Lower panel depicts the real-ear saturation response (RESR) as measured with a 90 dB swept pure-tone signal.

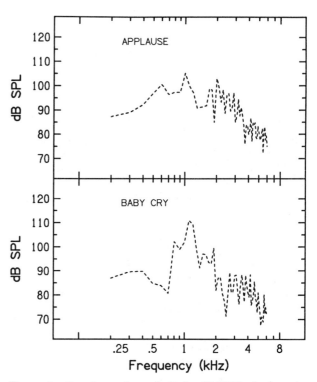

Figure 6. 2-cm³ coupler output (in dB SPL) of a broadband hearing aid (Phonak Audinet PPC-L™) in response to applause (top panel) and a baby cry (lower panel).

situations. Alternatively, while we do listen to a wide variety of complex signals, we rarely listen to the *long-term* speech spectrum.

In order to gain a better understanding of how complex signals are processed by a hearing aid operating in saturation, a series of measurements were made with a variety of complex input signals. The stimuli used were a range of environmental signals either prerecorded on compact disc or digitized speech samples stored on computer (PDP 11/23). Signals were amplified and routed to a hearing aid test chamber (Fonix 6500™). The broadband hearing aid at the settings described in the legend of figure 3 were used for all measures. An FFT with an integration time of 10 ms was used to generate the spectra shown in figures 6 through 8. In all cases, it was empirically verified that the hearing aid was in saturation. The top panel in figure 6 illustrates the saturated maximum output in response to applause. In this case, the peak output is 105 dB SPL, considerably lower than the 117 dB SPL seen with a pure-tone input. Thus, with this type of relatively broadband input, the output is similar to that obtained with a speech-shaped complex. The lower panel depicts the saturated output in response to a baby cry. Here, the spectrum is considerably nar-

rower and the peak output is 112 dB SPL. Figure 7 illustrates similar measures for a telephone ring and a hairdryer. In both cases, the maximum output approaches that observed in the pure-tone case in the frequency region of highest energy. Figure 8 illustrates the saturated output in response to two digitized speech samples. The top panel depicts the response to the vowel /u/ which has a rather broad spectrum. The peak output is 105 dB SPL, which lies between the output as measured with pure-tone and complex signals. The lower panel represents the /ʃ/ portion of the utterance /uʃ/. Here, the energy is high-frequency in nature and the output peaks at 112 dB SPL. In all of these cases, the rms output ranged from 112 to 116 dB SPL. It is apparent from these examples that maximum output as defined by pure-tone and broadband inputs represent two extremes. These results suggest that, although broadband signals will produce lower maximum output on a frequency by frequency basis, spectrally narrower signals will produce outputs that approach those observed with pure-tone signals. In the case of the child with the high-gain hearing aid, setting the maximum output with a broadband input resulted in loudness discomfort. Clearly, the most conservative approach to setting maximum output would be to obtain LDLs using pure-tone

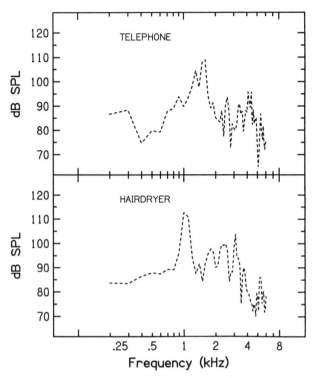

Figure 7. Similar to figure 6, hearing aid output in response to a telephone ringing (top panel) and a hairdryer (lower panel).

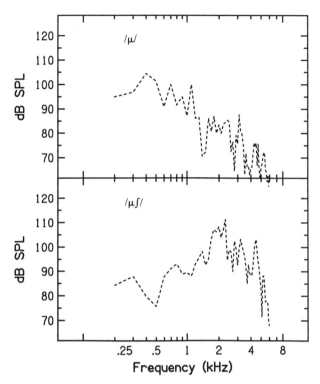

Figure 8. Similar to figure 6, hearing aid output in response to the phoneme /μ/ (top panel) and the /ʃ/ portion of the utterance /μʃ/ (lower panel).

stimuli and to set the maximum output using the same signals. Using this approach will ensure that no incoming signals, regardless of spectral content, will result in loudness discomfort.

Real-Ear Measures of LDLs

The remainder of this chapter describes the methodology used to obtain real-ear LDLs as a function of frequency. Although this approach was suggested first by Erber in 1973, the technology to implement it clinically was not yet available. At present, many clinical probe-tube microphone systems allow direct measures of ear-canal SPL for either internally or externally generated signals. These systems can be used to measure the SPL in the ear canal at the loudness discomfort threshold for each test frequency. The primary advantage of this approach is that these values can be directly compared to the real-ear saturated output of a hearing aid. When LDLs are obtained using supra-aural earphones, insert earphones, or with a precalibrated hearing aid or hearing-aid receiver (Cox 1983; Dillon, Chew, and Deans 1984; Hawkins 1980; Hawkins et al. 1987), the sound pressure reference is usually a

2-cm³ or 6-cm³ coupler. It is well known that these couplers do not estimate accurately the SPL in the ear canal. Transforms can be applied to account for the *average* coupler-to-real-ear differences as a function of frequency, but large individual differences will still exist. The use of probe-tube microphone measures for this purpose eliminates the errors associated with transducer differences and data transformation based on average values. Furthermore, previous investigators have shown good test-retest reliability of LDLs as measured with a probe-tube microphone system (Gagne et al. 1989; Zelisko et al. 1990).

From a practical standpoint, there are a number of ways in which these measures can be obtained. It is outside the scope of this paper to review various psychophysical methods for the measurement of LDLs. Numerous investigators have proposed instructional sets and procedures both for adults (Morgan and Dirks 1974; Cox 1981; Hawkins et al. 1987) and for children (Kawell, Kopun, and Stelmachowicz 1988; Gagne et al. 1989; Zelisko et al. 1990) and any of these can be used in conjunction with probe-tube microphone measures. Here, we focus primarily on issues related to the sound delivery system and the measurement of the associated SPL in the ear canal. We take a conservative approach, consistent with the previous discussion, using frequency-specific signals only.

The first point involves the issue of probe-tube placement. When measuring insertion gain, it is assumed that the exact location of the probe tube within the ear canal is not crucial as long as the tube remains in the same place for the measurement of the unaided and the aided responses. Because gain is a relative measure, it does not matter that the SPL measured at a given point in the ear canal is not equivalent to the SPL at the tympanic membrane. For LDL measures, however, we are concerned with *absolute measures* of SPL rather than *gain* and probe-tube placement becomes more critical. From the model of Gilman and Dirks (1986), it is clear that the SPL measured at a remote point in the ear canal can deviate substantially from that developed at the tympanic membrane. Based upon their work and estimates of average ear canal length (Shaw 1980; Zemplenyi, Gilman, and Dirks 1985; Kruger 1987; Kruger and Ruben 1987), an insertion depth of approximately 15 mm from the ear canal entrance in children under five years of age and 20 mm for older children and adults should provide reasonably accurate predictions of the SPL at the tympanic membrane. At these insertion depths, probe-tube measures should agree with eardrum SPLs within +2 dB for frequencies up to 4,000 Hz.

Crucial to this discussion is the fact that, at any given frequency, the SPL in the ear canal at any criterion-based reference (auditory threshold, MCL, or LDL) should be constant regardless of how the signal is introduced to the ear (Killion 1978). While it may take a greater voltage to drive a given sound-delivery system compared to another, the SPL at the tympanic membrane required to obtain the same behavioral response should be the same in both cases. As such, LDLs can be obtained with signals transduced using any of the methods shown in table I. Because the SPL is being measured directly in the ear canal, it is not essential for the stimulus delivery system to be calibrated to any particular reference. Of these methods, soundfield presentation via a loudspeaker is probably the least desirable. Factors such as standing wave patterns, limited output, and measurement variability with

head movement introduce problems that are not inherent with other methods. Although supra-aural earphones should yield more reliable results than soundfield measurements, the configuration of some probe-tube microphone assemblies may interfere with proper placement of the earphone cushion. In addition, because earphones are calibrated in a 6-cm^3 coupler, direct comparison to hearing aid specification data is not possible.

The three remaining stimulus delivery methods have distinct advantages over the two discussed thus far. All three systems can be referenced to a 2-cm^3 coupler, allowing for quick calculation of coupler-to-real-ear differences when necessary.[1] Additionally, any type of earmold can be used, because the SPL in the ear canal at the loudness discomfort threshold should not vary with the coupling method. Unfortunately, the maximum output of the most widely used insert earphone (e.g., Etymotic ER-3A™), is limited to below 120 dB SPL (as measured in a Zwislocki coupler), and thus cannot be used on individuals whose LDLs exceed this level. Button type hearing aid receivers or broadband, high-gain BTE hearing aids usually will provide a higher maximum output. In the latter case, signals should be introduced via direct audio input to avoid the problems inherent in soundfield presentation of signals.

If the particular probe-tube microphone system being used does not allow for gated presentation of frequency-specific signals in small enough intensity increments (e.g., 2 dB), an external sound generation system may be needed. In our clinic, a portable audiometer is used for this purpose. The output of the audiometer is coupled to a high-gain hearing aid with direct audio input capabilities.[2] Signal output from the probe-tube microphone system should be disabled, and the loudspeaker should be disconnected in systems where the reference microphone is in an active feedback loop. If the system makes frequency-by-frequency probe-tube corrections or employs a tracking filter, it may be necessary to change frequency in the probe-tube system manually to correspond with the test frequency. After an LDL is established (using any method), the

Table I. Stimulus Delivery Systems Used to Measure Loudness Discomfort Levels

Loudspeaker
Supra-aural earphone (e.g., TDH-39, TDH-49)
Insert earphone (e.g., Etymotic ER-3A™)
Button-type hearing-aid receiver
Hearing aid (direct audio input)

[1]Cox (1981) has cautioned that 2-cm^3 coupler-to-real-ear differences will depend upon the source impedance of the receiver. As such, the acoustic impedance of the receiver used during LDL measurements should be the same as that in the hearing aid if accurate coupler measures are needed. Dillon, Chew, and Deans (1984) have suggested using a high-impedance miniature receiver (Knowles, CI-2955™) mounted in a hearing aid case.

[2]Depending upon the impedance of the hearing aid, an impedance-matching device may be needed at the audiometer output.

probe-tube microphone can be used to measure the corresponding SPL in the ear canal. As recommended by Zelisko et al. (1990), 5 dB of attenuation can be introduced before presenting a steady-state signal for measurement purposes in order to avoid loudness discomfort. This 5 dB will need to be added to the measured value at each frequency. To a first approximation, these real-ear SPLs represent the maximum tolerable RESR levels with any hearing aid. Figure 9 illustrates how these values can be used to adjust the maximum output of a hearing aid to an appropriate level. The asterisks represent the real-ear SPLs at LDL as a function of frequency. In this case, the RESR was adjusted to occur at or below these values.

Clinical Measures of RESR

At present, the measurement of real-ear SSPL90 or RESR values seems to be a controversial issue. Sullivan (1987) has suggested that the direct measurement of this response in an aided real ear increases "the likelihood of emotional and acoustic trauma to the patient, resulting in economic trauma to the dispenser" (p. 36). He suggests an alternative approach that entails computation of 2-cm³ coupler-to-real-ear differences for a low-level (60 dB SPL) signal. This transfer function is then added to the 2-cm³ coupler SSPL90 curve to estimate the RESR. This indirect method can be time consuming and does not include the acoustic effects of various earmold configurations. The concern that direct RESR measures using high-level input increase discomfort to the hearing aid user and/or create a liability situation is unwarranted. If the LDLs as a function of frequency

are known and the hearing aid is set appropriately, the loudness discomfort threshold should not be reached regardless of the stimulus input level. The setting of hearing aid maximum output should be approached conservatively. That is, the maximum output should be increased gradually until the RESR approaches the LDL values. When swept pure-tone signals are used, the actual exposure time to high SPLs is extremely short at any given frequency and is well within published guidelines for risk from noise exposure (Kryter et al. 1966). Clinically, the goal should be to ensure that the RESR does not exceed the user's LDLs and does not exceed some predetermined levels that may pose a risk to residual hearing. The most valid method for attaining this goal is to make direct measures of the RESR at the time of the hearing aid fitting.

Summary

In summary, it is unrealistic to expect any one type of input signal to predict hearing aid performance under all listening conditions. For measures of hearing aid gain, the choice of signal type will depend upon both hearing aid characteristics and the question to be answered. For measures of hearing aid maximum output, the use of pure-tone signals is the most conservative approach. Probe-tube microphone estimates of ear canal SPL at loudness discomfort threshold then can be used to set the RESR to appropriate levels as a function of frequency.

References

Cox, R.M. 1983. Using ULCL measures to find frequency/gain and SSPL90. *Hearing Instruments* 34:17–21, 39.

Cox, R.M. 1981. Using LDLs to establish hearing-aid limiting levels. *Hearing Instruments* 32:16, 18, 20.

Dillon, H., Chew, R., and Deans, M. 1984. Loudness discomfort level measurements and their implications for the design and fitting of hearing aids. *Australian Journal of Audiology* 6:73–79.

Erber, N. 1973. Body-baffle and real-ear effects in the selection of hearing aids for deaf children. *Journal Speech and Hearing Disorders* 38:224–31.

Frye, G. 1987. Crest factor and composite signals for hearing aid testing. *Hearing Journal* 40:15–18.

Gagne, J.-P., Seewald, R., Zelisko, D., and Hudson, S. 1989. Procedure for defining the auditory area of hearing-impaired children. *ASHA* 31:151(A).

Gilman, S., and Dirks, D. 1986. Acoustics of ear canal measurement of eardrum SPL in simulators. *Journal of the Acoustical Society of America* 80:783–93.

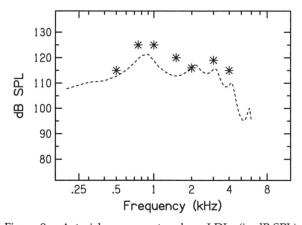

Figure 9. Asterisks represent real-ear LDLs (in dB SPL) as a function of frequency. The dashed line represents RESR of a high-gain hearing aid, adjusted not to exceed the LDLs.

Hawkins, D. 1980. Loudness discomfort levels: A clinical procedure for hearing aid evaluations. *Journal of Speech and Hearing Disorders* 45:3–15.

Hawkins, D., Walden, B., Montgomery, A., and Prosek, R. 1987. Description and validation of an LDL procedure designed to select SSPL90. *Ear and Hearing* 8:162–69.

Kawell, M., Kopun, J., and Stelmachowicz, P. 1988. Loudness discomfort levels in children. *Ear and Hearing* 9:133–36.

Killion, M.C. 1978. Revised estimate of minimal audible pressure: "Where is the missing 6 dB?" *Journal of the Acoustical Society of America* 63:1501–1508.

Kinghorn, W. 1976. Linear and nonlinear systems. Are some new evaluation procedures for hearing aids needed? *Hearing Instruments* 27:15.

Kruger, B. 1987. An update on the external ear resonance in infants and young children. *Ear and Hearing* 8:333–36.

Kruger, B., and Ruben, R. 1987. The acoustic properties of the infant ear. *Acta Otolaryngologica (Stockholm)* 103:578–85.

Kryter, K.D., Ward, W.D., Miller, J.D., and Eldredge, D.H. 1966. Hazardous exposure to intermittent and steady-state noise. *Journal of the Acoustical Society of America* 39:451–64.

Morgan, D.E., and Dirks, D.D. 1974. Loudness discomfort level under earphone and in the free field: The effect of calibration methods. *Journal of the Acoustical Society of America* 56:172–78.

Preves, D.A., Beck, L.B., Burnett, E.D., and Teder, H. 1989. Input stimuli for obtaining frequency responses of automatic gain control hearing aids. *Journal of Speech and Hearing Research* 32:189–94.

Shaw, E.G. 1980. Acoustics of the external ear. In *Acoustical Factors Affecting Hearing Aid Performance*, eds. G. Studebaker and I. Hochberg. Baltimore: University Park Press.

Stelmachowicz, P.G., Lewis, D.E., Seewald, R., and Hawkins, D. 1990. Complex and pure-tone signals in the evaluation of hearing-aid characteristics. *Journal of Speech and Hearing Research* 33:380–85.

Studebaker, G. 1979. Utilization of real-time spectral analyzers for the electroacoustical evaluation of hearing aids. In *Auditory and Hearing Prosthetics Research*, eds. V. Larson, D. Egolf, R. Kirlin, and S. Stile. New York: Grune and Stratton.

Sullivan, R.F. 1987. Aided SSPL 90 response in the real ear: A safe estimate. *Hearing Instruments* 38:(10)36.

Zelisko, D., Seewald, R., Gagne, J.-P., and Hudson, S. 1990. Evaluation of a procedure for measuring loudness discomfort levels in children. Paper presented at the 15th Annual Conference of the Canadian Association of Speech-Language Pathologists and Audiologists, Vancouver, British Columbia, Canada.

Zemplenyi, J., Gilman, S., and Dirks, D. 1985. Optical measurement of ear canal length. *Journal of the Acoustical Society of America* 78:2146–2148.

CHAPTER 12

New Developments in Hearing Aid Measurements

James M. Kates

Electroacoustic hearing aid measurements are needed for many reasons. One obvious need is to be able to characterize the device behavior, that is, to develop a physical description of the linear and nonlinear characteristics of the instrument. A second reason for measuring a hearing aid is to determine if a given hearing aid is suitable for the desired application, which is done by performing a set of physical measurements that enable one to predict to what degree the hearing aid will benefit the user. A third reason is quality control, that is, to ensure that all hearing aids having the same specifications are similar enough in their electroacoustic behavior to be interchangeable when making a fitting. These needs have led to the development of standardized measurement techniques, and motivate the development of other new techniques.

Identifying the need for measurements, however, still leaves unanswered the question of what quantities are most appropriate to measure and how the measurements should be performed. Several factors are important in the selection of the measurement procedure. One factor is the type of hearing aid being measured, because the expected behavior will influence the selection of the test signal and procedure used to analyze it. For example, one would not feel the need to measure the compression characteristics of a linear hearing aid, but may want a special set of tests to determine the unique characteristics of an adaptive noise-canceling instrument.

The ease of making the measurement is also a factor in selecting the procedure. A complicated set of measurements may be appropriate for a laboratory but impractical for a clinic. Ease of use includes the equipment needed to make a measurement, the time required to acquire and analyze the data, and the special knowledge needed to interpret the results. Extraordinary demands made in any of these areas will limit the practical application of any new

technique. The best measurements are fast, inexpensive, and have an obvious intuitive connection with the user's experience.

The last factor to be considered is standardization. One feels safest using an established technique having a clear set of rules. The existence of a standard technique, however, does not guarantee that it is appropriate to the hearing aid under test, because standard test procedures often lag behind the advances in hearing aid technology. The manufacturer's specifications for a hearing aid, for example, are commonly determined in accordance with the American National Standards Institute S3.22 procedure (ANSI 1987). But the ANSI standards are not meant to be all-inclusive; rather, they are primarily quality-control standards for the manufacture of the instruments, and were originally developed for single-channel hearing aids containing linear or compression processing. More complicated processing, such as two-channel compression or automatic signal processing (Kates 1986), cannot be tested adequately using the ANSI S3.22 procedures. Thus, new tests are needed for the newest generation of hearing aids.

The emphasis in this chapter is on procedures that can be implemented in a standard test box using a 2-cc coupler; the same basic techniques can also be used for in-situ measurements with an anthropometric manikin or used in an individual ear.

Hearing Aid Signal Processing

Linear Processing

The basic linear hearing aid consists of a microphone, amplifier, and receiver (output transducer). Additional shaping of the frequency response to match the individual audiogram can also be provided, either through tone controls, selection of the microphone characteristics, or by modifications of the acoustic response via a vent in the earmold or hearing aid shell (Kates 1988). The linear hearing

The preparation of this chapter was supported by Grant No. G00830251 from the National Institute on Disability and Rehabilitation Research.

aid is linear only in the sense that no nonlinear processing has been designed intentionally into the instrument. In normal operation, an intense input signal can require more output power than the amplifier can provide, leading to amplifier clipping or saturation distortion. Thus, the typical measurements for a linear hearing aid are the frequency response as a function of the input signal level and the distortion of the instrument.

Compression

A common option in hearing aids is automatic gain control (AGC), or compression, in which the gain of the hearing aid is constant for low-intensity signals and is reduced for signals above a preset threshold. In most hearing aids the action of the compression is broadband; the compression affects the overall gain of the hearing aid but does not affect the shape of the frequency response. In addition to frequency response and distortion, measurements of a compression instrument are intended to describe the transient and steady-state behavior of the compression circuit. Among the differences in compression circuits are variations in the attack and release times (Burnett and Schweitzer 1977), release times that are dependent on the signal level (Smriga 1986), compression ratios that vary from mild compression to compression limiting, and variations in the rules giving the change in gain with signal level (Killion 1988).

Compression also can be implemented in a multichannel system, in which the compression acts independently in each frequency channel (Hodgson and Lade 1988; Waldauer and Villchur 1988). In a two-channel system, for example, the compression parameters include the crossover frequency between the two channels and the gain, compression threshold, and compression ratio in each channel. Increasing the number of channels greatly increases the complexity of the instrument, and the measured behavior can depend strongly on how the instrument is adjusted. The distortion depends on the compression parameters that have been selected, and the measured compression characteristics depend on the gains in the two channels since the channel having the higher gain will dominate the overall system behavior (Kates 1990a).

Adaptive Processing

In an adaptive system, the signal processing changes in response to the input signal characteristics. Thus, the measured behavior of an adaptive hearing aid depends on the test signal, and two signals that give identical results for a linear instrument may give substantially different results when used to measure the performance of an adaptive instrument. Adaptive processing has been proposed for modifying the frequency response of the hearing aid to reduce the effects of low-frequency noise (Ono, Kanzaki, and Mizoi 1983; Kates 1986), to reduce feedback (Bustamante, Worrall, and Williamson 1989; Kates 1991), and to modify the directional pattern of a microphone array in the presence of interference (Weiss 1987).

In each of these applications, the adaptive processing will cause the system behavior to change in response to specific characteristics of the applied signal. For example, the Bustamante, Worrall, and Williamson (1989) feedback cancellation system treats a continuous sinusoid as evidence of feedback and will try to remove it from the hearing aid output. Thus, using a sinusoid to measure distortion with this system will lead to inaccurate results because the test tone will be eliminated by the adaptive processing. The Kates (1991) feedback cancellation system, on the other hand, reacts to a continuous sinusoid by turning off the normal hearing aid processing and injecting a special probe signal to measure the feedback path characteristics. Using a continuous sinusoid to measure distortion with this approach will lead to a different set of inaccurate results, because the hearing aid output, depending on exactly when the measurement is made, may be a noise burst instead of a sinusoid.

Digital Processing

Digital signal processing in hearing aids does not pose any special measurement problems in and of itself. The potential for difficulty does not arise from digital versus analog processing, but rather from the greater complexity that can be designed into a digital processing system. Many adaptive processing systems will be digital, and measurement problems due to the interaction of the test signals and the hearing aid processing are to be expected. Sophisticated nonlinear algorithms, such as the detection and modification of specific speech features, also can be implemented using digital technology. In such nonlinear systems, the system frequency response in the presence of a single tone may be very much different from the response to two simultaneous tones, and this may in turn differ from the responses to varying spectra of noise. The more complicated the system, the more difficult it will be to obtain a simple unambiguous measurement of its performance.

Standard Procedures

The need for new measurement procedures is best understood in the context of the established procedures embodied in the ANSI S3.22 standard (ANSI 1987). The purpose of the ANSI S3.22 standard is not to measure every possible characteristic of a hearing aid. Rather, the major objective is production line quality-control tests used by manufacturers. But because the procedures are standardized, they also constitute the typical battery of hearing aid tests made in research and clinical settings.

Frequency Response

The test signal and analysis procedure used to measure the hearing aid frequency response is not actually specified in the ANSI S3.22 (ANSI 1987) standard; one is requested only to "record or otherwise develop the frequency response curve" (p. 17). The assumption, however, is that the frequency response of the hearing aid is measured with a swept sinusoid because there are specifications as to the accuracy of the frequency of the sound source, strip recorder paper rulings, paper speed, and pen accuracy. The input excitation is required to have a flat spectrum, so the hearing aid output gives the frequency response. The gain of the hearing aid then can be computed as the output frequency response less the amplitude of the excitation signal.

For an ideal linear hearing aid, the swept sinusoid is an effective test signal for obtaining the frequency response. In fact, for an ideal linear device having no noise or distortion, all test signals that cover the desired frequency range are equivalent and will yield the same frequency response as long as compensation is provided in the analysis for the shape of the excitation spectrum.

All test signals are not equivalent, however, for a nonlinear device such as an AGC hearing aid or an instrument having amplifier saturation. The use of a swept sinusoid to test these instruments leads to an effect called "blooming." The problem, as pointed out by Preves et al. (1989), is that a swept sinusoid at a constant amplitude may activate the compression circuit over only part of the frequency range if the

AGC threshold (or amplifier saturation) is itself frequency-dependent. For example, the AGC detection circuit is often designed to be most sensitive to high frequencies. As the input level of a swept sinusoid is increased, the behavior of the instrument may appear to be linear at low frequencies where the signal level is always below the compression threshold, and compressive at high frequencies where the AGC threshold is lower. A similar effect can be caused by amplifier saturation, because the gain often is lower at lower frequencies than at high frequencies, resulting in more headroom for a low-frequency tone, e.g., a higher input level can be tolerated before saturation occurs. In either case, the frequency response of the hearing aid appears to emphasize low frequencies as the input level is increased, since the full gain of the instrument is available at low frequencies but only reduced gain available at high frequencies.

AGC Characteristics

The ANSI S3.22 standard requires measurement of the temporal behavior of an AGC instrument only at the frequency of 2 kHz. One measurement is the attack and release time for a sinusoid that starts at 55 dB SPL, jumps to 80 dB SPL, and then returns to 55 dB SPL. Measurements at other frequencies, which would be needed for a two-channel hearing aid, are not specified, although the ANSI test signal can easily be extended to other frequencies (Kates 1990a). And although the ANSI S3.22 standard defines the compression threshold or kneepoint, it does not contain a procedure for estimating the signal envelope from which the attack and release times are estimated, other than to indicate that an oscilloscope trace "or other appropriate means" (p. 22), should be used. The ANSI S3.22 procedure for determining the input/output characteristics uses a 2 kHz sinusoid stepped in increments of 10 dB from 50 to 90 dB SPL; the single test frequency and the large steps in signal level may also be inadequate for accurately characterizing a compression instrument.

Distortion

The only distortion measurement specified in the ANSI S3.22 standard is harmonic distortion measured at three frequencies (500, 800, and 1600 Hz for a standard instrument). The interpretation of harmonic distortion data in hearing aids can be quite confusing, however. One of the problems is caused by the frequency response of the hearing aid. Consider, for example, an instrument having 0 dB gain at low frequencies and 30 dB gain at high frequencies, which is representative of a hearing aid prescribed for a moderate high-frequency loss. If the distortion mechanism occurs before the frequency-response shaping in the circuit, then the high-frequency emphasis will result in more gain being given to the distortion components than to the test tone itself. In general, distortion and gain are distributed throughout the hearing aid circuitry, so the harmonic distortion measurement intertwines the nonlinear distortion and the linear frequency shaping of the instrument.

A second problem is the incompleteness of harmonic distortion measurements in characterizing the system under test. In particular, harmonic distortion indicates that the presence of a tone causes additional higher-frequency components to be generated. The measurement does not give any indication of how distortion at high frequencies—where many hearing aids have their highest amount of gain and therefore most easily go into amplifier saturation—will affect the reproduction of lower-frequency speech sounds occurring at the same time.

Intermodulation distortion (IM) measurements, typically performed by sweeping a pair of sinusoids having a constant separation in hertz, are capable of measuring the generation of low-frequency distortion products. Interaction of the two tones with the nonlinearities will cause a distortion product at the fixed difference frequency. The weakness with IM distortion measurements, however, is that they can be defeated by placing a notch in the system frequency response at the frequency of the expected difference tone, thereby reducing the measured distortion while leaving all of the distortion problems intact, and the two-tone test signal may not be sufficiently complex to completely characterize the distortion mechanism. Thus, new procedures for measuring distortion are needed.

New Measurements

New measurement techniques are being developed because of dissatisfaction with the ability of the standard procedures to characterize accurately hearing aid processing, as in the case of swept-sinusoid frequency-response measurements, or to produce meaningful data, as in the case of harmonic distortion. The advent of new hearing-aid signal processing is also a motivating factor, since measurement

techniques that are adequate for simple hearing aids may not be adequate for the more complex instruments now being developed.

Frequency Response

The swept sinusoid typically used for frequency-response measurements is a highly artificial signal. Although this makes the analysis quite simple, it also means that the test signal itself has very little to do with speech. Burnett, Bartel, and Roland (1987) have proposed using a speech-shaped noise signal instead of a swept sinusoid to measure the frequency response of a hearing aid. The stimulus consists of white Gaussian noise that has been band-limited to the range 200 Hz to 5000 Hz, and then shaped with a one-pole low-pass filter (roll-off of 6 dB per octave) at 900 Hz to give an approximation to the long-term spectrum of speech. The spectrum that results from a digital version of the shaped-noise test signal (Kates 1990a) is shown in figure 1. Although the envelope fluctuations of speech are not reproduced by this test signal, the signal comes closer to a speech-like stimulus than does a swept sinusoid.

The analysis of this test signal is more complicated than merely recording the hearing aid output on a chart recorder. One analysis procedure (Kates 1990a) involves dividing 2 sec of the hearing aid output into windowed blocks of approximately 50 ms duration and having 50% overlap. The magnitude-squared spectrum of each windowed block is computed using the FFT algorithm, and the spectra are averaged together. The resultant estimated power spectrum is then smoothed in frequency by combining the frequency points into overlapping one-third octave bands. This reduces the fluctuations in the frequency-response measurement, although it will broaden sharp spectral peaks in the frequency response. Other procedures for smoothing the spectral data over different bandwidths also can be used. The output power spectrum is divided by the smoothed spectrum of the excitation signal, also smoothed in one-third octave bands, to give the gain of the hearing aid as a function of frequency. The level of the input signal in dB can then be added to the gain in dB of the hearing aid to get a family of offset gain curves.

The frequency-response measurement produces a family of gain curves for shaped-noise input signals ranging from 60 dB SPL to 90 dB SPL in steps of 10 dB. As an example, sets of offset gain curves were generated for two simulated hearing aids (Kates 1990b). The linear hearing aid has 0 dB

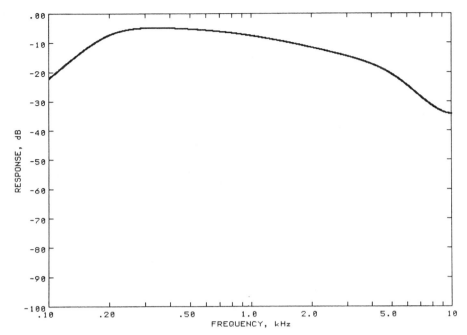

Figure 1. Spectrum of the shaped-noise test signal used for the frequency-response measurements.

gain at high frequencies, a relative gain of −20 dB at low frequencies, and amplifier clipping at an input-referred level of 85 dB SPL. The compression hearing aid is a two-channel compression instrument having a compression ratio of 2:1, a threshold of 65 dB SPL, and 0 dB relative gain in the high-frequency channel and a compression ratio of 4:1, a threshold of 75 dB SPL, and a gain of −20 dB in the

low-frequency channel. The outputs of the two channels are summed and then processed by an amplifier having clipping at an input-referred level of 85 dB SPL. The frequency-response curves have been normalized by removing the amplifier gain from the output.

The response for the linear hearing aid in figure 2 clearly shows the linear behavior at low input

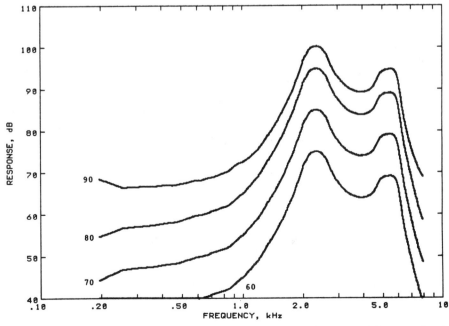

Figure 2. Set of offset gain curves for the simulated linear hearing aid for input levels from 60 to 90 dB SPL.

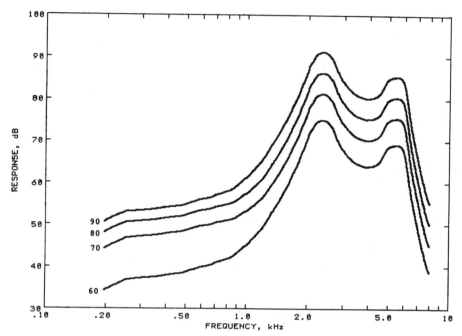

Figure 3. Set of offset gain curves for the simulated compression hearing aid for input levels from 60 to 90 dB SPL.

levels because the lower three curves have a uniform separation of 10 dB. The amplifier saturation becomes apparent for the 90 dB SPL input level because the last 10 dB increment in the input produces only a 4 dB increment in the hearing aid output at high frequencies; the greater increment in output at low frequencies is the result of less amplifier saturation for the low-frequency content of the test signal. The response for the compression hearing aid in figure 3 shows the 4:1 compression behavior and the 75 dB SPL threshold in the low-frequency channel because the curve spacing is 10 dB between the 60 dB and 70 dB SPL curves and then reduces to 2.5 dB between the remaining curves. At high frequencies, the lower threshold causes the separation between all the curves to be similar, and the spacing of 5 dB between the curves is a result of the 2:1 compression ratio in the high-frequency channel. The shaped-noise test signal is therefore very effective in determining the frequency response of a hearing aid under varying conditions, including linear instruments with amplifier saturation and two-channel instruments with different compression parameters in each channel.

AGC Characteristics

The AGC circuit measurements proposed by Kates (1990a) are the hearing aid input/output characteristics and the attack and release times. In a multi-

channel instrument the input/output characteristics are measured at or near the geometric center of each frequency band, whereas in a single-channel instrument the measurement is made at the 2 kHz center frequency specified in the ANSI S3.22 standard (ANSI 1987) because many single-channel compression instruments are most sensitive at this frequency. The test signal is a sinusoid of fixed frequency having segments stepped in level from 40 dB SPL to 95 dB SPL in increments of 5 dB; the initial portion of each segment is discarded to allow for transients in the response of the hearing aid, and the signal amplitude is determined from the average over the latter portion of the segment.

The input/output characteristics for the linear hearing aid are given in table I. The linear operation is indicated clearly by the compression ratio of 1.0:1 for inputs up to 80 dB SPL. The amplifier saturation is starting to have an effect for the 85 dB SPL input, since the compression ratio has increased to 1.11:1, and the saturation is strongly evident for inputs at the higher levels since the effective compression ratio increases rapidly. Note that this test cannot distinguish between compression and saturation since either effect causes a reduction in gain with increasing signal level.

The input/output characteristics for the compression hearing aid are given in table II for the test frequencies of 800 and 3150 Hz used for the low-frequency and high-frequency channels, respec-

Table I. Input/Output Measurements for the Simulated Linear Hearing Aid

| Input dB SPL | Frequency = 2000 Hz | |
	Output dB SPL	Comp Ratio
40	48.93	—
45	54.00	0.99
50	58.94	1.01
55	64.03	0.98
60	69.03	1.00
65	74.03	1.00
70	79.03	1.00
75	84.03	1.00
80	89.02	1.00
85	93.52	1.11
90	94.32	6.20
95	94.90	8.63

Table II. Input/Output Measurements for the Simulated Compression Hearing Aid

| Input dB SPL | Frequency = 800 Hz | | Frequency = 3150 Hz | |
	Output dB SPL	Comp Ratio	Output dB SPL	Comp Ratio
40	23.27	—	45.77	—
45	26.85	1.40	50.77	1.00
50	31.75	1.02	55.75	1.00
55	36.43	1.07	60.76	1.00
60	41.52	0.98	65.45	1.07
65	46.54	1.00	67.95	2.00
70	51.49	1.01	70.46	2.00
75	55.41	1.28	72.96	1.99
80	58.28	1.74	75.47	1.99
85	61.94	1.37	77.98	2.00
90	65.19	1.54	80.47	2.01
95	67.49	2.17	82.97	2.00

tively. The compression ratio of 1.40:1 for the 45 dB SPL input signal is an artifact caused by measurement noise effects at the low signal level. The compression ratio then becomes near unity over the linear range of the instrument, and then increases as the signal rises above threshold in each channel. The high-frequency channel shows a compression ratio close to the specified 2:1, but the compression ratio in the low-frequency channel is far from the specified 4:1. This difference is the result of the relative gains in the two channels; because the gain in the low-frequency channel is 20 dB below that of the high-frequency channel, the signal level in the lower channel is dominated by the tail of the high-frequency channel high-pass filter response. Thus, the measurements of the behavior of each channel may be corrupted by the presence of the other channel; the most accurate measurements of one channel will be made with the other channel turned off, and as the gain of one channel is increased relative to the other channel, the hearing aid will behave increasingly like a single-channel instrument.

The attack and release times use a measurement procedure quite similar to the ANSI S3.22 standard (ANSI 1987). The only change is to perform the measurement at the one-third octave frequency closest to the geometric center of the frequency band. A procedure for estimating the signal envelope has also been developed (Kates 1990a), because an explicit procedure is not provided in the ANSI S3.22 standard.

Distortion

The new distortion measurements are based on using a test signal more complicated than a simple sinusoid. A particularly attractive signal is broad-

band noise, because all frequency components are present at the same time. Distortion measured using such a test signal will combine the effects of the noise present in the hearing aid circuitry, harmonic distortion, and intermodulation distortion. Hearing aid distortion measurements using a noise signal were originally proposed by Burnett (1967), who developed an analog system having a shaped noise excitation containing a single notch that was swept in frequency. The noise distortion was computed by estimating the amount of energy that was found in the notch, but the accuracy of the system was limited by the available instrumentation.

A more recent notched-noise distortion-measurement system has been proposed by Kates (1990a), in which digital signal-processing techniques are used to overcome the limitations of the earlier analog procedure. The test signal is the shaped noise of figure 1, which is then sent through a comb filter to create a series of interleaved peaks and valleys. The comb-filter response, shown in figure 4, suppresses the frequency regions contained in the notches by over 60 dB, enabling distortion to be measured at the 0.1% level; the notches are spaced every 625 Hz.

The distortion-measurement procedure is based on determining how much energy from the peaks of the comb-filtered shaped noise spills over into the valleys. The distortion energy is computed as the mean-squared energy in the center of the valley, and the signal energy is computed as the mean-squared energy in the peaks to either side of the valley with the bias equal to the distortion energy removed. The transition regions between the peaks and valleys are not used. The signal-to-distortion ratio (SDR) is the square root of the ratio of the com-

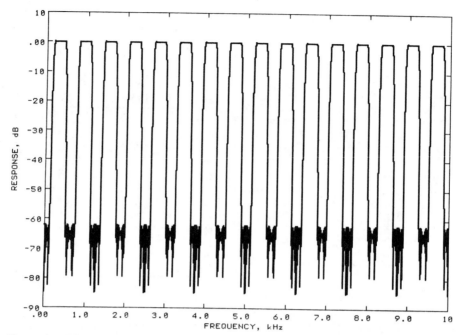

Figure 4.   Filter used for placing notches in the shaped-noise excitation to give the distortion test signal.

puted signal energy to the distortion energy, expressed in dB for each valley center frequency. The relative distortion can also be expressed as a percent of the signal level in the adjacent peaks.

In addition to expressing the distortion as a function of frequency, there is a need for a single figure of merit to indicate the overall effect of the distortion on speech intelligibility. The figure of merit proposed by Kates (1990a) is a weighted signal-to-distortion ratio index, computed using a procedure similar to the Articulation Index (French and Steinberg 1949; Kryter 1962). The SDR in dB at each valley center frequency is limited to the range of 0 to 30 dB, divided by 30, and the ratios are then combined using the weights given in table III to get a number between 0 and 1.

A set of broadband distortion measurements for the simulated linear instrument is presented in table IV. The percent root-mean-squared distortions in the valleys from 625 through 5000 Hz are given for input signal levels from 60 through 90 dB SPL, along with the weighted SDR index. The distortion values at an input of 60 dB SPL show the effects of noise in the measurement procedure itself, and thus the lowest distortion values are found for the input at 70 dB SPL. The frequency response of the linear instrument to the notched noise at 70 dB SPL is shown in figure 5, where the energy in the valleys falls below the frequency axis.

Increasing the signal level above 70 dB SPL results in increased distortion caused by the amplifier

clipping. At the highest test-signal level, 90 dB SPL, distortion is quite large at the low test frequencies, and the weighted SDR has been reduced to 0.472. This is caused by the high-frequency input being clipped by the amplifier and the distortion products being splattered to all frequencies; the lower gain at the low frequencies means that the relative level of the distortion products will be greater than at high frequencies. The relative distribution of signal and distortion for the linear hearing aid is illustrated in figure 6, where the distortion products for the 90 dB SPL input have filled in the valley almost completely at 625 Hz.

The distortion measurements then were repeated for the simulated compression hearing aid. The results are given in table V. The compression processing in the hearing aid results in an increase in the measured distortion at low signal levels, al-

Table III.   Weights for Combining the Signal-To-Distortion Ratios into a Single Distortion Index

Band	Valley Center Frequency, Hz	Band Edges Hz	Weight
1.	625	312.5–0937.5	0.258
2.	1250	937.5–1562.5	0.209
3.	1875	1562.5–2187.5	0.180
4.	2500	2187.5–2812.5	0.121
5.	3125	2812.5–3437.5	0.084
6.	3750	3437.5–4062.5	0.063
7.	4375	4062.5–4687.5	0.047
8.	5000	4687.5–5312.5	0.038

though the amount of distortion is not enough to affect the weighted SDR index. At high signal levels, the compression reduces the probability of amplifier clipping, resulting in a small increase in the measured distortion to about 2%, but no change in the weighted SDR index. These distortion effects are shown in figures 7 and 8 for input levels of 70 and 90 dB SPL, respectively; the compression tends to generate a small amount of distortion at both signal levels, but the valleys are not filled in for the more intense test signal.

Coherence

Another procedure that can be used for measuring the amount of noise and distortion in the response of a hearing aid is the magnitude-squared coherence function. The phrase *coherence function* normally is used to indicate the magnitude-squared coherence function, and is used with that meaning here as well. The coherence function determines the amount of output signal that is linearly related to the input signal as a function of frequency. The value of the coherence function can vary from one to zero; a coherence function value of one indicates that the output is a linear transformation of the input and that no noise or nonlinear distortion is present, and a coherence function value of zero indicates that the output has no relationship to the input at all. Any test signal can be used as the excit-

Table IV. Ratio of RMS Distortion to Signal Level and the Weighted SDR Index for the Simulated Linear Hearing Aid

Frequency, Hz	Input Signal Intensity, dB SPL			
	60	70	80	90
625	0.16%	0.15%	6.11%	46.32%
1250	0.08	0.07	3.01	25.54
1875	0.06	0.04	1.07	9.51
2500	0.12	0.07	1.44	12.82
3125	0.13	0.06	1.44	11.06
3750	0.17	0.08	1.54	13.18
4375	0.21	0.09	1.66	14.09
5000	0.22	0.09	1.78	15.42
Index	1.000	1.000	0.951	0.472

ation when computing the coherence function as long as it contains adequate power in all frequency regions that are of interest.

The coherence function is computed in the frequency domain by computing the magnitude-squared cross-spectral density of the output and input signals and normalizing by the product of the spectral densities of each of the two signals (Benignus 1969; Carter, Knapp, and Nuttall 1973). Because the shape of the spectrum is normalized out of the calculation, the coherence function gives a measure of the phase variations from segment to segment of the output signal relative to the phase of the input signal. If the phase shift remains constant

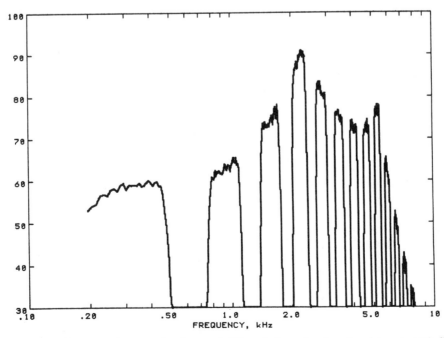

Figure 5. Output spectrum for the comb-filtered shaped noise signal input at 70 dB SPL for the simulated linear hearing aid.

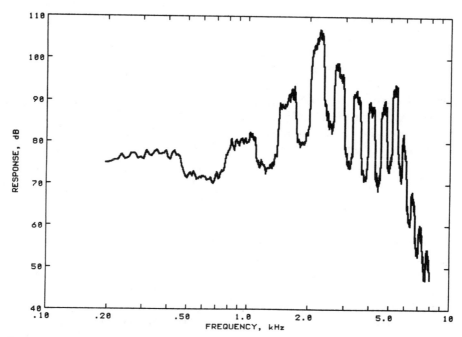

Figure 6.   Output spectrum for the comb-filtered shaped noise signal input at 90 dB SPL for the simulated linear hearing aid.

from segment to segment, then the coherence function approaches one, but if there are random fluctuations in the output phase shift, then the coherence function will be reduced.

Estimates of the coherence function are subject to several sources of error. One error is a bias in the estimated coherence function towards a value of one (Carter, Knapp, and Nuttall 1973); this can be understood on an intuitive basis because the coherence for a single data segment is identically unity (no phase fluctuations can be detected if only one sample of the phase difference is available), so the results from many segments will have to be averaged together in order to get an accurate esti-

mate of a low coherence function value. This effect can be reduced, for a given amount of data, by using short data segments in order to average the computation over as many segments as possible. Using short segments, however, leads to a different problem, because a time delay between the input and the output, or the presence of a reflection having a long time delay in the output, leads to an error that is inversely proportional to the segment length (Carter 1980). A related problem is caused by the length of the impulse response of the system being measured, and this also leads to an error that is inversely proportional to the segment length (Kates 1990a). Thus, the value of the coherence function may contain errors caused by the parameters of the computational procedure in the context of the system being measured.

The signal-to-distortion ratio can be derived from the magnitude-squared coherence function using the relationship

$$SDR = \frac{\gamma^2(f)}{1 - \gamma^2(f)} \qquad (1)$$

where $\gamma^2(f)$ is the magnitude-squared coherence function. The equation represents the ratio of the coherent to the noncoherent power as a function of frequency. This procedure was applied to the same simulated linear and compression hearing aids that were used to illustrate the notched-noise distortion-measurement procedure. The segment length for

Table V.   Ratio of RMS Distortion to Signal Level and the Weighted SDR Index for the Simulated Compression Hearing Aid

Frequency, Hz	Input Signal Intensity, dB SPL			
	60	70	80	90
625	0.09%	1.03%	2.08%	2.15%
1250	0.07	1.17	1.47	1.40
1875	0.06	0.71	0.79	0.76
2500	0.13	0.93	0.95	0.95
3125	0.13	0.89	0.90	0.90
3750	0.17	0.92	0.92	0.92
4375	0.20	1.01	1.01	1.02
5000	0.23	1.01	1.01	1.01
Index	1.000	1.000	1.000	1.000

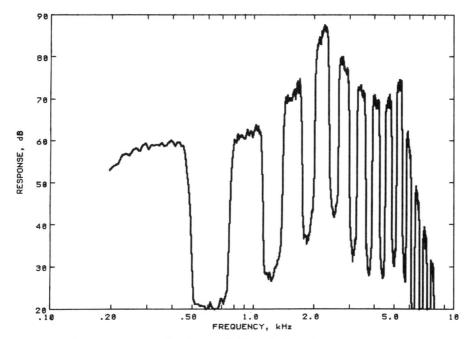

Figure 7.   Output spectrum for the comb-filtered shaped noise signal input at 70 dB SPL for the simulated compression hearing aid.

computing the coherence function was 102.4 ms (2048 samples) at a sampling rate of 20 kHz, and the excitation was the shaped-noise test signal.

The SDRs derived from the coherence function are presented in figures 9 and 10 for the linear and compression hearing aids, respectively. The curves for the input levels of 60 and 70 dB SPL overlap for the linear hearing aid, and give a SDR of about 34 dB in the vicinity of 1.25 kHz. The notched noise measurement, at the same frequency for the same linear instrument, gave a distortion level of 0.08%, which corresponds to a SDR of about 62 dB. Thus, the coherence function is in error by 28 dB in this example, and the SDR curves for the compression

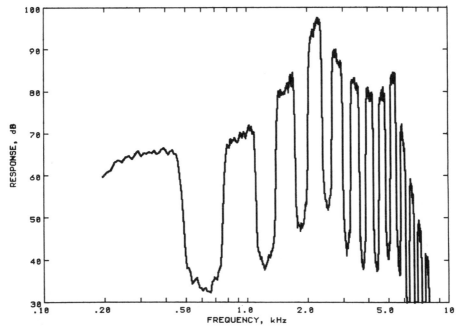

Figure 8.   Output spectrum for the comb-filtered shaped noise signal input at 90 dB SPL for the simulated compression hearing aid.

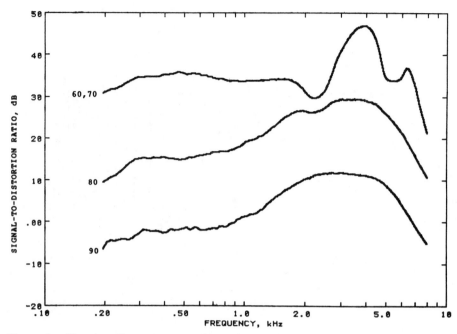

Figure 9. Signal-to-distortion ratio (SDR) derived from the magnitude-squared coherence function as the input level goes from 60 to 90 dB SPL for the simulated linear hearing aid.

instrument show a similar error. Measurements on actual hearing aids performed by Dyrlund (1989) and Bareham (1990) also show a maximum SDR of about 30 dB. Given that there is essentially no noise or distortion in the simulated hearing aid for the low input levels, the error is most likely caused by the duration of the ringing of the hearing aid impulse response relative to the 100 ms analysis segment. This interpretation is reinforced by the fact that doubling the length of the analysis segment

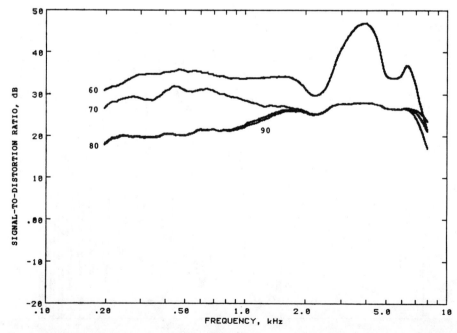

Figure 10. Signal-to-distortion ratio (SDR) derived from the magnitude-squared coherence function as the input level goes from 60 to 90 dB SPL for the simulated compression hearing aid.

size while processing the same amount of data from simulated hearing aids resulted in an increase of 6 dB in the SDR derived from the coherence function (Kates 1990a). Thus, the use of the coherence function, as typically implemented, may lead to a substantial overestimation of the amount of distortion and/or noise in a hearing aid.

Type of Processing

The type of processing and the number of processing channels can be determined by observing how a bias tone modifies the frequency response of the instrument. In the system proposed by Kates (1990a), the response of the hearing aid is measured for an excitation consisting of the 60 dB SPL shaped noise combined with an 80 dB SPL swept sinusoid. The response of the instrument to the noise alone and to the swept tone alone also are measured. The purpose of the swept sinusoid is to bias the nonlinear processing that may be present in the hearing aid; the power in the swept tone is detected by the control circuitry that then changes the hearing aid response. The shaped noise signal is used to determine the frequency response of the hearing aid while the processing changes take place.

As the swept bias tone moves through different frequency regions, it will change the gain and/or frequency response of a hearing aid containing nonlinear processing such as AGC, ASP, or amplifier saturation. Most commercially available single-channel AGC hearing aids, for example, have a band-pass filter tuned to the region around 2 kHz in front of the compressor control circuit and a threshold above 65 dB SPL in the most sensitive frequency region. An input at 80 dB SPL will be processed linearly if it is far enough removed from 2 kHz, but will cause a reduction in gain if it is near 2 kHz. The swept tone thus reduces the gain while it is present in the frequency region or regions that control the nonlinear processing. The gain will be unchanged from the linear value, however, when the swept tone is either too low or too high in frequency to be detected by the control circuitry.

To determine the changes in the frequency response caused by the nonlinear processing, the hearing aid response to the swept tone alone is subtracted from the response to the swept tone plus noise. This leaves the shaped-noise output as modified by the presence of the sweep. The spectrum of this noise is then compared to the spectrum of the hearing-aid response to the shaped noise alone; the difference in the spectra indicates the degree of nonlinear processing in the hearing aid caused by

the presence of the bias tone. The changes in the spectral difference as a function of the sweep frequency indicate the frequency regions controlling the nonlinear processing. A linear hearing aid will result in no recorded gain changes at any frequency of the swept tone; different realizations of equivalent linear processing, such as single-channel or multi-channel frequency shaping, will thus be indistinguishable by this procedure.

The change in the system frequency response is determined from the shaped noise spectrum each time the swept tone crosses the boundary of a third-octave frequency band, and again at the end of the sweep. In order to simplify the presentation, the frequency response is calculated only at the frequencies corresponding to each edge of the third-octave bands and is replaced by a blank if the reduction in gain is less than 3 dB and by a solid character if the reduction in gain is equal to or greater than 3 dB. This leads to a square two-dimensional grid in which the gain change in each third-octave frequency region is indicated each time the sweep crosses a third-octave boundary.

A set of idealized system-identification patterns is presented in figure 11 for a one- or two-channel hearing aid with various types of signal processing. A perfectly linear system, as shown in the upper left-hand pattern, results in a blank pattern because the swept tone does not cause any gain change at any frequency.

The next pattern is for an ASP circuit (Kates 1986). In this type of processing, the cutoff frequency of a high-pass filter moves lower in frequency as the amount of low-frequency energy decreases. The detection circuit that controls the high-pass filter tends to be most sensitive to energy around 250 to 300 Hz. This processing leads to a pattern in which the lower left-hand corner is blacked out on a diagonal because raising the sweep frequency causes a reduction in the amount of energy detected by the control circuit, and as a result the ASP cutoff frequency moves lower.

A broadband AGC circuit results in the pattern shown in the upper right-hand corner of figure 11. This pattern has a horizontal stripe blacked out because the gain at all frequencies is reduced as soon as the sweep goes above the threshold most sensitive to energy at 2 kHz. The processing is linear at low frequencies because the energy detected by the control circuit is still below the AGC threshold. Combining ASP and AGC results in a pattern where both the ASP and the AGC areas are blacked out, as shown in the lower left-hand corner.

A two-channel hearing aid having compres-

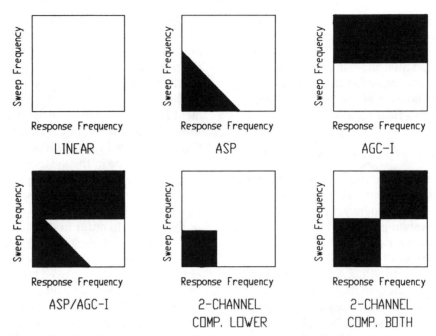

Figure 11.   Idealized system-identification patterns for determining the type of processing in a hearing aid.

sion only in the lower-frequency channel results in the next pattern. When the swept tone is in the low-frequency channel, the AGC detects the energy and causes a reduction in the gain in the channel. The gain in the high frequency is unchanged. Thus, the lower left-hand corner is blacked out because the gain at low frequencies is reduced as long as the sweep is in the lower-frequency channel. The low-frequency gain returns to the linear value as soon as the sweep moves out of the low-frequency channel.

A two-channel instrument having compression in both channels results in the checkerboard pattern shown in the lower right-hand corner of figure 11. The gain at low frequencies is reduced while the sweep is in the low-frequency channel, and the gain at high frequencies is kept at the linear value because the AGC in that channel has not been engaged. The gain at high frequencies is then reduced when the sweep moves into the high-frequency channel, and the gain at low frequencies returns to the linear value for the channel.

The test program compares the actual system-identification pattern for the hearing aid under test with each of the idealized patterns shown in figure 11 to form a pattern-match score. In determining the scores for the processing options, all possible cross-over frequencies are tried for each option, with the program indicating the score for the best frequency match and the cross-over frequency at which it occurs. The indicated processing is that which corre-

sponds to the highest score among all the processing options, and the final cross-over frequency is the frequency at which the highest test score was found.

Conclusions

There are two significant trends apparent in the development of new hearing aid test methods. One trend, the use of computer-based systems and associated digital signal-processing techniques, is leading toward the development of sophisticated yet practical measurement strategies. In particular, measurement systems are no longer tied to the oscillators, voltmeters, and chart recorders that represented the state of the art in the 1970s. Spectrum analysis based on the FFT algorithm, the ability to perform cross-correlations or cross-spectral measurements, easily implemented and extremely sharp digital filters, and adaptive algorithms now form the basic set of analysis tools. Many of the new tests described in this chapter, including frequency response computed from a shaped-noise test signal, broadband distortion using a notched noise test signal, distortion computed from the coherence function, and the test for the type of processing, require extensive computational capability in the measurement equipment.

The second trend is the use of test stimuli that

are closer to speech. The assumption is that speech is an appropriate signal for testing the performance of a hearing aid, and signals that deviate from speech may be of more limited predictive value. The use of shaped noise is one step in this direction, because a broadband excitation is closer than a single sinusoid to a speech-like stimulus. But there will always be a need for carefully specified and easily described and interpreted artificial test signals such as sinusoids; in the past such signals were used for every hearing-aid test, whereas in the future there will be a better matching of the test signal to the measurement objective.

References

ANSI S3.22 1987. *American National Standard Specification of Hearing Aid Characteristics.* New York: American National Standards Institute.

Bareham, J. 1990. Part 2: Hearing instrument measurements using dual channel signal analysis. *Hearing Instruments* 41(1):32–33.

Benignus, V.A. 1969. Estimation of the coherence spectrum and its confidence interval using the fast Fourier transform. *IEEE Transactions on Audio and Electroacoustics* 17:145–50.

Burnett, E.D. 1967. A new method for the measurement of nonlinear distortion using a random noise test signal. *Bulletin of Prosthetics Research* Spring 1967.

Burnett, E.D., and Schweitzer, H.C. 1977. Attack and release times of automatic-gain-control hearing aids. *Journal of the Acoustical Society of America* 62(3):784–86.

Burnett, E.D., Bartel, T.W., and Roland, W.R. 1987. NBS hearing aid test procedures and test data. In *Handbook of Hearing Aid Measurement 1987* IB 11–78 (revised). Washington, DC: Veterans Administration.

Bustamante, D.K., Worrall, T.L., and Williamson, M.J. 1989. Measurement of adaptive suppression of acoustic feedback in hearing aids. Proc. 1989 International Conference on Acoustics, Speech and Signal Processing, Glasgow.

Carter, G.C. 1980. Bias in magnitude-squared coherence estimation due to misalignment. *IEEE Transactions on Acoustical Speech and Signal Processing* 28:97–99.

Carter, G.C., Knapp, C.H., and Nuttall, A.H. 1973. Estimation of the magnitude-squared coherence function via overlapped fast Fourier transform processing. *IEEE Transactions on Audio and Electroacoustics* 21:337–44.

Dyrlund, O. 1989. Characterization of non-linear distortion in hearing aids using coherence analysis: A pilot study. *Scandinavian Audilogy* 18:143–48.

French, N.R., and Steinberg, J.C. 1949. Factors governing the intelligibility of speech sounds. *Journal of the Acoustical Society of America* 19:90–119.

Hodgson, W.A., and Lade, K.P. 1988. Digital technology in hearing instruments. *Hearing Journal* 41(4):28–34.

Kates, J.M. 1986. Signal processing for hearing aids. *Hearing Instruments* 37(2):19–22.

Kates, J.M. 1988. Acoustic effects in in-the-ear hearing-aid response: Results from a computer simulation. *Ear and Hearing* 9(3):119–32.

Kates, J.M. 1990a. A test suite for hearing aid evaluation. *Journal of Rehabilitation Research and Development* 27(3): 255–78.

Kates, J.M. 1990b. A time domain simulation of hearing aid response. *Journal of Rehabilitation Research and Development* 27(3):279–94.

Kates, J.M. 1991. Feedback cancellation in hearing aids. *IEEE Transactions on Signal Processing* 39(3):553–62.

Killion, M. 1988. Principles of high fidelity hearing aid amplification. In *Handbook of Hearing Aid Amplification Volume I: Theoretical and Technical Considerations,* ed. R.E. Sandlin. Boston: College-Hill Press; Little, Brown and Company.

Kryter, K.D. 1962. Methods for the calculation and use of the Articulation Index, *Journal of the Acoustical Society of America* 34:1689–1697

Ono, H., Kanzaki, J., and Mizoi, K. 1983. Clinical results of a hearing aid with noise-level-controlled selective amplification. *Audiology* 22:494–515.

Preves, D.A., Beck, L.B., Burnett, E.D., and Teder, H. 1989. Input stimuli for obtaining frequency responses of automatic gain control hearing aids. *Journal of Speech and Hearing Research* 32:189–94.

Smriga, D. 1986. Modern compression technology, developments, and applications, Part II. *Hearing Journal* 39(7):13–16.

Waldauer, F., and Villchur, E. 1988. Full dynamic range multiband compression in a hearing aid. *Hearing Journal* 41(9):29–32.

Weiss, M. 1987. Use of an adaptive noise canceller as an input preprocessor for a hearing aid. *Journal of Rehabilitation Research and Development* 24(4):93–102.

CHAPTER 13

Application of Acoustic Impedance Measures to Hearing Aid Fitting Strategies

Vernon D. Larson, David P. Egolf, and William A. Cooper, Jr.

Not long ago, the relationship of audiologists to hearing aid manufacturers was clear-cut. The manufacturers supplied a stock of hearing aids to satisfy a wide range of fitting requirements and the audiologist selected or adjusted these instruments to achieve the desired result. Today, however, as a consequence of miniaturized conventional hearing aids and prescriptive fitting strategies, a different relationship has evolved.

All too often a clinical scenario exists wherein the audiologist, convinced of the reliability and validity of his or her measurements, provides the manufacturer with certain real-ear, coupler, and/or behaviorally estimated data that may or may not include elements of existing prescriptive fitting formulae. The manufacturer designs and assembles a device according to experience and/or "best estimate" criteria and records its gain and spectrum shape using one of the commercially available ear simulators or couplers.

When the dispenser fits the aid, if the requirements have not been satisfied, another hearing aid configuration is assembled, presumably based on the knowledge of the shortcomings of the previous attempt, and the process is repeated. This process may be repeated several times until the requirements are met or, unfortunately, until it is concluded that the fitter has come as close to the amplification target as is possible.

Clearly, in many of these cases, insofar as ear-simulator measurements indicate, the requested response requirements have, in fact, been met by the manufacturer for a particular hearing aid configuration. An obvious question then arises: are the recordings made in a simulator indicative of what that particular hearing aid will actually deliver to the patient? Probably not, according to the preponderance of contemporary literature on the subject (c.f.,

Bratt, Sanders, and Larson 1980; Cooper, Larson, and Ahlstrom 1986; Egolf 1980; Egolf et al. 1985; Gilman, Dirks, and Stern 1981; Kates 1988; Kennedy and Egolf 1985; Larson, Harrell, and Talbott 1984; Larson, Studebaker, and Cox 1977; and Sanborn 1990). A generalization that could be made from the results reported by these investigators is that the sound spectrum in the aided ear is dependent on geometry of the ear canal and on eardrum impedance. Thus, real-ear simulators designed to represent the "average" normal adult ear are likely to yield spectral data that are different from that produced in a particular patient's ear using the same hearing aid. These differences could be especially pronounced if the patient has small ear canals or if eardrum impedance differs significantly from the average.

The purpose of this chapter is to discuss the development of a possible augmentative approach to current prescriptive fitting procedures. In practice, the approach would be an integral part of a comprehensive computer-based model (c.f., Kates 1988) to select hearing-aid components for the individual patient. We are aware of several manufacturers who use modeling techniques to some extent for the selection of hearing aid components to "prescription fit" the patient. However, clinicians have not had technology available that would allow them to provide the manufacturer with the missing component to their models: estimates of aural acoustic impedance across the range of frequencies important to hearing aid fitting.

Transformation of Sound by Hearing Aids

Description

Sound transformation by hearing aids may be explained by referring to the in-the-ear (ITE) hearing

---

Work supported by VA Rehabilitation Research and Development Service (Project 337-RA).

aid depicted in figure 1. As shown, the sound pressure P of waves at some distant point in the sound-field is transformed by transfer function I to sound pressure P_i at the microphone inlet port. The microphone M then transduces sound pressure P_i to an electrical signal that undergoes amplification and then drives receiver R. The receiver output sound pressure P'_R is transformed to sound pressure P'_T at the eardrum via the serial connection of sound tube T_1 and the residual ear canal T_2.

Some sound leaks through the earmold vent T_3, so that sound pressure P'_o at the earmold tip becomes P'_v at the vent outlet. Waves of sound pressure P'_v emerging from the vent traverse an external "feedback" path F, returning to the microphone with sound pressure P_F. Upon reaching the microphone inlet port, these waves then combine with incident waves of sound pressure P_i, a process denoted by the left-hand dashed circle labeled SUM in figure 1. Such a summation process, producing either constructive or destructive interference, naturally results when two sound-pressure waves occur together at the same point in space.

Also illustrated in figure 1 is an alternate, direct path E to the eardrum via the earmold vent. By traversing this different incident path, the sound pressure P of waves in the free field becomes sound pressure P''_v as these waves arrive at the vent exit.

Sound pressure P''_v is then transformed to sound pressure P''_T at the eardrum via the serial connection of the earmold vent T_3 and ear canal T_2. The total pressure at the eardrum is the sum of sound pressures P'_T and P''_T, denoted by the right-hand dashed circle in figure 1.

Need for Computer-Based Plan

The foregoing description reminds us that the transformation of sound by a hearing aid is governed by an almost bewildering array of variables. Such variables include, for example, (1) orientation of the head in the sound-field, (2) type and location of the microphone, (3) amplifier design, (4) type of receiver, (5) dimensions of the sound tube and earmold vent, (6) existence of an external feedback path, (7) geometry of the ear canal, and (8) eardrum impedance. Consequently, a priori determination of the sound spectrum at the eardrum of an aided patient would be difficult, if not impossible, without the assistance of some type of computer-based, analytical plan to keep track of all of these variables. For detailed treatments of the various acoustic and electroacoustic elements, the reader is referred to articles that have contributed directly or indirectly to the mathematical characterization of one or more parts of a hearing aid (among others, c.f., Bade et al. 1984; Bauer 1987; Carlson 1974, 1980; Dalsgaard, Johansen, and Chisnall 1976; Egolf 1976; Egolf 1977; Egolf, Haley, and Larson 1986; Egolf, Haley, Howell, and Larson 1988; Egolf, Haley, Bauer, Howell, and Larson 1988; Egolf, Haley, Howell, Legowski, and Larson 1988; Egolf and Leonard 1977; Grossman and Molloy 1944; Lybarger 1972; Kates 1988; Kuhn 1977, 1985; Kuhn and Greller 1984; and White et al. 1980).

The Elusive Components: Impedance of the Residual Ear Canal and Impedance of the Eardrum

It is almost axiomatic to state that the logical plane of reference in the ear canal for sound pressure and for impedance determinations is at the eardrum. However, in order to refer measurements to the eardrum location, an accurate and valid determination must be made of the contribution of the ear canal to estimates of eardrum quantities made at a remote site in the ear canal.

Since the early work of Wiener and Ross (1946), it has been common practice to treat the ear canal mathematically as though it were a single, right-circular, cylindrical tube terminated at right angles by the eardrum (c.f., Rabinowitz 1981). More recent

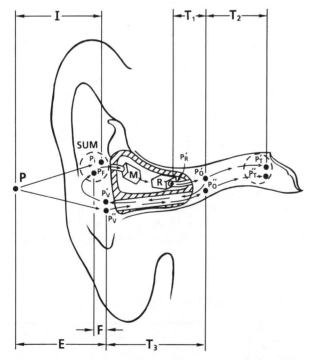

Figure 1. Illustration of the transformation of sound by an in-the-ear hearing aid from the soundfield to the eardrum.

observations by Stinson (1985) and Stinson and Shaw (1983), among others, have shown that this model is inadequate at least for frequencies in the range above approximately 4 to 5 kHz. Later investigators, therefore, have used other models.

Khanna and Stinson (1985) and Stinson (1985), for example, treated the ear canal mathematically as a serial connection of tapered cylinders, called "horns," spaced along a meandering centerline. Kuhn's (1985) mathematical treatment was similar in that he approximated the ear canal as a serial connection of cylinders, but with uniform, rather than tapered sides. Stevens et al. (1987) represented the ear canal as a single uniform cylinder terminated by an off-axis tapered section.

In analytical treatments, models of the ear canal are terminated by the acoustical impedance of the eardrum. If ear canal geometry is correctly determined, then impedance of the eardrum can, in turn, be accurately estimated. Acoustic impedance data for normal ears has been collected in laboratories for many years. In fact, a number of years ago Shaw (1974) summarized eardrum impedance data for normals collected by several investigators. Zwislocki (1963) published eardrum impedance data recorded on several subjects with pathologic middle ears. Rabinowitz (1981) and Larson, Egolf, Cooper, and Oliver (1989) and Larson et al. (1990)

reported more recent acoustic impedance data for normal ears.

Despite the existence of these models, and the ability to measure aural acoustic impedance quantities in the laboratory, a clinically viable yet accurate method for acquiring data that could be used in the context of hearing aid prescriptive fitting methodologies has not evolved. Moreover, until the relatively recent advent of fast personal computers and associated signal processing hardware and software, the implementation of algorithms to obtain both input and eardrum impedance data lacked clinical feasibility.

The remainder of this chapter is devoted to (1) describing present efforts toward implementing a clinically feasible aural acoustic impedance measurement system (Larson et al. 1989; Larson et al. 1990) and (2) the applicability of using the measurements obtained from such a system to prescription fit hearing aids (Larson, Cooper, and Oliver 1990).

A Personal Computer Based System

System Description

The measurement system employed to make these measurements uses a relatively low-cost, two-channel spectrum analyzer (Rapid Systems, Inc. Model 1200 with a Texas Instruments 320-10 signal processor) controlled by an IBM compatible, AT computer.[1] The system is menu-driven, using the data-base handling capability of dBase III+ (Ashton-Tate, Inc.). Menus call 'C' software routines (Microsoft C, V.5.1), which, in turn, pass parameters to assembly language routines in residence in the signal processor. Although an algorithm for precisely quantifying the geometry of the ear canal has been implemented in software, a clinically viable method for obtaining the dimensions of the ear canal has not yet evolved.

Illustrated in figure 2 is the probe assembly, composed of an ER-3A earphone (Etymotic Research, Inc.) and an ER-7C probe microphone (Etymotic Research, Inc.) that was used. The tubing associated with these transducers terminates in an apparatus suited for coupling to the ear canal (Grason-Stadler, 1733 probe tip).

To initiate a measurement sequence, the as-

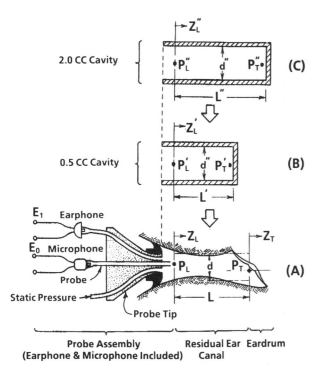

Figure 2. Illustration of the probe-tube assembly as sealed or mounted on (A) the ear canal, (B) a 0.5 cc cavity, and (C) a 2.0 cc cavity.

---

[1] An earlier version (Larson et al. 1989) used a Hewlett-Packard 3582A spectrum analyzer. Data reported herein with that system are so annotated.

sembly is hermetically sealed in the measurement environment and a waveform synthesizer produces a train of brief clicks. Three sets of measurements are made because the method is based on a two-load method (note the two calibration cavities and the ear canal in figure 2). The electrical input to the earphone (E_i) and the electrical output (E_0) from the probe microphone are fed through anti-alias filters to the input of the spectrum analyzer that is bidirectionally interfaced with the computer. Cross and auto-spectra are computed from the signals monitored by the two channels and transfer functions E_0/E_i (magnitude and phase) are computed for each of the three measurements. These calculations, together with the calculation of magnitude-squared coherence functions, as described by Kates this volume, Chapter 12, are made using locally developed software routines. The transfer function data (E_0/E_i) are used to compute impedance quantities at the plane of measurement in the ear canal (Z_L).

Computations Implemented in Software

The real and imaginary parts of acoustic input impedance (Z_L) are computed using the expression in figure 3 where E_0''/E_i'', E_0'/E_i', and E_0/E_i are the measured probe-assembly transfer functions when coupled to the 2.0 cc cavity, the 0.5 cc cavity, and the outer ear canal, respectively. The quantities S'', L'', S', and L' are the cross-sectional areas and lengths of the 2.0 cc and 0.5 cc cavities, respectively. The term k is the wavenumber $2\pi f/c$, where f is frequency, and c is the speed of sound. Air density is represented by the symbol r and j is the imaginary operator $\sqrt{.1}$.

A distributed-parameter model for estimating the acoustic impedance of the ear canal itself was developed and implemented, treating the dimensions of the canal in a manner similar to that of Kuhn (1985). As mentioned earlier, however, due to the lack of a clinically expedient and accurate method to estimate the actual dimensions of the canal, the eardrum impedance data reported herein were obtained by treating the ear canal as a circular cylinder terminated at right angles by the eardrum.

Nevertheless, the algorithm calls for the residual ear canal to be cut up into n hypothetical sag-

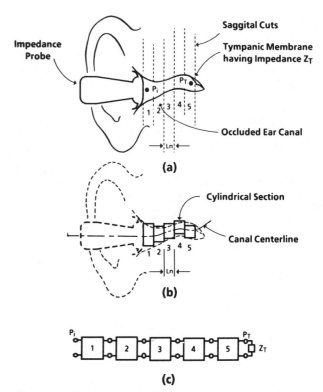

Figure 4. Diagram and illustration of a distributed parameter model for estimating the acoustic impedance of the ear canal.

gital cuts as shown in figure 4a. Each nth slice has a measured cross-sectional area S and thickness L (length corresponding to the centerline distance between saggital cuts) as shown in figure 4b. In order to compute eardrum impedance (Z_T), the multiple-cylinder characterization of figure 4b is represented by a serial connection of two-port electrical analog networks (see figure 4c), each corresponding to one cylinder.

Eardrum impedance (Z_T) is then calculated by the equation

$$Z_T = \frac{Z_L D_S - B_S}{A_S - Z_L C_S}, \qquad (2)$$

where the terms in equation (2) are given by

$$\begin{bmatrix} A_S B_S \\ C_S D_S \end{bmatrix} = \begin{bmatrix} A_1 B_1 \\ C_1 D_1 \end{bmatrix} \begin{bmatrix} A_2 B_2 \\ C_2 D_2 \end{bmatrix} \cdots \begin{bmatrix} A_n B_n \\ C_n D_n \end{bmatrix}, \qquad (3)$$

and

$$Z_L = j \frac{rc(E_0/E_i)[(E_0''/E_i'') - (E_0'/E_i')]}{S''(E_0''/E_i'')[(E_0'/E_i') - (E_0/E_i)]\tan(kL'') - S'(E_0'/E_i')[(E_0''/E_i'') - (E_0/E_i)]\tan(kL')} \qquad (1)$$

Figure 3. Equation (1).

$$A_n = D_n = COS\ (kL_n),$$
$$B_n = j\ (rc/S_n)\ SIN\ (kL_n), \quad (4)$$
$$C_n = j(S_n/rc)\ SIN\ (kL_n).$$

System Validation

Studies of Cylindrical Cavities As a part of a series of studies conducted in order to validate measurements and computations made with the system described herein, input acoustic impedance (Z_L) measurements were made on a variety of cylindrical tubes, up to 1.65 cm inner diameter and 19.8 cm in length with rigid terminations. Transfer function measurements were accomplished as described above with the coherence function for each being very nearly 1.0 at all frequencies. Input impedance calculations of a rigidly terminated cylindrical tube of 1.65 cm inner diameter and 6.0 cm length were made using the software developed to implement equation (1). The result is shown in the illustrations of figure 5 for the real and the imaginary components. Also shown in figure 5 are data calculated using a well-known expression for the input impedance of a hard-wall circular tube with a rigid termination, which is:

$$Z_L = R_L + jX_L \quad (5)$$

where

$$R_L = 0 \text{ and }$$
$$X_L = -j(rc/s)\cot KL$$

Figure 5 shows that there is close agreement between the measured (i.e., utilizing equation [1]) and the computed (i.e., via equation [7]) values of reactance (X_L) except very near the resonance frequencies. Similarly, there is close agreement between the measured (equation [1]) and computed (equation [6]) values of resistance (R_L) except near the resonance frequencies. Resonance peaks in the measured resistance (R_L) curve of figure 5 are artifacts that can be attributed to mathematical anomalies called "poles" that originate in equation (1) when measurements are made on rigidly terminated cylindrical tubes (Ross 1976). There is sufficient justification in the literature (Ross 1976) to allow investigators to neglect these peaks. If these peaks are neglected, then the agreement between measured and computed values of R_L is quite good. Such close agreement between measured and computed values of input acoustic impedance (Z_L) of a rigidly terminated cylindrical tube, as illustrated in figure 5, serves to demonstrate validity of the measurement technique described herein.

Comparison to Published Data Figure 6 shows a comparison to published data of data (Larson et al.

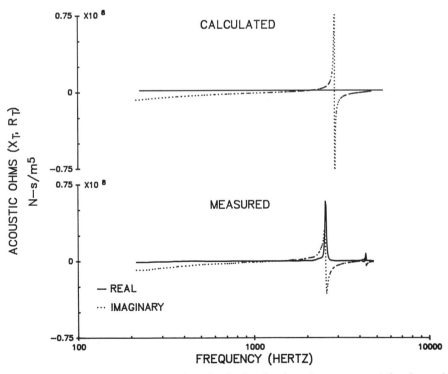

Figure 5. Measured (lower curves) and calculated values (upper curves) for the real and imaginary components of the acoustic impedance of a 1.65 (i.d.) by 6.0 cm cavity with a rigid termination.

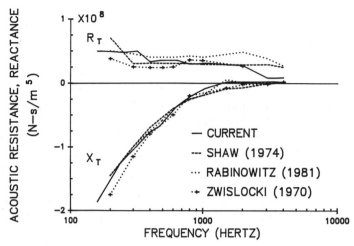

Figure 6.   Comparison of four sets of data (real and imaginary) reported by Larson et al. (1989), Shaw (1974), Rabinowitz (1981), and Zwislocki (1970).

1989) collected on normal ears (N = 6) with the impedance measuring system described herein (Hewlett-Packard spectrum analyzer). The published data in figure 6 include Shaw's (1974) composite curve, mean data reported by Rabinowitz (1981) on four male subjects, and data reported by Zwislocki (1970) on 22 ears. The current data are plotted in 80 Hertz intervals from 160 to 4800 Hz, whereas the data for comparison were taken from illustrations in the cited publications. The ear canal was treated as a single right-circular cylinder, as is common practice. Input impedance (Z_L) was computed from the transfer function measurements using equation (1) and eardrum impedance (Z_T) was computed using equations (2) through (4). Although some of the differences among these sets of data are of theoretical interest, very close agreement is seen.

Repeatability of Measurements   Test-retest comparisons of input-impedance (Z_L) quantities were conducted on four subjects (Larson et al. 1990). After the first transfer function measurements were made, the probe assembly was removed from the ear canal and re-inserted. Excellent agreement between the two sets of means was seen for both the real and the imaginary components, with only slight differences appearing in the imaginary component in the lower frequency region. These were attributed to the difficulties associated with inserting the probe to the same depth in the ear canal and maintaining an hermetic seal. The inter-subject standard deviations associated with both trials were low, on the order of 40 acoustic ohms, across the frequency range for both the real and the imaginary components.

Impedance Measurements and Hearing Aid Fittings

Assuming that the measurement technique described herein is accurate and reliable, and the data collected to date suggest that it is, its application is one in which the manufacturer has implemented the "front-end" of a computer-based hearing aid designing procedure and the audiologist-dispenser then provides the "back-end" or missing-link to the manufacturer: individual aural acoustic impedance data. At the very least, the front-end would need to include a knowledge of the characteristics of the microphone (M), receiver (R), and sound tube (T_1). Receiver characteristics could be provided through component product specifications (Carlson 1974, 1980) or through the use of the two-load method to estimate these quantities (Egolf and Leonard 1977; Bade et al. 1984, Larson and Cooper 1988). Then, within this context, rather than having the manufacturer deliver a product based on "averaged" data, these measurements would allow the manufacturer to account for individual differences in ear canal geometry and eardrum impedance.

Constant-Volume-Velocity Sound Sources and Ear Impedance

Hearing aids, especially in-the-ear (ITE) and in-the-canal (ITC) aids, are commonly assumed to behave as constant-volume-velocity sound sources. That is, they are assumed to have very high acoustic impedances relative to the input impedance of the ear (c.f., Barry and Larson 1980; Egolf, Haley, and Larson 1986). Under this condition, the sound-pressure

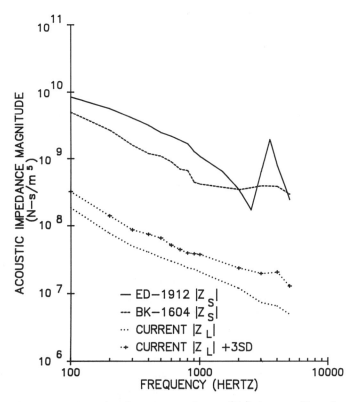

Figure 7. Acoustic Source impedance ($|Z_S|$) for two Knowles Hearing Aid Receivers and for two sets of Acoustic Load ($|Z_L|$) impedance data (Mean and Mean + 3 SD, $N=15$ subjects).

level (SPL) in the ear canal changes in direct proportion to changes in the input or load impedance (Z_L) of the ear, a situation that is problematic to both the audiologist and the manufacturer. Conversely, if the impedance of the source were very low relative to the impedance of the ear, the SPL developed in the ear canal would be independent of the input impedance of the ear. Unfortunately, this is not the case.

To illustrate the importance of ear impedance measurements within this context, reference is made to figure 7 in which the source ($|Z_S|$) and ear ($|Z_L|$) impedance relationships for two receivers (Knowles Electronics, Inc.) *located at the earmold tip*[2] used in a typical ITE hearing aid are shown. The solid line in the upper part of the illustration shows ($|Z_S|$) for an ED-1912 receiver and the dashed line shows ($|Z_S|$) for a BK-1604 receiver at selected frequencies. The lower part of the graph shows mean data (dotted line) for 15 subjects involved in the present study. The remaining set of data in the lower part of the illustration represent values calculated by adding three standard deviations to the mean data ($|Z_L|$ + 3 SD).

With two curves for $|Z_S|$ and two curves for $|Z_L|$,

four source-load combinations are depicted. Observe that, over the entire frequency range, $|Z_S|$ for both receivers is much greater than either set of ear impedance data, exceeding the rule-of-thumb (10 × $|Z_L|$) for judging a constant-volume-velocity condition (Egolf, Haley, and Larson 1986). To further illustrate that the four combinations qualify as constant-volume-velocity conditions, calculations were made of the SPL at a midcanal location that would be developed across $|Z_L|$ (by assuming an arbitrary sound pressure developed across $|Z_S|$ and an arbitrary voltage [E_i] driving the receiver). Figure 8A shows the ear canal sound pressures that would result from the interaction of the ED-1912 receiver with the two ear loads. Not surprisingly, lower sound pressures were developed across the mean load ($|Z_L|$) and higher pressures are developed across the higher impedance load ($|Z_{L3}|$). The difference in sound pressure developed across the two loads can be predicted closely by the expression

$$20 \log_{10} |Z_L|/|Z_{L3}|. \qquad (6)$$

That is, sound pressure in the ear canal changes in direct proportion to the change in load impedance. Figure 8B shows the same comparisons for the BK-1604 receiver. Again, sound pressure changed

---

[2]Tube T_1 as shown in figure 1 is set to zero, a condition that may result in higher $|Z_S|$.

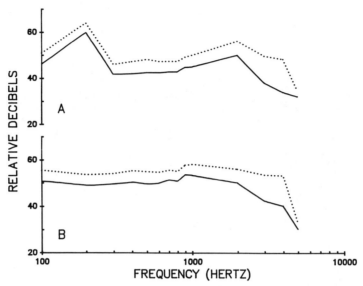

Figure 8. Calculated sound pressures resulting from the four source-load combinations illustration in figure 7.

as a function of ear impedance but, in this case, the difference in SPL was not exactly proportional.

The Hearing Aid Prescription and Acoustic Impedance Measurements

Although the foregoing illustrations served to demonstrate source-load interactions and, thus, the problem created for the manufacturer and the fitter, for purposes of improving hearing aid prescriptions, the appropriate utilization of individual ear impedance data is more illustrative.

Figure 9A shows ear impedance ($|Z_L|$) data (solid line) for a "normal" male ear. The ear is otoscopically normal and the subject had normal hearing and no history of middle ear pathology. Also, for purposes of comparison, the curve for the average ($|Z_L|$) of 15 normal subjects from figure 7 (dashed line) has been redrawn.

Let these data serve as the basis for a hypothetical hearing aid patient and a hypothetical order for an ITE or ITC hearing aid. Assume that data sent to the manufacturer will allow the audiologist/dispenser to meet a specific prescriptive "amplification target," an NAL prescription, perhaps. Recall also that either the audiologist or the manufacturer or both assumed average ear impedance (i.e., the dotted line in figure 9A) at some stage in the ordering and delivery process.

The manufacturer then delivers a response curve based on averaged impedance data and this is verified by both the audiologist and the manufacturer using ear-simulator or corrected 2-cc coupler

measures. The "response" of the ITE or ITC hearing aid with the ED-1912 receiver working into the "average" ear is shown in figure 9B (dotted line). The audiologist, upon receipt of the hearing aid, fits the instrument and does real-ear, probe-tube measures. The solid curve in figure 9B is the "response" of the hearing aid working in the individual ear (impedance data shown as a solid line in figure 9A). The difference, of course, between the average curve and the individual curve in figure 9B is the amount by which the target-gain curve has been incorrectly estimated. The relevance of these data to

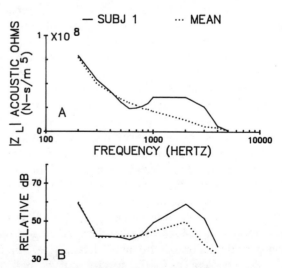

Figure 9. (A) Acoustic impedance data ($|Z_L|$) and (B) calculated sound pressure data for one normal ear for an ED-1912 receiver.

hearing aid prescription and fitting protocols seems obvious: if individual data were provided to the manufacturer, closer approximations to target gain values would result.

Summary

Appropriate use of broad-band acoustic impedance data may serve to improve hearing aid prescription fittings. With the advent of personal computers and associated signal processors, the acquisition, clinically, of such data is feasible. To this end, a personal computer-based measurement system has been developed. Additional research, including an analysis of the applicability of applying broad-band aural impedance data to the various prescriptive hearing aid fitting approaches, is under way. Clinical trials involving the audiologist and the manufacturer in the ordering and dispensing loop are planned.

References

Bade, P.F., Engebretson, A.M., Heidebreder, A.F., Niemoller, A.F. 1984. Use of a personal computer to model the electroacoustics of hearing aids. *Journal of the Acoustical Society of America* 75:617–20.

Barry, S.J., and Larson, V. 1980. Acoustic couplers. *Monographs in Contemporary Audiology.* 2:1–26.

Bauer, K.M. 1987. Mathematical simulation and experimental verification of the closed-loop frequency response of an "in-situ" hearing aid including feedforward. Unpublished M.S.E.E. thesis, Univ. of Wyoming, Laramie, WY.

Bratt, G., Sanders, J., and Larson, V. 1980. Occluded ear canal volume and SPL in children. *ASHA* 22:753.

Carlson, E.V. 1974. Smoothing the hearing aid frequency response. *Journal of the Audio Engineering Society* 22:426–29.

Carlson, E.V. 1980. Electrical analogs for Knowles Electronics, Inc. receivers. Report 10531-1, Industrial Research Products Inc.

Cooper, W.A., Larson, V.D., and Ahlstrom, C.J. 1986. Relationships among admittance, ear canal spectra and body position. *Abstracts of XVIII International Congress on Audiology.* Prague, Czech., 46.

Dalsgaard, S.C., Johansen, P.A., and Chisnall, L.G. 1966. On the frequency response of ear-moulds. *Journal of Audiological Technology* 5:126–39.

Egolf, D. P. 1976. A mathematical scheme for predicting the electroacoustic frequency response of hearing aid receiver-earmold-ear systems. Unpublished doctoral dissertation, Purdue University, West Lafayette, IN.

Egolf, D.P. 1977. Mathematical modeling of a probe-tube microphone. *Journal of the Acoustical Society of America* 61:200–205.

Egolf, D.P. 1980. Techniques for modeling the hearing aid receiver and associated tubing. In *Acoustical Factors Affecting Hearing Aid Measurement and Performance,* eds. G.A. Studebaker and I. Hochberg. Baltimore: University Park Press.

Egolf, D.P., Feth, L.L., Cooper, W.A., and Franks, J.R. 1985. Effects of normal and pathologic eardrum impedance on sound pressure in the aided ear canal: A computer simulation. *Journal of the Acoustical Society of America* 78:1281–1285.

Egolf, D.P., Haley, B.T., and Larson, V.D. 1986. The constant volume velocity nature of hearing aids: Conclusions based on computer simulations. *Journal of the Acoustical Society of America* 79:1592–1602.

Egolf, D., Haley, B., Howell, H., and Larson, V. 1988. A technique for simulating the amplifier-to-eardrum transfer function of an *in-situ* hearing aid. *Journal of the Acoustical Society of America* 84:1–10.

Egolf, D., Haley, B., Bauer, K., Howell, H., and Larson, V. 1988. Experimental determination of cascade parameters of a hearing-aid microphone via the two-load method. *Journal of the Acoustical Society of America* 83:2439–2446.

Egolf, D., Haley, B., Howell, H., Legowski, S., and Larson, V. 1988. Simulating the open-loop transfer function as a means for understanding acoustic feedback in hearing aids. *Journal of the Acoustical Society of America* 85:1, 454–67.

Egolf, D.P., and Leonard, R.G. 1977. Experimental scheme for analyzing the dynamic behavior of electroacoustic transducers. *Journal of the Acoustical Society of America* 62:1013–23.

Gilman, S., Dirks, D.D., and Stern, R. 1981. The effect of occluded ear impedances on the eardrum SPL produced by hearing aids. *Journal of the Acoustical Society of America* 70:370–86.

Grossman, F.M., and Molloy, C.T. 1944. Acoustical sound filtration and hearing aids. *Journal of the Acoustical Society of America* 16:52–59.

Kates, J. 1988. Computer simulation of hearing aid response and the effects of ear canal size. *Journal of the Acoustical Society of America* 83:1952–1963.

Kennedy, W.A., and Egolf, D.P. 1985. Programmable artificial ear incorporating a desk-top scientific computer. *Journal of the Acoustical Society of America* 77:S105.

Khanna, S.M., and Stinson, M.R. 1985. Specification of the acoustic input to the ear at high frequencies. *Journal of the Acoustical Society of America* 77:577–89.

Kuhn, G.F. 1977. Model of the interaural time differences in the azimuthal plane. *Journal of the Acoustical Society of America* 62:157–67.

Kuhn, G.F. 1985. Acoustic pressure distributions in cadaver ear canals. *Journal of the Acoustical Society of America* 78:S12.

Kuhn, G.F., and Greller, L.D. 1984. Sound pressure distributions and resonances in the human ear canal in the presence of a measuring microphone. *Journal of the Acoustical Society of America* 75:S11.

Larson, V., and Cooper, W. 1988. Variables affecting hearing aid performance. *Rehabilitation R&D Progress Reports* 25 (Suppl.):331–32.

Larson, V., Cooper, W., and Oliver, J. 1990. Predicting SPLs in the Ear Canal by Acoustic Impedance Measurements. *ASHA* 32:10.

Larson, V., Cooper, W., Oliver, J., and Egolf, D. 1990. Validation of an aural impedance measurement system. *Audiology Today* 2:32.

Larson, V., Egolf, D., Cooper, W., and Oliver, J. 1989. Estimates of aural acoustic impedance quantities. *ASHA* 31 10:123.

Larson, V.D., Harrell, D.M., and Talbott, R.E. 1984. Ear canal volume and spectra in adults and children. *ASHA* 26:175.

Larson, V., Studebaker, G.A., and Cox, R.M. 1977. Sound levels in a 2-cc cavity, a Zwislocki coupler and occluded ear canals. *Journal of the Acoustical Society of America* 3:63–70.

Lybarger, S.F. 1972. Ear molds. In *Handbook of Clinical Audiology*, ed. J. Katz. Baltimore: Williams and Wilkins.

Rabinowitz, W.M. 1981. Measurements of the acoustic input immittance of the human ear. *Journal of the Acoustical Society of America* 70:1025–1035.

Ross, D.F. 1976. An experimental investigation of the normal specific acoustic impedance of an internal combustion engine. Unpublished doctoral dissertation, Purdue University, West Lafayette, IN. 100–113.

Sanborn, P. (1990). Hearing aid to ear impedance-matching: A literature survey. 1990. *Teknisk Audiologi Report TA 118*. Stockholm: Karolinska Institutet.

Shaw, E.A.G. 1974. The external ear. In *Handbook of Sensory Physiology*, eds. W.D. Keidel and W.D. Neff. Berlin: Springer-Verlag.

Stevens, K.N., Berkovitz, R., Kidd, G., and Green, D.M. 1987. Calibration of ear canals for audiometry at high frequencies. *Journal of the Acoustical Society of America* 81:470–484.

Stinson, M.R. 1985. The spatial distribution of sound pressure within scaled replicas of the human ear canal. *Journal of the Acoustical Society of America* 78:1596–1602.

Stinson, M.R., and Shaw, E.A.G. 1983. Sound pressure distribution in the human ear canal. *Journal of the Acoustical Society of America* 73:559–60.

White, R.E.C., Studebaker, G.A., Levitt, H., and Mook, D. 1980. The application of modeling techniques to the study of hearing and acoustic systems. In *Acoustical Factors Affecting Hearing Aid Measurement and Performance*, eds. G.A. Studebaker and I. Hochberg. Baltimore: University Park Press.

Wiener, F.M., and Ross, D.A. 1946. The pressure distribution in the auditory canal in a progressive soundfield. *Journal of the Acoustical Society of America* 18:401–408.

Zwislocki, J.J. 1963. An acoustic method for clinical examination of the ear. *Journal of Speech and Hearing Research* 6:303–314.

Zwislocki, J.J. 1970. An Acoustic Coupler for Earphone Calibration. Report LSC-S-7. Institute for Sensory Research, Syracuse University, Syracuse, NY.

CHAPTER 14

Complex Signal Testing of Hearing Aids
Limitations and Improvements

Edwin D. Burnett

Kates (this volume, Chapter 12), has summarized the problems with existing standardized techniques for hearing aid testing and has presented new methods for measurement using a random noise signal. This chapter discusses some additional aspects of random noise testing for determining frequency response, for making distortion measurements, and for finding directionality. It also presents the use of speech as a test signal when measuring hearing aids with signal processing circuits whose behavior changes with the temporal nature of the signal.

One fact should be clearly stated at the outset. There is no one measurement technique that indicates the "real" frequency response of a device such as a hearing aid, because there is no one unique frequency response for nonlinear systems. The frequency response obtained with a swept sinusoid is indeed a correct frequency response—for a swept sinusoid. The response may not be useful for predicting performance with speech signals, but it is valid.

Usually, for Automatic Gain Control (AGC) hearing aids, the desired relative frequency response has been considered to be that which would be obtained for the hearing aid when it is operated in the region below the threshold of AGC operation (Preves et al. 1989). In view of this, why go to extreme lengths to measure the frequency response above this threshold, instead of just remaining in the linear region for the measurement? First, the threshold may not be known. If it is know, it may be so low in level that accurate measurements are not possible. Not only the relative response, but the absolute response for a given input level is needed.

This work was supported by the Department of Veterans Affairs.

V. Nedzelmitsky is participating in the study of speech statistics.

Random Noise Tests

Frequency Response The spectrum of the random noise should be shaped to resemble that of speech. This is true because a signal with more relative high-frequency energy than speech, such as a white noise, will cause overload to occur at a lower input level than does speech. This overload occurs because of the high-frequency emphasis used in almost all hearing aids. Accurate measurements then cannot be made, especially at higher input levels. If a shaped input spectrum is used, measurements made with 2-channel analyzers will still show the frequency response directly, because the output spectrum is compared to the input spectrum as part of the 2-channel process. Measurements made with single-channel analysis must be corrected for the input spectrum.

The particular speech weighting referred to by Kates originally was developed for the purpose of obtaining random-noise distortion measurements on hearing aids (Burnett 1967) and then adapted to obtain a single-number saturation sound pressure level. It was based on the data for peak speech levels in the classic study of Dunn and White (1940). In recent years, several studies, using advanced equipment, have made determinations of long-term average speech spectra. The work of Cox and Moore (1988) and the summary by Olsen, Hawkins, and Van Tassell (1987) were especially useful in our studies. These studies tend to show somewhat less high-frequency energy than is found in the random noise spectrum. For comparison, digital speech recordings were made in the large anechoic chamber in our laboratories. These recordings also will be used in the future for determining statistics more detailed than long-term spectra. The recordings were obtained at distances of 1 m and 5 m from the speaker's mouth. These distances are more realistic than the 30 cm spacing that has been used in many studies. The spectrum of a two-minute sample of speech at 1 m, averaged for five male and five female speakers, is shown in figure 1. The averaging is done after normalizing the speech sample from each speaker to the overall sound pressure level for that sample. If this normalization is not done, the spectra of the highest level speakers dominate the average. The spectra at 5 m do not show significant differences from the 1 m spectra, other than the overall level difference expected from the inverse distance law. A determination of the slopes from 500 Hz to 10 kHz, based on a least-squares regression fit was made. The value of the slope was 6.5 dB, a value only slightly greater than the 6 dB per octave originally chosen for the random noise spectrum. the starting frequency for the slope frequency, at least for these samples, is lower, at about 600 Hz.

Many studies of speech spectra have determined the relative levels in one-third octave bands. For comparison with such data, figure 2 shows the averaged levels in one-third octave bands for the same speech samples as in figure 1.

Directionality   A number of different methods have been used for expressing the directional behavior of hearing aids. Some of these, such as the ratio of the sensitivity at 0 degrees to the sensitivity at 180 degrees, are essentially meaningless because they depend upon the sensitivity to an interfering signal at one particular angle, instead of averaging over the entire field. Unless it is known that the undesired noise will occur at one particular position in an acoustically dead environment, basing the measurement on a random arrival angle for the interfering signal is more useful. This type of directivity measurement is commonly used for electroacousti-

cal devices (Beranek 1954). It expresses the ratio of the sensitivity of the device at a particular angle to its sensitivity averaged over all angles. When the ratio is expressed as a level difference it is called the *directivity index*.

The listener will usually be looking at the talker. Thus, the assumption may be made safely that the desired signal is at 0 degrees azimuth and nearly 0 degrees elevation. This assumption will break down in the cases where two people are walking side-by-side and talking or are seated side-by-side and looking ahead. In such situations, a directional hearing aid may not be significantly better than a nondirectional device.

The directional pattern of a hearing aid is very different on a head than in free space. Because the latter condition gives misleading results, directivity should be measured on an anthropometric manikin.

The directivity of a hearing aid varies a great deal with frequency. By using the speech weighted random noise as the test signal, a single number directivity index is obtained that has been weighted by the directivity at various frequencies and by the energy content at those frequencies. This method gives a useful result as long as the desired signal and interfering signal have spectra resembling those of the speech weighted noise. This may not always be the case, and it is sometimes useful to know the directivity index versus frequency. This can be done by using the speech weighted noise as the test signal, and using a turntable whose rotation is halted every 10 degrees while an FFT frequency response measurement is made. The data are then combined to show the directivity index as a function of frequency. Notice that the directivity at any given frequency will not change if tone controls, or other set-

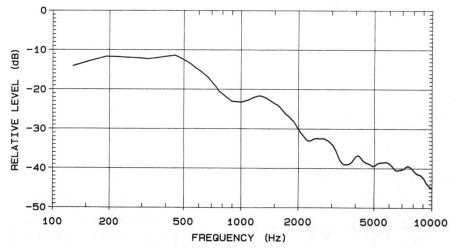

Figure 1.   Spectrum of a two minute sample of speech, relative to the overall level of each speaker, averaged for five male and five female speakers.

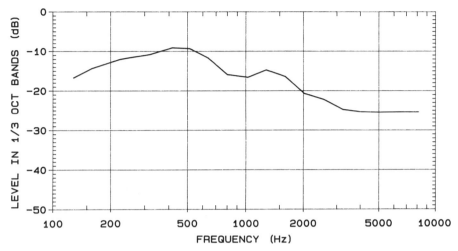

Figure 2. Spectrum of the averaged speech sample of figure 1, determined in one-third octave bands.

tings, are varied, as long as the hearing aid is in linear operation. The random noise directivity will vary as tone settings are changed, because it depends on the integration of the signal with frequency.

Figure 3 shows the directivity index as a function of frequency for two directional hearing aids, a nondirectional hearing aid, and for the open manikin ear. The results for the broad-band speech weighted noise are also shown at the upper frequency end of each plot. Notice that the unaided ear is most directional at high frequencies, whereas the hearing aids are most directional at low frequencies, and may have little directionality in the region where the ear is most directional.

Speech Tests

As useful as random noise is for testing certain types of hearing aids, it is not the ultimate test signal. Random noise, by definition, has a Gaussian amplitude distribution that is exceedingly different from the distribution for a sinusoid. Speech has an amplitude distribution that is neither that of a Gaussian signal nor a sinusoid (figure 4). Speech lingers more at or near zero amplitude (representing quiet intervals) and spends some time at amplitudes greater than a Gaussian signal of the same long-term rms level ever reaches. This is not surprising. After all, not all speech sounds are emitted at the

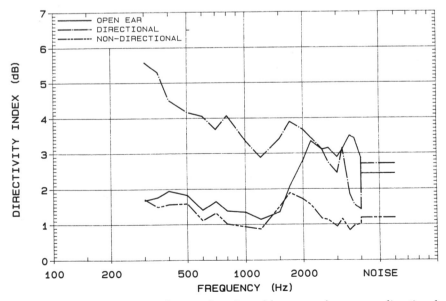

Figure 3. The directivity index as a function of frequency for one nondirectional and two directional hearing aids and for the manikin open ear. The legends are shown on the graph.

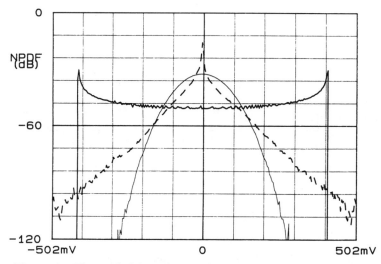

Figure 4. The probability density function (expressed logarithmically) of a sinusoid, of random (Gaussian) noise, and of a sample of male speech. Light trace: random noise. Dark trace: sinusoid. Dashed line: male speech.

same amplitude. Random noise represents speech better than do sinusoids, but still differs in important ways.

The short-term level and spectrum of a random noise signal can be quite different from those of the long-term average signal. Thus, the AGC circuits of a hearing aid may cause a short-term response that is different from the long-term average response that is ultimately determined. This will be especially true for hearing aids with short attack and release times. This may be of enough perceptual significance in some cases that both short- and long-time frequency responses should be measured.

Hearing aids have been developed whose processing depends upon the temporal nature of the signal in order to distinguish speech from noise. Hearing aids incorporating the Zeta Noise Blocker™ circuitry are an example. We have taken an approach to testing these hearing aids that is based on the premise that nothing will simulate the desired characteristics of speech as well as speech itself. A 30-second speech sample, spoken by I. Hirsh as the commentary for track 22 (Houtsma, Rossing, and Wagenaars 1987), was used as the test signal.[1] Measurements were made using a 2-channel FFT analyzer.

Some precautions must be taken when using speech as the input signal for 2-channel FFT analysis. The signal must be continuous in both time and frequency. Time continuity is assured by triggering to the speech signal, so that analysis occurs only when speech is present. This triggering must be done at the lowest level possible without false triggering, or else low-level, high-frequency components will be represented inadequately in the input signal. Frequency continuity can be assured by adding low-level broad-band random noise to the signal, about 60 or 70 dB below the peak speech levels.[2] Further references to "speech alone" should be taken to mean speech plus this very low level "continuity" noise.

Insertion frequency responses for a hearing aid using the Zeta Noise Blocker™ are shown in figures 5A and 5B. The response with speech alone is shown, as are the responses obtained with various levels and frequency bands of added noise, simulating interfering signals.

This method is a general one, because speech is the signal for which a hearing aid, regardless of its type, is designed. Given the present ease of storing signals digitally—especially with compact disc (CD) and CD ROM techniques—a standard speech signal can be conveniently stored and played back with exact repeatability.

---

[1]This particular sample was used because it was on hand at the time the work was done. The compact disc was intended for an entirely different purpose. It would be desirable to use a sample for which complete documentation concerning acoustic environment, talker levels, and microphone type and placement was available.

---

[2]In fact, it is difficult to avoid having extraneous signals of this nature.

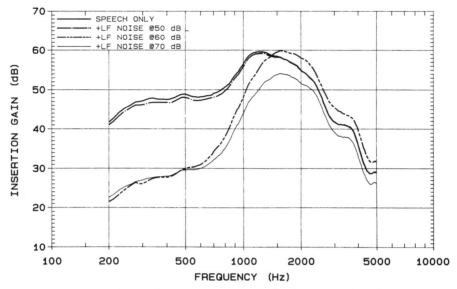

Figure 5A. The insertion frequency response of a hearing aid with Zeta Noise Blocker™ circuitry with speech at an input level of 60 dB, and with several added amounts of low-frequency noise of 400 to 600 Hz. The legends are shown on the graph.

Distortion Measurements

Measures of harmonic distortion have long been used to characterize the nonlinearity of hearing aids. Equipment to make these measurements is readily available and easy to use, but harmonic distortion gives obvious correlations with intelligibility only for large amounts of distortion. For any partic-

ular amplifying system, perceptual effects can be determined empirically for a given amount and type of harmonic distortion, but the results are difficult or impossible to extrapolate to different systems. When many frequencies are present in a signal, the harmonic distortion produced is trivial compared to the intermodulation distortion occurring at sum and difference frequencies of the components of the input signal (Brockband and Wass

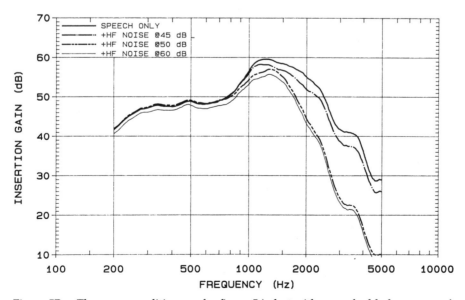

Figure 5B. The same conditions as for figure 5A, but with several added amounts of high-frequency noise of 3000 to 3200 Hz.

1945). Nor do simple two-frequency intermodulation tests adequately model the distortion produced when speech and background noises with many simultaneous frequencies are present. Burnett (1967) suggested that measuring the amount of distortion produced at various frequencies with a random noise input signal would be helpful in predicting the objectionability of distortion. Peters and Burkhard (1969) showed that the effects of distortion depended not only upon the amount of distortion, but also upon the nature of the nonlinear process. With measurements of distortion using noise as the signal, information about the nature of the distortion process is lost. Bell-Northern Research has prepared several reports for the International Telegraph and Telephone Consultative Committee (CCITT) (1983a, 1983b, 1987) concerning work using a synthetic speech signal. The output range is divided into four quartiles. This method predicted perceptive results reasonably well for those distorting processes studied. The work has not been extended to systems having various sorts of frequency response, such as hearing aids, nor to listeners with hearing losses.

It is not clear at the present time that other measures of distortion, including coherence, have been developed to the point where reliable predictions can be made, although methods such as Kates (this volume, Chapter 12) go a long way in this direction. There may well be interactions between nonlinearity and certain frequency response effects (e.g., peaks in the response), which would require very complicated algorithms for exact evaluation. This should not be taken to disparage investigation of advanced techniques: it is clear that harmonic distortion measurements cannot be predictive of speech degradation in hearing aids, and other methods are needed.

Given the complications of distortion evaluation, it is easy to see why it is considered desirable to keep distortion low, at least at the gain setting and input level used for evaluation. If the distortion is low enough, then the functional relation of distortion to perception is trivial. Zero times any multiplier is still zero. Unfortunately, in the real world, overload will always occur at some point, if not in the output circuits because of AGC, then in the input circuits. Its occurrence may be dictated by economy of circuitry, battery drain, vanity (small size), or by the need for ear protection. Given that saturation must occur at some level, is it better for it to occur abruptly, as indicated by a transfer function like the dark line of figure 6, or gradually, as shown in the light line of the same figure? If the signal is always below the ultimate overload level, it would appear that abrupt clipping is superior. However, if higher levels do occur, abrupt clipping will produce high order components with an objectionable quality.

Thus, a device that shows low distortion for an input level of say 70 dB, but abrupt overload at 75 dB, may be more objectionable than one that shows higher distortion at 70 dB because of a gradual overload characteristic. This overload property cannot be addressed by measurements at only one level. A meaningful measure might consist of distortion

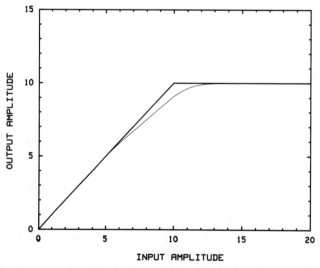

Figure 6. Two hypothetical output versus input level functions. Dark trace: abrupt overload. Light trace: gradual overload.

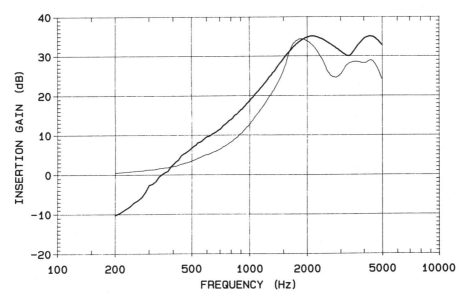

Figure 7A.   Insertion frequency response of two in-the-ear hearing aids, intended to be similar in frequency response. Dark trace: hearing aid with a closed ear mold. Light trace: hearing aid with an open ear mold.

measurements at more than one level, or of input/ output curves near the overload point combined with distortion measurements.

It is not true that the high-frequency cutoff of a hearing aid will eliminate high-order components produced by abrupt clipping. There will be as many difference-frequency components falling at low frequencies as there are sum-frequency components falling at high frequencies. This is shown for second-order distortion in Corliss et al. (1968).

In fact, many hearing aids, if they are used with a closed-mold fitting, will have low-frequency outputs that consist of more spurious components than of the actual input signal. Figure 7A shows the insertion frequency responses of two in-the-ear hearing aids, one with a closed ear mold and one with an open ear mold. They are intended to have similar frequency responses, within the constraints of the two types of molds. Figure 7B shows the coherence functions of the same hearing aids. Notice

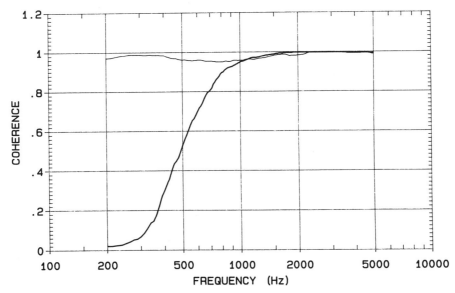

Figure 7B.   Coherence functions for the same hearing aid and test conditions, showing the low coherence function (high relative amount of incoherent power) at low frequencies when a closed mold design is used.

that with the closed mold design the low frequency output below 500 Hz consists of incoherent signals, which in this case are a mixture of distortion products and the internal noise of the hearing aid. Although the gain of the hearing aids is low in this region, a subject fitted for one of these hearing aids would likely have sufficient sensitivity in these low frequencies for these components to be audible. Thus, the venting produces not only frequency shaping, but by this shaping, and by passing the direct acoustic signal, it is also produces a significant low-frequency distortion reduction. However, only so much distortion reduction can be achieved by this technique. Many distortion components will fall in the midst of the actual midrange speech components, and these cannot be eliminated.

References

Bell-Northern Research 1983. Objective evaluation of non-linear distortion effects on voice transmission quality. CCITT COM XII-131.

Bell-Northern Research 1983. Evaluation of non-linear distortion using simulated speech signals. CCITT COM XII-132.

Bell-Northern Research 1986. Objective evaluation of non-linear distortion effects on voice transmission quality. CCITT CAN COM XII-8.

Bell-Northern Research 1987. Re-evaluation of the objective method for measurement of non-linear distortion. CCITT COM XII-175.

Beranek, L.L. 1954. *Acoustics.* New York: McGraw-Hill Book Company.

Brockband, W.A., and Wass, C.A.A. 1945. Non-linear distortion in transmission systems. *Journal of the Institution of Electrical Engineers* 92(Pt III):45–56.

Burnett E.D. 1967. A new method for the measurement of nonlinear distortion using a random noise test signal. *Bulletin of Prosthetics Research* Spring.

Corliss, E.L.R., Burnett, E.D., Kobal, M.T., and Bassin, M.A. 1968. The relative importance of frequency distortion and changes in time constants in the intelligibility of speech. *IEEE Transactions in Audio and Electroacoustics* AU-16:36–39.

Cox, R.M., and Moore, J.N. 1988. Composite speech spectrum for hearing aid gain prescriptions. *Journal of Speech and Hearing Research* 32:102–107.

Dunn, H.K., and White, S.D. 1940. Statistical measurements in conversational speech. *Journal of the Acoustical Society of America* 11:278–88.

Houtsma, A.J.M., Rossing, T.D., and Wagenaars, W.M. 1987. *Auditory Demonstrations.* Compact disc Phillips: 1126–061. New York: Acoustical Society of America. Prepared at the Institution for Perception Research for the Acoustical Society of America.

Olsen, W.O., Hawkins, D.B., and Van Tassell, D.J. 1987. Representations of the long-term spectra of speech. *Ear and Hearing* 8:100S.

Peters, R.W., and Burkhard, M.D. 1968. *On Noise Distortion and Harmonic Distortion Measurements.* Industrial Research Products, Inc. Report No. 10350-1 (Preliminary).

Preves, D.A., Deck, L.D., Burnett, E.D., and Teder, H. 1989. Input stimuli for obtaining frequency responses of automatic gain control hearing aids. *Journal of Speech and Hearing Research* 32:189-94.

PART IV
Evaluation Procedures

CHAPTER 15
Measures of Intelligibility and Quality

Gerald A. Studebaker

This chapter discusses aspects of intelligibility and quality measures as they relate to hearing aid selection and the measurement of hearing aid performance. The literature on the measurement of speech intelligibility is extensive, with several books (e.g., Konkle and Rintelmann 1983; Martin 1987) and many chapters devoted to the subject. For these reasons, a comprehensive review of the area is not attempted. Instead, I first discuss a few selected issues concerning the reliability of intelligibility and quality measures. The chapter concludes with some remarks about models of speech recognition and their potential utility in the areas of hearing aids, hearing impairment, and rehabilitation needs assessment.

Definitions

The terms used in the title of this chapter perhaps require some discussion. It is generally assumed that the term *speech intelligibility* refers to the recognition *and* understanding of meaningful speech units. *Recognition* is taken to mean the identification of meaningful or nonmeaningful speech elements, including phonemes and nonsense syllables. Understanding is not implied. Thus, the term *recognition* is more appropriate in some applications, such as speech recognition testing. *Intelligibility* is used in the title, however, because the chapter includes a discussion of judgments of speech intelligibility as well. In the text, both words are used as seems appropriate.

The term *quality*, in the title of this chapter, is assumed to mean the overall "goodness" of an electronically processed signal. It thereby includes all of the characteristics that might contribute to overall quality, such as intelligibility, pleasantness, clarity, quietness, or other features. Often investigators have asked subjects to judge the quality of hearing aid processed signals. One problem with the use of the word *quality* in this application is that it is uncer-

tain which features a subject will use as a basis for his or her judgment or whether all subjects will use the same criteria or criterion. Thus, the word *quality* in the title does not necessarily mean exactly the same thing as what is assessed when a subject is asked to judge quality in a laboratory or clinic procedure.

Speech intelligibility and speech recognition can be directly measured using either objective or subjective methods. Quality, as used here, can be tested only with subjective methods. In this context, objective procedures are those wherein the responses of the subject are scored right or wrong by the examiner. Subjective procedures are those wherein the subject is asked to make a judgment about some aspect of a signal.

Reliability Issues

Monosyllabic Word Tests

It was not very many years ago that speech recognition testing dominated at least the audiological segment of the hearing aid selection business. Now that has changed. One of the reasons for the change is that these tests are seen as not very reliable. Although speech tests have a substantial degree of face validity, validity without reliability is meaningless. Given these conditions, one of two courses of action was available. Investigators could attempt to improve the reliability of the speech recognition tests, or they could substitute other, more reliable, procedures. One hoped that the validity of these procedures would be established in the laboratory. Both approaches have been tried.

What can be done to improve the reliability of the speech recognition test? Thornton and Raffin (1978) effectively demonstrated that the reliability of the monosyllable word recognition test, although perhaps not very good, was, in fact, close to what was predicted by the binomial theorem, at least

185

when interlist differences in difficulty are reduced to a minimum. One implication of these results may be that little can be done to improve the reliability of a recognition test other than to (1) reduce the interlist differences in difficulty and (2) increase the number of scorable items. The effects of interlist differences are discussed first.

Correcting For List Difficulty Differences   Over the past few years, our group has used the Technisonics W-22 monosyllabic word test in several experiments. This test consists of four lists of 50 words each. It soon became apparent to us that the four lists were not equally difficult. In addition, it was noted that the relative difficulty of the four lists varied with masker and filter conditions. To compensate for this, we presented all four lists an equal number of times under each listening condition, a procedure in line with common experimental practice.

While often necessary, it should be noted that counterbalancing does have a negative effect—it increases the observed intersubject and/or test-retest variance by an amount equal to the interlist variance. The relation is shown in equation 1.

$$Var_{obs} = Var_{true} + Var_{list} \qquad (1)$$

The equation suggests that one way to obtain a more accurate picture of the true intersubject or test-retest variance in a counterbalanced study is to subtract the list variance from the observed variance. We found that the effect of this operation in the case of the W-22 test was to reduce the apparent test–retest or intersubject standard deviation by about 0.3% to 1.5%, depending on the size of the list difficulty difference under the listening condition in question.

In some experiments, and frequently in clinical situations, counterbalancing cannot be done. In these cases, a correction for list difficulty difference might be helpful. A possible method to do this is to use the proficiency factor. The proficiency factor could prove to be a powerful tool in this application because it permits correction for the list effect under essentially all listening conditions.

The proficiency factor is an articulation index concept designed to account for differences in the proficiency of talkers and listeners (Fletcher and Galt 1950). In this case, lists are treated as though they were different talkers. In order to obtain a proficiency factor, it is necessary to know the transfer function, the relation between score and the articulation index, for the test material being used. Unfortunately, transfer functions are now available for only a few test materials. However, at least one appeared in 1991 (Studebaker and Sherbecoe 1991), and more should become available in the next several years.

As one check on the validity of the procedure, the proficiency factor correction was applied to a set of counterbalanced word recognition data that included a substantial list difficulty effect. The reduction in variability obtained was compared to the reduction determined by subtracting variances, as described previously. The comparison is shown in figure 1. It can be seen that the reduction in intersubject standard deviation produced by the two methods was similar in magnitude and pattern. The somewhat smaller reductions produced by the proficiency factor correction probably were due to the fact that the list proficiency values used in the calculation were based on data from a separate study.

Another check on the proficiency factor in this application was carried out using data from another study in which the W-22 word lists had been always presented in the same order, a procedure used because we were primarily interested in the distribution of the subjects' performances. The subjects were inexperienced listeners, so it was expected that performance would improve over trials. Average performance over three presentations of four lists without a correction for list difficulty is shown as the line labeled *Unadjusted* in figure 2. In this case, performance varied so greatly that the learning effect could be discerned only with difficulty. The line labeled *Adjusted* in the figure shows the same data after correction for list difficulty using list proficiency factors. The factor values were obtained in an earlier study in which conditions were counterbalanced and highly experienced subjects were used. The adjustment caused the data to be more

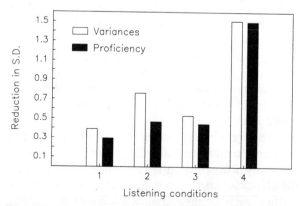

Figure 1.   A comparison of the reduction in intersubject standard deviations produced by (1) subtracting the list variance from the observed variance and (2) correcting individual scores for list difficulty based on list proficiency factors obtained in a separate study.

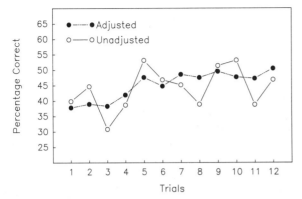

Figure 2. A comparison of learning curves before and after correction for list difficulty effects using list proficiency factors obtained in a separate study.

regular, and made the learning effect more obvious. Some residual irregularity remains, possibly because the relative difficulty of the lists differs for experienced and inexperienced subjects.

Increasing Scorable Units Although adjusting for interlist differences is difficult and produces relatively small rewards in the case of a well-designed test, making a test longer and/or adding subjects is simple to do and produces substantial rewards. Unfortunately, these methods can be time consuming. The basic relation is well known, but for completeness it is presented in equation 2.

$$SD_n = \frac{SD_o}{\sqrt{N_p}} \qquad (2)$$

The equation says that, as data are added, the proportionate decrease in the standard deviation is equal to the reciprocal of the square root of N, where N is the proportion of additional data. The critical difference is decreased to the same extent. Thus, in order to reduce the critical difference by half, it is necessary to collect four times as much data.

Adding subjects and replications are not normally practical solutions to the reliability problem in clinical applications for the reason that they take too much time. Two alternatives that have been put forward to increase scorable elements while not significantly increasing testing time are phoneme scoring (Boothroyd 1968) and tri-word testing (Harris 1980). In a tri-word test, three words are presented to the subject at a time. Although the method has been little studied, the work of Sergeant, Atkinson, and LaCroix (1979) indicates that multiple word presentations do not produce improved reliability. Possibly the added complexity for the subject offsets the increased number of scorable items.

The picture with phoneme scoring is more positive. For example, in 1976, Walker and Booth-

royd found that phoneme scoring of an NU-6 monosyllabic word test improved the reliability of the test by an amount approximately equal to that predicted by the relation shown in equation 2. In the case of the NU-6 test, which has three phonemes per word, the expected reduction in the critical difference would thus be the reciprocal of the square root of three, or about 0.58 of the critical difference for word scoring of the same test. This appears to be a substantial gain in reliability with no increase in testing time and only a slight increase in scoring effort.

Up-Down Tests

The literature suggests another method for improving the reliability of speech tests. This is the adaptive, or up-down method. In contrast to conventional speech testing, where the speech and noise levels are held constant, the adaptive tests vary the intensity of the speech or the noise in order to estimate the level at which a predetermined percentage of correct recognition will be achieved (Dubno, Dirks, and Morgan 1984; Plomp 1986; Van Tasell and Yanz 1987; Walker and Byrne 1985). The results of these tests are given in dB rather than in percent correct.

Several researchers have described the reliability of these adaptive speech recognition tests as "high" (Dubno, Dirks, and Morgan 1984, p. 95), "quite good" (Plomp 1986, p. 147) and "excellent" (Walker and Byrne 1985, p. 24). This is high praise for a speech test, particularly when contrasted to the words often used to describe the reliability of 50-item word recognition tests. However, the difference in the reliability of these two types of tests probably is not so great as the differences in adjectives might suggest.

In order to make a comparison, the results of one type of procedure need to be converted into units that can be compared with the other. First, convert typical monosyllabic word test-retest variability, expressed in percent, into variability in dB using the following relation:

$$SD_{dB} = \frac{SD_\%}{(\% / dB)} \qquad (3)$$

That is, the standard deviation in dB is assumed to equal the standard deviation in percent divided by the slope of the performance-intensity function in percent per dB.

According to the binomial theorem, the within-subject variability of a single 50-word test is 7.07%. Thus, the test-retest standard deviation would be 10%. This gives a 95% confidence interval of about

±20%, or a 40% range. This is exactly the kind of result that has caused many to conclude that the reliability of the speech recognition test is poor. According to Bess (1983) the performance-intensity function slope for the NU-6 monosyllabic word test is about 5.6%/dB. Thus, according to the relation shown in equation 3, the predicted test-retest standard deviation in dB for this material is 1.8 dB.

This result is compared with test-retest standard deviations reported for the up-down procedure in the literature in table I. The results at the top of the table are for the quiet listening condition. As shown, in quiet, Dubno, Dirks, and Morgan (1984) obtained a test-retest SD of 1.3 for low probability SPIN sentences, and Van Tasell and Yanz (1987) obtained 1.7 dB for spondee words.

At the bottom of table I are shown results for the noise masked condition. In each case, the noise used was either the same as, or was similar to, the spectrum of the talker's speech. Under these conditions, the P-I function slope for monosyllables is at least 8%/dB (Studebaker and Sherbecoe 1991). Using this slope in our calculation produces a value of 1.2 dB as the test-retest variability of a 50-item test expressed in dB. This is the same as the value reported by Walker and Byrne (1985) for an up-down procedure and only slightly larger than that reported by Plomp (1986). It is, however, substantially larger than that reported by Dubno, Dirks, and Morgan (1984).

Although test-retest variability of monosyllable word lists perhaps looks somewhat larger in these comparisons, conversion of the up-down results into percentages, using the same method in reverse, produces a somewhat different picture. In this conversion it was assumed that spondee P-I

function in quiet is 13%/dB, based on the data of Hudgins et al. (1947) and Harris (1948). The spondee function in speech spectrum noise is about 18%/dB as determined from the 1983 summary of Wilson and Margolis (1983, p. 88). The P-I slope for sentences in speech shaped noise is about 15%/dB according to Plomp and Mimpen (1979) and Walker and Byrne (1985). The low probability SPIN sentences used by Dubno, Dirks, and Morgan (1984) have a slope of about 6.3%/dB and the high probability sentences a slope of about 14%/dB, according to our reading of the 1977 Kalikow, Stevens, and Elliot curves (Taylor 1991). Using these values, the test-retest variability of the adaptive tests reported in several studies, converted to percent, are shown in table II. Again, the results in quiet are recorded at the top of the table and the results in noise are at the bottom. In each case, the test-retest standard deviations for monosyllables were assumed to be 10%, as suggested by the binomial theorem. Note that while the Dubno, Dirks, and Morgan results generally reveal smaller test-retest standard deviations than monosyllables, the range of results across the various up-down studies is substantial, with some producing values considerably larger than 10%.

Obviously, care should be taken not to overinterpret these comparisons because of the differences in test materials and listening conditions used in various studies. Also, one should not jump to the conclusion that the reliability of the up-down procedures is poor. Perhaps it is our view of 50-item tests that needs modification. But in either case, the comparison seems adequate to make the point that the variabilities of the 50-item tests and the up-down procedures may not be so different as a casual reading of the literature might suggest.

Table I. The Test-retest Variability (in dB) Reported in Several Investigations for the Up-down Speech Threshold Procedure†

Quiet	
Dubno et al. (1984), SPIN-PL	1.3 dB
Van Tasell & Yanz (1987), spondees	1.7 dB
Binomial Theorem, 50 monosyllabic words	1.8 dB*
Noise	
Dubno et al. (1984), SPIN-PL	0.7 dB
Plomp (1986), sentences	1.0 dB
Binomial Theorem, 50 monosyllabic words	1.2 dB**
Walker & Byrne (1985), speech passage	1.2 dB

　*assumes slope of 5.6%/dB

　**assumes slope of 8.0%/dB

†Also included is an estimate of the test-retest variability (in dB) of a 50-item monosyllabic word test in quiet and in noise. See text for a discussion of the transformation.

Table II. The Estimated Test-retest Variability (in %) Based on Several Up-down Results Originally Reported in dB†

Binomial Theorem	
Monosyllabic words, 50 items	10%
Quiet	
Dubno et al. (1984), SPIN-PL	8%
Dubno et al. (1984), SPIN-PH	16%
Van Tasell & Yanz (1987), spondees	22%
Noise	
Dubno et al. (1984), SPIN-PL	4%
Dubno et al. (1984), SPIN-PH	6%
Plomp (1985), sentences	15%
Walker & Byrne (1985) speech passage	18%

†See text for a discussion of the transformation. Also reported is the text-retest variability (in %) of a 50-item test based on the binomial theorem.

Subjective Judgments

Recently, subjective judgments of hearing aid quality and intelligibility have been put forward as possible clinical procedures because they can be done quickly and because early evidence from experiments using paired comparisons indicated they are reasonably reliable and valid. More recent evidence (e.g., Punch et al. 1980; Studebaker et al. 1982) supported the conclusion of Zerlin (1962) that the paired comparison procedure was reliable. It was also demonstrated that the reliability of paired comparisons of both quality and intelligibility was somewhat better than that of nonsense syllables by Punch and Parker (1981) and slightly better than a 50-item monosyllabic test by Studebaker et al. (1982). An additional advantage of these procedures, noted by Zerlin (1962), Studebaker et al. (1982), and Tecca and Goldstein (1984) was that they reliably differentiated among aids even in cases where differences in objectively measured recognition scores were not significant. Unfortunately the literature also suggests that the reliability of hearing-impaired listeners may be less than that of normal-hearing subjects (Schwartz et al. 1980 versus Punch et al. 1980 and Studebaker et al. 1982).

The reliability of subjective methods other than paired comparisons may not be as good as objectively scored tests. Cox, Alexander, and Rivera (in press) compared objective and subjective measures of intelligibility using the Connected Speech Test (CST). Subjective scores were obtained using a rating technique. The objective scores were based on 150 key words. (The results of this experiment were expressed in rationalized arcsine units, or rau [Studebaker 1985]. Over most of the score range, rau may be thought of as comparable to percentage.)

The objective score test-retest critical difference reported by Cox and colleagues (in press) was 10.3 rau for the normal-hearing subjects. It should be noted that the critical difference predicted for a 150-item test by the binomial theorem is 10.5 rau. This close agreement suggests that the reliability of the objectively scored CST is as good as any well-designed test with 150 scorable items. The critical difference of the objective scores of the hearing-impaired subjects was somewhat greater at 12.5 rau. The critical differences for the subjective ratings ranged from 15.7 rau for normal hearers to 22.5 rau for the hearing impaired. Thus, the test-retest variability of the subjective estimates was 1.5 to 1.8 times greater than for the objective scores, while the test-retest variability of the older hearing-impaired subjects was about 20% to 40% greater than for normal-hearing subjects.

In a 1988 report, Studebaker and Sherbecoe noted that in addition to substantial test-retest variability, magnitude estimations were subject to nonlinear practice effects. That is, some subjects would give relatively similar estimations on repeated trials on one day, but then give a quite different set of somewhat internally consistent results on another day. Only 30% of the variance in the second day's results could be predicted from a knowledge of the first day's results.

In spite of these problems, in applications where the reliability problem can be dealt with adequately, magnitude estimations and ratings of quality and intelligibility can be quite useful because they have unique features. They are fast, thereby permitting research designs with a greater number of factors and levels in one experiment. They can be used under conditions in which objective scores are at or near 100%. In addition, they can be used to evaluate qualitative aspects of speech that cannot be evaluated by objective tests such as those done by Gabrielsson and his colleagues (e.g., Gabrielsson, Schenkman, and Hagerman 1988). Finally, in contrast to paired comparison data, magnitude estimations and ratings have good statistical characteristics.

Models

Acoustical Methods and Models

Another possible way to improve the reliability of intelligibility and quality measures is to assess them indirectly based on more reliable measures such as pure tone or noise thresholds or sound pressure levels in the ear canal. Then, based on what we think we know about the relationship between these quantities and intelligibility and quality, decide which values will result in the best intelligibility and quality for the subject. Most modern hearing aid selection methods are of this type. Although none of these methods actually provides quantitative predictions of intelligibility or quality, it is assumed, in each case, that the subject will perform best under the amplification conditions calculated to be optimal for him or her. This assumption is based on connections made in the laboratory and/or by logical argument.

Some of these procedures can be thought of as simplified models in that they include elements that are mathematical representations of a real system. The system being modeled, in most cases, is the acoustical system consisting of the characteristics of the source signal and the pathway it follows in going from the talker's lips to the listener's eardrum. Factors taken into consideration may include an assumed speech spectrum at the source and various elements of the signal transmission pathway including hearing aid, earmold, and subject's ear canal. It also may include some necessary ancillary aspects such as 2-cc coupler-to-real-ear transfer functions, and so forth.

Speech Recognition Models

Principles   Although these methods have proved very useful, more fully developed models probably could be used to even greater advantage. For example, a model that estimated the speech recognition performance of a patient based on his or her pure tone thresholds would have considerable potential. I will call models of this type *speech recognition models*. Some of the possible applications of these models are described later, but first some of the characteristics of models in general are noted.

One characteristic of any mathematical model is that it is absolutely reliable. That is, it gives exactly the same answer every time it is run with a particular set of input values. Unfortunately, however, the results may not be valid in that the answer may not be correct for some particular set of conditions. This could occur because either the model is incomplete or an assumption made in the creation of the model is in error or does not apply in a particular case. For example, the model may not take some effect of hearing loss into account or the effects of hearing loss might be quantitatively incorrect in the model.

Although measurements on human beings have greater face validity than the output of a model, such measurements are valid only to the extent that they are reliable. I would suggest also that there is the real possibility that we will not be able to make intelligibility measures on people much more reliable than they are now, a conclusion suggested by the earlier discussion. However, it seems likely that we will be able gradually to improve our models almost indefinitely. This reasoning appears to justify further work on models for future applications.

It seems self-evident that, when dealing with systems that can be measured with only relatively low reliability, a model may be a better predictor of long-term average ("true") performance of the system than will one or two measurements made at a particular time on the real thing. This statement would appear to apply in the case of speech recog-

nition testing where the test-retest variability of the measurement is large relative to differences that are thought to be significant.

Of course, this statement will be true only if the model is valid for the application in which it is being used. A valid model is one that predicts a result within acceptable limits of the true measured value over the major part of the range of expected input conditions. Given this definition, perhaps no one would argue that the statement is wrong but would argue instead that we do not have an adequate model now and that one is not likely to appear anytime soon. I would agree that we do not have one now, but recent work by Ludvigsen (1985, 1987), Leijon (1989), and work in my laboratory suggests that useful models could be produced now with the promise of rapid improvements if the approach were to be taken up by larger numbers of workers.

An Implementation   To test some of these ideas, I developed a prototypical model that predicts average speech recognition scores for the Technisonics W-22 monosyllabic word test under a wide range of acoustical conditions. This test material was used because we have the necessary information about it, in the form of frequency importance and transfer functions, to make the speech recognition predictions. The model is based on an extension of articulation theory which I have labeled *audibility theory*. A basic premise of audibility theory, like articulation theory, is that long-term average speech recognition scores can be predicted based on the derived weighted audibility of the speech signal.

I am promoting the use of the term *audibility theory* in these applications for several reasons. First, this term seems to describe more accurately the fact that it is the audibility of the signal that such models use in making their calculations. Also, it places emphasis on the activity of interest to us, that is, audition. The term *articulation* is thereby left to describe the act of producing speech.

Audibility theory differs from articulation theory principally in that it takes the effects of hearing loss and hearing aids into account. The current prototype does not include a provision for inputting modulation transfer function data, but it could easily be modified to do so.

One of the outputs of the model is an index called the weighted audibility index or WAI. This abbreviation helps differentiate it from the Articulation Index, or AI, and makes it clear that in making the calculations audibility has been weighted. The weighting factors include, for example, the frequency importance function for the speech material being used and two desensitization factors, one based on the absolute intensity of the signals and the other on the extent of the subject's hearing loss in each frequency band (Pavlovic, Studebaker, and Sherbecoe 1986). The model includes a calculation for high- and low-frequency spread of masking and widened critical bands. It incorporates several of the current threshold based hearing aid selection procedures, including the revised NAL, POGO, and others. The audibility calculation takes into account the hearing aid's frequency response and the frequency response of the test system, as well as any masking noise spectrum and level specified by the user. Another output of the model is the word recognition performance score. In making this calculation, the model takes the listening experience of the subject into consideration.

The model also calculates the loudness of the combined speech and noise signal. It uses the Zwicker method referred to as *Method B* in ISO standard 532-1977 (International Standards Organization 1977). We modified a basic program by Zwicker, Fastl, and Dallmayr (1984) to allow for the input of hearing loss and to obtain an output of the value of gain needed to produce a desired loudness level in phons. The Zwicker, Fastl, and Dallmayr program already included a provision for normal recruitment, that is, a recruitment that behaves like that seen in normal ears at low and high test tone frequencies. If a hearing-impaired subject's individual overall loudness function is available from a procedure like that recently demonstrated by Hellman and Meiselman (1988, 1990), the coefficient for that function can be used. However, if the subject's coefficients vary across frequency in a manner different from that assumed by the program, substantial reprogramming would be required.

In a 1989 dissertation, Leijon suggested that a hearing aid's characteristics should be chosen using a cost-benefit optimization model. That is, each change made in a hearing aid's response must be evaluated both in terms of the benefits gained and the costs incurred. In the case of frequency response, for example, adding energy in the high frequencies might increase audibility and thereby increase intelligibility. This represents the benefit side of the equation. However, this manipulation might also increase sound power and loudness, thereby making the sound less acceptable. The effect of the increased loudness probably would cause the subject to turn down the hearing aid's gain in order to re-establish an acceptable loudness. This, of course, has the effect of *reducing* audibility and intelligibility, and is the cost of the frequency modification.

The question is, do the benefits outweigh the costs? More precisely, was weighted audibility greater before or after the frequency response adjustment, assuming that gain is reset to achieve the same loudness in each case? Based on this reasoning it seems evident that the goal of any audibility-based hearing aid selection procedure should not be to maximize the audibility index only, but rather to maximize the index while holding loudness, or some other relevant variable, constant.

It also follows from this that anyone who evaluates the relative merits of hearing aid selection procedures on the basis of the size of the AI, or the WAI, without taking loudness or another relevant variable into account, as was recently reported in one of the trade journals (Berger 1990), is misguided. If loudness is not considered, then it is perfectly obvious that the hearing aid prescription method that calls for the most gain will be deemed the best method, a result that is often not true.

An Example   I would now like to show an example of the kinds of things that a speech recognition model can do. Although these results might be considered interesting and suggestive, they must, at this time, be considered preliminary. Although the model worked quite well in a recently completed validation test, there are many important aspects that have yet to be tested.

Figure 3 shows the calculated effect of variations in frequency response slope on weighted audibility under the constraint of a constant calculated loudness. Results for three different hearing losses taken from the literature are shown. Along the abcissa is relative frequency response slope. In this example, zero slope is that frequency response determined using the revised National Acoustics Lab-

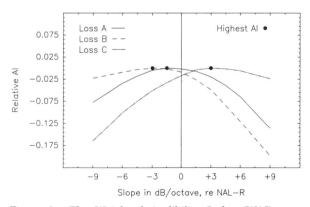

Figure 3.   The Weighted Audibility Index (WAI) as a function of frequency response slope for three cases. The dots indicate the slope producing the maximum WAI in each case.

oratories method (NAL-R) described by Byrne and Dillon (1986). Many other procedures could be used to produce a starting condition.

The other slopes along the abcissa are obtained by adding plus or minus 1.5, 3.0, 4.5, 6.0, and 9.0 dB/octave to the reference response. More sophisticated ways of making this adjustment are now under development. The ordinate records the weighted audibility index (WAI) obtained under each slope condition with calculated loudness held constant. In this figure, the WAI values were plotted relative to the maximum value obtained for each hearing loss, though in practice we plot out absolute values.

The procedure was: (1) calculate the audibility index obtained with the NAL-R response; (2) calculate the loudness of the amplified speech for an average person with the hearing loss in question; (3) modify the slope by 1.5 dB/oct; (4) adjust the gain of the modeled hearing aid until the calculated loudness was returned to its original value; and (5) calculate the weighted audibility index at this new gain setting. This procedure was then repeated at each of the other slopes.

If one were to use an audibility index as a basis for selecting a frequency response slope, presumably it would be done by choosing the slope that produced the highest index value for that subject. That value is represented by a dot for each subject in figure 3. As you can see, the best slope, in relation to that recommended by the NAL-R, varied somewhat with subject. According to this method, Subject A would do better with 1.5 dB less high frequency slope than NAL-R prescribes, while Subject B seems to need 3 dB less, and subject C about 3 dB more high frequency emphasis. It should be noted that, although these are three real hearing losses, they were chosen from a larger group to show that different outcomes are possible. The fact is, however, that the two methods agree within ±1.5 dB/oct in most cases, a result that supports the validity of both approaches. When the methods do differ, we do not know which is more nearly right, but we are very much aware that the NAL-R method has a great deal more data to back it up than has the weighted audibility index.

Even if speech recognition models do produce the same slope recommendation as other methods, they should be developed in any case because they have the potential to provide substantial *additional* information. For example, data such as those displayed in this figure can tell us *how much* performance will likely change as a function of any frequency response change or error. It should be noted that absolute WAI values can be converted into percent recognition scores at any time. From such results, one can estimate the cost of not hitting a prescription target or of purposefully choosing a less-than-optimal frequency response because of budget or availability constraints or the user's personal preference. Figure 3 indicates that the cost is quite low unless one misses the best response by ±3 dB or more. Another thing revealed by this display is that some subjects would be hurt more by errors in one direction than the other. In addition, the model can quickly estimate performance at different assumed input signal levels, speech spectra, type of speech material, noise spectra, and signal-to-noise ratios, a set of results that could be quite useful when selecting the optimal response for each of the several different settings that are available for different listening conditions in a digital hearing aid.

Speech recognition models can provide additional useful information when the results are expressed in absolute terms, something that is simple to do once adequate information about a speech test is available. For example, absolute WAI values would make it possible to estimate a person's hearing impairment both with and without a hearing aid. The difference would provide a quantitative estimate of the extent of the benefit provided by a hearing aid. Such information would be useful in patient counseling and decision making. It could also serve as an objective descriptor of the likely benefit of a hearing aid prescription under average conditions, a measure of possible use for third party payers and similar applications.

Even in cases where the model's result is not correct for a particular individual, the result can be useful. It might indicate that the individual was not performing as well as he or she should considering the extent of his or her hearing loss and the nominal benefit provided by his or her hearing aid. This information could have implications for counseling the patient about what to expect in the real world or whether the patient needs additional training or special help. Discrepancies that reflect a defect in the model would be equally useful in that they would indicate needed avenues for research and, ultimately, improvements in the model.

In those clinical and research applications where adequate data can be obtained from a subject, absolute WAI values would permit comparisons of a subject's observed performance with that expected using the proficiency factor. After transforming the subject's performance into a WAI, the subject's proficiency as a listener can be estimated by noting the ratio of the observed WAI to the expected WAI. This measure could prove useful because it remains constant over a range of performance values and permits estimations of the individual's performance under other listening conditions. It also permits comparison of a subject's performance with that of others, even when the extent of the hearing losses differ. Comparison of a subject's aided proficiency and unaided proficiency would provide an estimate of whether the subject was performing as well with his or her hearing aid as might be expected given the aided versus unaided audibility difference and the subject's underlying ability to process speech as revealed by his or her unaided proficiency.

In conclusion, even in its present primitive state, the speech recognition model described here has suggested a number of interesting and probably important research questions and clinical applications. More fully developed, such models could prove to be a valuable clinical tool furnishing the clinician with information that goes well beyond what is available today.

References

Berger, K.W. 1990. The use of an Articulation Index to compare three hearing aid prescriptive methods. *Audecibel* 39(Summer):16–19.

Bess, F. 1983. Clinical assessment of speech recognition. In *Principles of Speech Audiometry*, eds. D. Konkle and W. Rintlemann. Baltimore, MD: University Park Press.

Boothroyd, A. 1968. Developments in speech audiometry. *Sound (British Journal of Audiology)* 2:3–10.

Byrne, D.J., and Dillon, H. 1986. The National Acoustics Laboratories' (NAL) new procedure for selecting the gain and frequency response of a hearing aid. *Ear and Hearing* 7:257–65.

Cox, R.M., Alexander, G.C., and Rivera, I.M. In press. Comparison of objective and subjective measures of speech intelligibility in elderly hearing-impaired listeners.

Dubno, J.R., Dirks D.D., and Morgan, D.E. 1984. Effects of Age and mild hearing loss on speech recognition in noise. *Journal of the Acoustical Society of America* 76: 87–96.

Fletcher, H., and Galt, R.H. 1950. The perception of speech and its relation to telephony. *Journal of the Acoustical Society of America* 22:89–151.

Gabrielsson, A., Schenkman, B., and Hagerman, B. 1988. The effects of different frequency responses on sound quality and speech intelligibility. *Journal of Speech and Hearing Research* 31:166–77.

Harris, J.D. 1948. Some suggestions for speech reception testing. Report No. 2, Project NM-003-021, New Haven Connecticut. Naval Medical Research Laboratory as reported in Hirsh, I. 1951. *The Measurement of Hearing*.

Chapter 5, The intelligibility of speech. New York, NY: McGraw-Hill.

Harris, J.D. 1980. On the use of three words per item format in tests for hearing of speech. *Journal of the Acoustical Society of America* 67:345–47.

Hellman, R.P., and Meiselman, C.H. 1988. Prediction of individual loudness exponents from cross-modality matching. *Journal of Speech and Hearing Research* 31: 605–615.

Hellman, R.P., and Meiselman, C.H. 1990. Loudness relations for individuals and groups in normal and impaired hearing. *Journal of the Acoustical Society of America* 88:2596–2606.

Hudgins, C.V., Hawkins, J.E., Karlin, J.E., and Stevens, S.S. 1947. The development of recorded auditory tests for measuring hearing loss for speech, *Laryngoscope* 57:57–89.

International Standards Organization. 1977. Method of calculating loudness level. ISO 532-1975. International Standards Organization.

Kalikow, D.N., Stevens, K.N., and Elliot, L.L. 1977. Development of a test of speech intelligibility in noise using sentence materials with controlled word predictability. *Journal of the Acoustical Society of America* 61: 1337–1351.

Konkle, D.F., and Rintlemann, W.F. Eds. 1983 *Principles of Speech Audiometry*. Baltimore, MD: University Park Press.

Leijon, A. 1989. Optimization of hearing-aid gain, and frequency response for cochlear hearing losses. Technical Report 189, Goteborg, Sweden: Chalmers University of Technology.

Ludvigsen, C. 1985. Relations among psychoacoustic parameters in normal and cochlearly impaired listeners. *Journal of the Acoustical Society of America* 78:1271–1280.

Ludvigsen, C. 1987. Prediction of speech intelligibility for normal-hearing and cochlearly-impaired listeners. *Journal of the Acoustical Society of America* 82:1162–1171.

Martin, M. Ed. 1987. *Speech Audiometry*. London, England: Taylor and Francis.

Pavlovic, C.V., Studebaker, G.A., and Sherbecoe, R.L. 1986. An articulation index based procedure for predicting the speech recognition performance of hearing-impaired individuals. *Journal of the Acoustical Society of America* 80:50–57.

Plomp, R. 1986. A signal-to-noise ratio model for the speech-reception threshold of the hearing impaired. *Journal of Speech and Hearing Research* 29:146–54.

Plomp, R., and Mimpen, A.M. 1979. Improving the reliability of testing the speech reception threshold for sentences. *Audiology* 18:43–53.

Punch, J.L., and Beck, E.L. 1980. Low-frequency response of hearing aids and judgements of aided speech quality. *Journal of Speech and Hearing Disorders* 45:325–35.

Punch, J.L., and Parker, C.A. 1981. Pairwise listener preferences in hearing aid evaluation. *Journal of Speech and Hearing Research* 24:366–74.

Punch, J.L., Montgomery, A.A., Schwartz, D.M. Walden, B.E., Prosek, R.A., and Howard, M.T. 1980. Multidimensional scaling of quality judgments of speech signals processed by hearing aids. *Journal of the Acoustical Society of America* 68:458–66.

Schwartz, D.M., Montgomery, A.A., Punch, J.L., Walden, B.E., and Prosek, R.A. 1980. Quality judgements of hearing aid processed speech by hearing impaired listeners. Unpublished manuscript.

Sergeant, L., Atkinson, J.E., and LaCroix, P.G. 1979. The NSMRL tri-word test of intelligibility (TTI). *Journal of the Acoustical Society of America* 65:218–22.

Studebaker, G.A. 1985. A "rationalized" arcsine transform. *Journal of Speech and Hearing Research* 28:455–62.

Studebaker, G.A., and Sherbecoe, R.L. 1988. Magnitude estimations of the intelligibility and quality of speech in noise. *Ear and Hearing* 9:259–67.

Studebaker, G.A., and Sherbecoe, R.L. 1991. Frequency-importance and transfer functions for recorded CID W-22 word lists. *Journal of Speech and Hearing Research* 34:427–38.

Studebaker, G.A., Bisset, J.D., Van Ort, D.M., and Hoffnung, S. 1982. Paired comparison judgements of relative intelligibility in noise. *Journal of the Acoustical Society of America* 72:80–92.

Taylor, R. 1991. An investigation of the effects of audibility spectrum on speech recognition performance-intensity functions. Ph.D. Dissertation (in progress) Memphis State University, Memphis, Tennessee.

Tecca, J.E., and Goldstein, D.P. 1984. Effect of low-frequency hearing aid response on four measures of speech perception. *Ear and Hearing* 5:22–29.

Thornton, A.R., and Raffin, M.J.M. 1978. Speech dis-

crimination scores modeled as a binomial variable. *Journal of Speech and Hearing Research* 21:507–518.

Van Tasell, D.J., and Yanz, J.L. 1987. Speech recognition threshold in noise: Effects of hearing loss, frequency response, and speech materials. *Journal of Speech and Hearing Research* 30:377–86.

Walker, G., and Byrne, D. 1985. Reliability of speech intelligibility estimation for measuring speech reception thresholds in quiet and noise. *Australian Journal of Audiology* 1985:23–31.

Walker, J., and Boothroyd, A. 1976. Test-retest reliability of speech discrimination measures and the benefits of phoneme scoring. Paper presented at the annual meeting of the American Speech and Hearing Association, November 1976, Houston, Texas.

Wilson, R.H., and Margolis, R.H. 1983. Measurements of auditory thresholds for speech stimuli. In *Principles of Speech Audiometry*, eds. D.F. Konkle and W.F. Rintlemann. Baltimore, MD: University Park Press.

Zerlin, S. 1962. A new approach to hearing aid selection. *Journal of Speech and Hearing Research* 5:370–76.

Zwicker, E., Fastl, H., and Dallmayr, C. 1984. BASIC program for calculating the loudness of sounds from their 1/3-oct band spectra according to ISO 532 B. *Acustica* 55:63–67.

CHAPTER 16

Evaluation Measures of Speech Intelligibility and Quality
Research and Clinical Application

Denis Byrne

This chapter discusses some variations of the paired comparison judgments procedure for use in hearing aid evaluations. In the National Acoustic Laboratories (NAL), we have used this type of testing extensively in research and recently have developed a clinical procedure of this type. Our use of paired comparison judgments is strongly based on the work of others, but there are some differences both in research and clinical applications. It is these differences that are emphasized in this chapter.

Advantages of Paired Comparison Judgments

The best known advantage of the paired comparison judgments procedure for hearing aid evaluations is that it tends to be more sensitive than speech recognition testing for showing differences between amplification systems (Studebaker 1982). This certainly has been our experience in NAL research.

Figure 1 is based on data from four NAL studies (Byrne 1986; Murray and Byrne 1986; Byrne unpublished; Byrne, Parkinson, and Newall 1990) in which we used paired comparisons to evaluate differences in frequency response. It shows the percentage of comparisons for which one response was preferred to the other eight or more times out of ten. This corresponds approximately to a 5% significance level. The first three studies included four types of judgments but the fourth involved only speech intelligibility in quiet. First, consider the intelligibility in quiet judgments. These are shown by the cross-hatched bars. For the first, second, and fourth studies, between 70% and 80% of comparisons resulted in a significant preference for one frequency response over the other. These studies all involved

moderate sized differences in frequency response. The percentage of significant comparisons drops to about 55% for the third study, which involved smaller differences in frequency response. The first and fourth studies included extensive speech recognition testing. That testing showed very few significant differences in contrast to the high proportion shown for the intelligibility judgments.

Now consider the intelligibility in noise judgments. These are shown by the bars labeled "IN." Note that, for each of the three studies, the proportion of significant comparisons is less than the corresponding proportions for intelligibility in quiet. This highlights one reason for the greater sensitivity of the judgments procedure: there are fewer constraints on the conditions in which it can be used. For example, it often is not informative to perform speech recognition tests in quiet because most subjects will obtain very high scores over a wide range of amplification conditions. However, for some experimental purposes, it may be best to test in quiet because, for example, differences in frequency response tend to have more effect on speech intelligibility in quiet than in noise (Byrne 1986). The problem of ceiling effects is avoided largely with the judgments procedure because subjects can usually judge one sample of speech to be *more easily understood* than another, even when both are highly intelligible and would result in near perfect speech recognition scores. This means that we have greater freedom to select the test conditions to suit the experimental purposes whereas, with speech recognition testing, we may be severely constrained by the need to make the test suitably difficult.

Another advantage of the judgment procedure is that listeners may be asked to judge qualities other than, or in addition to, speech intelligibility. In many studies the required judgment has been

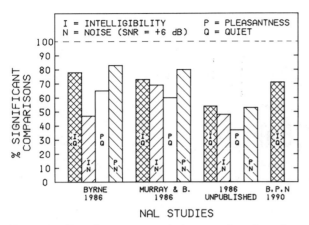

Figure 1. Paired comparison judgments data from four studies showing the percentage of times that one frequency response was preferred to the other for at least eight out of ten trials. The different bars indicate four different judgments.

overall quality (Jeffers 1960; Witter and Goldstein 1971; Punch 1978; Harris and Goldstein 1979; Punch and Beck 1980; Punch et al. 1980) but in others, the judgment has been specified as "intelligibility" (Zerlin 1962; Studebaker et al. 1982; Byrne, Parkinson, and Newall 1990) or "pleasantness" or "naturalness" (Byrne and Walker 1982). Several NAL studies have included both intelligibility and pleasantness judgments (Byrne and Walker 1982; Byrne 1986; Murray and Byrne 1986; Byrne and Cotton 1988). The range of required judgments can also be expanded by including two or more different types of materials. Most NAL studies have included speech-in-quiet and speech-in-speech spectrum noise with a signal-to-noise ratio of plus 6 dB.

An argument can be made for using overall quality judgments on the basis that this realistically indicates what a person would choose, regardless of the reasons for the choice. However, there are distinct advantages in obtaining judgments of at least two qualities, such as intelligibility and pleasantness, and of obtaining some judgments in quiet and some in noise. By using different qualities and different materials, we can determine whether different amplification characteristics would be optimal under different conditions or at different times, depending on the importance attached to particular qualities at the time in question. This is especially important when considering hearing aids that can automatically adapt their characteristics for different acoustic inputs or hearing aids that have multiple memories and can offer a choice of characteristics to the user.

Assessing the Need for Varied Amplification

We may ask the question: To what extent *do* listeners' requirements vary in different situations? This is addressed in figure 2 with data from a study that compared frequency response characteristics using judgments of intelligibility of speech in quiet, intelligibility in noise, pleasantness in quiet, and pleasantness in noise (Byrne 1986).

Figure 2 shows the results for two subjects. The letters on the horizontal axis, namely, N, M1, M5, and E designate different frequency responses. The four symbols show the score for each type of judgment. The score is the number of times, out of 20 trials, that each procedure was preferred to each of the other two procedures. First consider subject LU. For each frequency response, the scores for all four judgments are about the same. For this subject, the N response never was preferred, whereas the other two responses were preferred about equally. In other words, either of them would be equally good for both intelligibility and pleasantness and for speech in quiet and speech in noise. Now consider subject GB. The picture here is very different in that the score for any of the three frequency responses depends very much on which judgment is being made. For example, N was preferred only once for intelligibility in quiet, whereas it always was preferred for pleasantness in noise. Conversely, M1 was

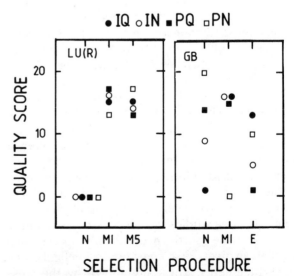

Figure 2. Paired comparison judgments data for two subjects (LU, GB) showing how the ranking of different frequency responses may or may not vary, depending on which judgment is being made (see text).

never preferred for pleasantness in noise, whereas it received the highest scores for the other three judgments. For this subject, if we ask: Which frequency response is best?, the answer depends on whether he is listening in quiet or in noise and on whether he attaches more importance to intelligibility or pleasantness.

These results are from a total sample of 14 test ears. Some of the other subjects showed almost as little variation as LU; others showed almost as much as GB. Other NAL studies have confirmed the general point that, for some listeners, the frequency response that is best for one condition is not best for another condition.

The judgment procedure could be extended to include other materials, such as music, or other conditions, such as listening plus lipreading. Such testing would seem very promising both for clinical evaluations and for research into how the need to vary amplification is related to listening conditions, hearing loss parameters, and personal preferences. At present, this issue has been addressed to only a limited extent. For example, one NAL study (Byrne and Cotton 1988) showed that the NAL frequency response was nearly always best for intelligibility in quiet but that a different response was better for pleasantness in noise for about 25% of subjects. That different response usually had more high frequency emphasis. However, it is not obvious how these 25% of subjects differed from the other 75% who found the NAL response best for pleasantness as well as intelligibility.

Clinical Use of Paired Comparison Judgments

In most research studies, speech or speech plus noise has been recorded through a number of hearing aids and the test procedure has involved comparing these recorded samples presented through earphones. This arrangement is convenient for testing a number of listeners with the *same* set of hearing aids but it obviously is not convenient if we want to test each person with a different set of hearing aids. A good solution is to present the speech through a master hearing aid that has filters that can be rapidly switched to simulate changing from one hearing aid to another. Such an approach has been used in research (Levitt et al. 1987) and is becoming feasible clinically with the development of hearing aids or fitting systems that have multiple

memories. However, the following is a different, and simpler, clinical procedure developed in NAL.

The basic strategy of the NAL procedure is the same as that adopted by Levitt and colleagues in that a reference frequency response is selected for each subject, according to a prescriptive procedure. That reference response is then compared with a series of variations that have either more or less relative gain in either the low or the high frequencies.

For example, in one of our studies (Byrne and Cotton 1988), the frequency response prescribed by the NAL procedure was compared with each of four variations. One variation had a 6 dB/octave low-frequency cut from 1.25 kHz to .25 kHz. Another had a 6 dB/octave low-frequency boost; the third had high-frequency cut, and the fourth a high-frequency boost. If any of the variations were superior to the NAL response, that variation was then compared with combinations of low and high-frequency cuts or boosts. The technique used was as follows: First, the client was fitted with a hearing aid that was adjusted to provide the NAL prescribed response as accurately as possible. This aid was worn throughout the experiment by the subject, who listened to samples of running speech presented through a loudspeaker. The different conditions were achieved by filtering the speech material as shown in figure 3.

The solid line shows the long-term average spectrum of speech. When the subject is presented with this, it represents *no* change in the hearing aid frequency response. In other words, he is listening with the response that has been fitted, namely the NAL response. When we present speech that has a low-cut, this is equivalent to putting a low-cut in the hearing aid. Similarly, if we present speech that is

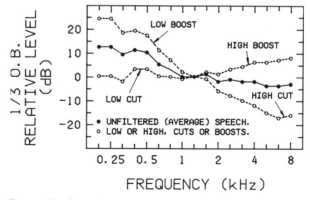

Figure 3. Long term average spectra of average (unfiltered) and filtered speech samples used for paired comparison evaluations in one study (Byrne and Cotton 1988) and in the NAL clinical evaluation procedure (Byrne 1987).

filtered to have a high-cut, that is equivalent to putting a high-cut in the hearing aid. The reason for using filtered speech instead of actually changing settings on the hearing aid is to avoid any delay in switching back and forth between the speech samples that are being compared. This is important because it would not only be inconvenient to change aid settings, but it has been found to make the procedure unreliable (Schum and Collins 1985).

The NAL clinical procedure is a simplification of the experimental procedure. There are only four comparison responses, namely, low-cut, low-boost, high-cut, and high-boost. This simplification is justified because we found, in the experiment, that the results for the combination responses were fairly predictable. For example, if the best response were a low-cut combined with a high-boost, we usually found that both the low-cut and the high-boost responses would show up as better than the NAL response. The evaluation procedure is described in detail in a report (Byrne 1987), but briefly it is as follows: In the first stage, each of the comparison responses is compared with the NAL response four times. The judgment is intelligibility and the speech is in quiet. If any comparison response is chosen two or more times, that response is retained for the next stage and the remainder are discarded.

Stage 2 is the same as stage 1, except there are unlikely to be more than one or two of the comparison responses left in it. If, at the end of stage 2 any comparison response has been chosen seven or more times, then that response is deemed to be the best response. If two comparison responses, such as the low-cut and the high-boost, have been chosen seven or more times, then the combination of those responses—that is a low-cut plus a high-boost—is deemed to be the best response. After carrying out these procedures with intelligibility judgments, they are repeated for pleasantness judgments of speech in noise.

The criteria used are such that a comparison response will be deemed to be better than the NAL response if it is significantly better at a level of approximately 5%. The idea is to identify those clients where a comparison response would be significantly better, either for intelligibility or pleasantness or both. This information may indicate the need for a change in aid fitting or it may be useful in advising the client. It would also have an obvious application in choosing the responses to include in a multiple-memory hearing aid.

The NAL evaluation procedure was developed from the work of others, notably Levitt and colleagues. However, there are important differences in philosophy and in practical implications. The basic difference is in the question addressed by each procedure. In the NAL procedure, the question is: Is any comparison response *significantly better* than the NAL response? In the Levitt procedure, the question is: Which response is *best*, out of a set of responses that include a reference response and number of variations? In the Levitt procedure, the reference response is treated simply as a starting point and, thereafter, an unbiased comparison is made of all the responses in the set. In the NAL procedure, the reference response has a special status in that it is deemed to be best unless something else can be demonstrated to be significantly better.

The philosophical justification for the NAL approach is that the NAL selection has been validated by a substantial body of research and it, therefore, should not be discarded unless the evidence for an alternative is conclusive. This recognizes that all evaluation procedures are of limited reliability and we are, therefore, not justified in attaching any significance to any small differences that may be found. Our philosophy is that the evaluation is for checking and refining the prescription rather than regarding the prescription as simply a starting point for the evaluation.

One practical advantage of the NAL procedure is that it will usually involve less testing than a procedure that searches for the best response. Another important advantage is that it *always* gives a clear result. Either there is, or there is not, a comparison response that is significantly better than the NAL response. In other words, there is never any problem of deciding which response is best if two or more result in similar scores.

One possible concern about the NAL approach could be: Will the reference response (i.e., the NAL response) emerge as best most of the time, simply because the procedure is not sensitive enough to show many differences? Our research has shown that this generally is not so. As shown earlier in figure 1, when we compare moderately different frequency response characteristics, we find that *most* of the time we do get a significant preference for one response over the other for both intelligibility and pleasantness judgments. Also, in the study from which the clinical procedure was developed (Byrne and Cotton 1988), there was a clear preference for the NAL response when it was compared with the low-cut, low-boost, or high-boost responses although the preference was far less clear when the comparison response was the high-cut response.

Conclusions

This chapter has presented some ideas for evaluating the intelligibility and quality of speech with different amplification options. The clinical procedure described could be varied in many ways, such as using a different prescriptive procedure to select the reference response, or conducting the evaluation through a master hearing aid instead of using filtered speech samples. The need for such evaluation is obvious and is becoming even more pressing with the ever-increasing range of amplification possibilities. Indeed, something of this kind may become a necessity if we are to make effective use of multiple memory hearing aids or aids that have individually selectable adaptive capabilities. So far, paired comparison judgment procedures have been used mainly in research but they are also practical for clinical use because they are relatively quick and can be done with fairly simple equipment. I am confident that methods of this type will be used increasingly and will prove highly valuable in clinical applications as well as in research.

References

Byrne, D. 1986. Effects of frequency response characteristics on speech discrimination and perceived intelligibility and pleasantness of speech for hearing-impaired listeners. *Journal of the Acoustical Society of America* 80: 494-504.

Byrne, D. 1987. *A Post-(Hearing Aid) Fitting Evaluation Procedure Using Speech Intelligibility and Pleasantness Judgments.* NAL Report No. 112. Canberra: Aust. Govt. Publishing Service.

Byrne, D., and Cotton, S. 1988. Evaluation of the National Acoustic Laboratories' new hearing aid selection procedure. *Journal of Speech and Hearing Research* 31:178-86.

Byrne D., Parkinson A., and Newall P. 1990. Hearing aid gain and frequency response requirements for the severely/profoundly hearing-impaired. *Ear and Hearing* 11:40-49.

Byrne, D., and Walker, G. 1982. The effects of multichannel compression and expansion amplification on perceived quality of speech. *Australian Journal of Audiology* 4:1-8.

Harris, R.W., and Goldstein, D.P. 1979. Effects of room reverberation upon hearing aid quality judgments. *Audiology* 18:253-62.

Jeffers, J. 1960. Quality judgments in hearing aid selection. *Journal of Speech and Hearing Disorders* 25:259-66.

Levitt, H., Sullivan, J.A., Newman, A.C., and Rubin-Spitz 1987. Experiments with a programmable master hearing aid. *Journal of Rehabilitation Research and Development* 24:29-54.

Murray, N., and Byrne, D. 1986. Performance of hearing-impaired and normal hearing listeners with various high frequency cut-offs in hearing aids. *Australian Journal of Audiology* 8:21-28.

Punch, J.L. 1978. Quality judgments of hearing aid processed speech and music by normal and otopathologic listeners. *Journal of the American Auditory Society* 3: 179-88.

Punch, J.L., and Beck, E.L. 1980. Low-frequency response of hearing aids and judgments of aided speech quality. *Journal of Speech and Hearing Disorders* 45:325-35.

Punch, J.L., Montgomery, A.A., Schwartz, D.M., Walden, B.E., Prosek, R.A., and Howard, M.T. 1980. Multidimensional scaling of quality judgments of speech signals processed by hearing aids. *Journal of the Acoustical Society of America.* 68:458-66.

Schum, D.J., and Collins, M.J. 1985. Test retest reliability of two paired-comparison hearing aid evaluations. ASHLA Annual Convention, Washington, DC.

Studebaker, G.A. 1982. Hearing aid selection: An overview. In *The Vanderbilt Hearing-aid Report: State of the Art-Research Needs* ed. G.A. Studebaker and F.H. Bess. Upper Darby, PA: Monographs in Contemporary Audiology.

Studebaker, G.A., Bisset, J.D., Van Ort, D.M., and Hoffnung, S. 1982. Paired comparison judgments of relative speech intelligibility in noise. *Journal of the Acoustical Society of America* 72:80-92.

Witter, H.L., and Goldstein, D.L. 1971. Quality judgments of hearing aid transduced speech. *Journal of Speech and Hearing Research* 14:312-22.

Zerlin, S. 1962. A new approach to hearing aid selection. *Journal of Speech and Hearing Research* 5:370-76.

CHAPTER 17

Objective and Self-Report Measures of Hearing Aid Benefit

Robyn M. Cox, Genevieve C. Alexander, and Christine Gilmore

Since the last Vanderbilt hearing aid conference, there has been continued strong interest in refining procedures for fitting hearing aids. Many different approaches for specifying electroacoustic characteristics have been put forward. At the same time, technological advances have made it possible to produce more sophisticated hearing aids than ever before. Many of these new approaches to designing and fitting hearing aids were discussed at the second conference.

With so many new ideas around, it is clear that methods are needed to evaluate their relative effectiveness. Without such methods, how can we determine whether, and with whom, fitting approach A is better than fitting approach B? How can we know which noise reduction scheme is likely to meet an individual's needs, or if any of them are? These and similar questions are encountered routinely in current audiological practice.

Several groups of researchers have been attempting to address these kinds of questions. In 1986 we began a research program, supported by the Department of Veterans Affairs, that has attempted to take a systematic approach to the study of benefit obtained from hearing aids. Overall, the goal is to develop methods to predict validly the benefit in daily life that will be obtained ultimately from a hearing aid fitting and to make this prediction on the day that the instrument is fitted and issued in the clinical setting.

Definition of Benefit   In our investigations, benefit is operationalized as a change between unaided and aided speech communication ability. This approach to benefit quantification has two positive aspects. First, it is a relatively pure measure of the advantage or disadvantage attributable to the hearing aid. Other variables, such as satisfaction or hours of use per day, have been used to measure hearing aid effect. However, these have been shown to be influenced by factors that are independent of the hearing aid such as lifestyle, extent of hearing loss, earmold discomfort, and dexterity (e.g., Hutton 1983; Haggard, Foster, and Iredale 1983; Kapteyn 1977; Hutton and Canahl 1985). Second, a concentration on speech communication is well supported by research. Wearers, or potential wearers, of hearing aids almost uniformly indicate that improved communication via speech is their primary need (Barcham and Stephens 1980; Golabek et al. 1988; Hagerman and Gabrielsson 1984). Thus, although hearing aid benefit may incorporate other significant factors, these are generally secondary to speech communication.

Listening Environments   To enhance our ability to generalize laboratory-measured benefit to daily life, and to facilitate comparison with daily life situations, three distinct, but typical, listening environments were defined, and these have been used throughout the studies. Environment A represents situations in which the speech level is normal or casual, background noise is low, and visual cues are fully available. Examples of Environment A include face-to-face conversation in a living room or quiet office. Environment B represents situations in which speech cues are reduced because of reverberation, low speech level, or limited visual cues. Examples of Environment B include communication over a distance or listening to a classroom lecture. Environment C represents communication situations with groups of people. The speech level is raised and there is a relatively high level of competing multitalker babble. Visual cues are available. This environment typifies the well-known "cocktail party" situation. For a more complete description of the listening environments, see Cox and Alexander (1991a).

This work was supported by funding from the Department of Veterans Affairs Rehabilitation Research and Development Service.

Hearing Aids Investigations to date generally have employed linear, nondirectional, monaural, ear-level hearing aid fittings. An important aspect of these early studies has been the establishment of a baseline for benefit derived from well-fitted, conventional amplification. This will provide a reference for future evaluations of innovative approaches.

Subjects The subject population consists of elderly individuals with bilateral sensorineural hearing loss of mild to moderately severe extent. The typical subject is 67 years old and has a gently or sharply sloping audiogram. Etiology of hearing loss is typically presbyacusis or noise exposure or a combination of these two.

Objective Measurement of Benefit in Typical Environments

Studies of objectively measured hearing aid benefit usually have been conducted within the confines of a laboratory or clinic. There appear to be few, if any, documented studies in which hearing aid benefit has been measured objectively in everyday listening environments. Because of the paucity of objective benefit data in daily life settings, we do not have a clear idea of the actual percentage of improvement in speech communication abilities that can be anticipated with hearing aid use. Furthermore, we cannot determine the extent to which clinical measurements of benefit can be generalized to daily life. In addition, unless hearing aid benefit is quantified objectively in typical settings, the relationship between objectively measured and self-assessed hearing aid benefit will remain obscure. To begin addressing these types of issues, we undertook to explore objectively measured benefit in the three everyday listening environments defined above.

The Connected Speech Test

To maximize face validity of the hearing aid benefit data, the test of speech communication ability needed the following features: (1) speech produced in a conversational manner; (2) a talker whose intelligibility is average; (3) availability of visual speech cues; and (4) speech that follows the same topic for several sentences and for which the topic is known to the listener. In addition, to be a useful research tool, the test needed: (5) objective scoring; (6) reasonable reliability so that small differences could be detected; and (7) quite a few equivalent forms so that test items would not have to be repeated.

We were unable to locate any test that met all of these requirements; consequently, we attempted to develop one. The final product is called the *Connected Speech Test*, or CST (Cox, Alexander, and Gilmore 1987; Cox et al. 1988, 1989). Although this test is less than perfect, it has proven quite useful. The CST consists of ten-sentence passages of connected speech about commonplace topics. The talker is a female who produces speech of average intelligibility, neither especially easy nor especially difficult to understand. Each passage is repeated one sentence at a time and is scored in terms of correct repetition of 25 key words. The score for a condition is based on results for six passages, or 150 key words. The test may be presented either audio-visually or audio-only, and there are eight equivalent forms.

Objective Measures of Benefit

Using the CST, we have developed two objective indices of hearing aid benefit. The first is a measure of improvement in speech intelligibility, defined as the aided CST score minus the unaided CST score. Intelligibility benefit has high face validity in that it appears to be a direct measure of improved speech communication ability.

The second benefit index measures the change in time required to respond to speech when the hearing aid is worn. It is defined as the unaided response time minus the aided response time.[1] The response-time measure was included in an attempt to tap the improved "ease of listening" that is reported by many hearing aid wearers. Previous research on response time has shown that it is highly related to intelligibility score; as intelligibility goes up, response time decreases (e.g., Wright, Spanner, and Martin 1981). It has been proposed that

---

[1]Response time was recorded using a microcomputer. After presentation of a CST sentence, the examiner hit a key as soon as the subject began to repeat the sentence. Response time for that sentence was measured from the end of the sentence playback to the beginning of the subject's response registered by the examiner's keystroke. This method of response-time measurement includes the examiner's reaction time in the measured response times. The examiner's reaction time is assumed to add a constant value to both aided and unaided response-time scores, and, therefore, does not affect the benefit score. The resolution of the microcomputer's measurements of response-time was ±50 msec. Sixty independent measurements were accumulated to produce each response-time score. Because positive and negative errors would cancel, the resolution of each score is estimated to be much better than 50 msec.

response-time measures may be more sensitive than intelligibility measures and, thus, more able to detect small differences between conditions (e.g., Hecker, Stevens, and Williams 1966; Pratt 1981; Gatehouse and Gordon 1990). We hypothesized that response-time benefit and intelligibility benefit would measure somewhat different dimensions of speech communication ability.

Cox and Alexander (1991a) measured hearing aid benefit, using both objective indices, for a group of hearing-impaired listeners. All subjects were carefully fitted with three hearing aids that were systematically varied in frequency response. Figure 1 illustrates the mean 2-cm³ coupler frequency-gain functions for these hearing aid fittings. The middle hearing aid (HAO) followed a prescription. The more positive emphasis hearing aid (HAP) varied from HAO by +4 dB/octave. The more negative emphasis hearing aid (HAN) varied from HAO by −4 dB/octave. Thus, the total range of variation across frequency response conditions was nominally 8 dB/octave.

With subjects wearing these hearing aids, benefit measurements were made in rooms representing each of the three typical listening environments described earlier. For intelligibility benefit data there were 33 subjects. For response-time benefit data there were 21 subjects. Any given subject served in only one of the listening environments. The investigation asked the following questions:

1. How much benefit are people really getting from well-fitted hearing aids in typical daily life settings?

2. Is the amount of benefit in daily life affected by moderate differences in the hearing aid's frequency response?
3. Is benefit dependent on visual cues to speech? That is, is benefit for speech presented audio-visually different from that for speech without visual cues? If so, is the optimal frequency response dependent on the presence/absence of visual input?

Effects of Environments, Frequency Responses, and Visual Cues

Figure 2 illustrates the effects of listening environments and frequency responses on both intelligibility and response-time benefit. This figure also shows the distribution of subjects across environments. Figures 2, 3, and 4 display response-time data for only 17 of the 21 subjects who were tested, because data for four subjects were judged to be invalid. This matter is discussed later. The upper panel of figure 2 describes the mean intelligibility

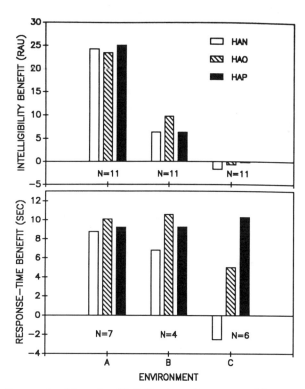

Figure 2. Mean intelligibility benefit measured in raus (upper panel) and mean response-time benefit measured in seconds (lower panel) for subjects listening in three different everyday environments. In each environment, data are given for three hearing aid conditions. (Adapted in part from Cox and Alexander [1991a], with permission from *Ear and Hearing*.)

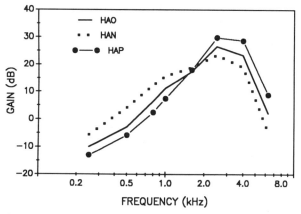

Figure 1. Mean 2-cm³ coupler frequency-gain functions for hearing aids fitted to 33 subjects. Each subject was fitted with three hearing aids that differed in frequency response slope. (From Cox and Alexander [1991b], with permission from *Ear and Hearing*.)

benefit obtained with each frequency response in each environment. Benefit is quantified in rationalized arcsine units (raus): these may be interpreted in a manner similar to percentages (Studebaker 1985). In Environment A (the living room), benefit was about 24 rau. In Environment B (the classroom lecture), benefit was 7 to 10 rau. In Environment C (the cocktail party), benefit was zero to −2 rau. The differences across environments were statistically significant, with A greater than both B and C ($p < .05$).

Analyses revealed that there were no significant differences due to hearing aid frequency response; i.e., in a given environment, each frequency response produced about the same average intelligibility benefit. However, note that in Environment C, although the differences among frequency response conditions were small, the results were ordered according to high frequency emphasis: the instrument with the least high-frequency gain (HAN) produced the poorest result, whereas the instrument with the greatest high-frequency gain (HAP) produced the best result.

The lower panel of figure 2 shows mean response-time benefit obtained with each frequency response in each environment. All environments yielded mean response-time benefit in the range from 4 to 9 seconds. There were no significant differences in benefit across environments. That is, about the same average response-time benefit was measured in all environments. Overall, there were again no significant differences due to frequency response. However, note that the Environment C results were once more ordered according to high frequency emphasis and that the differences across frequency responses were much greater than shown in the upper panel for intelligibility benefit. Taken alone, these data produced a statistically significant effect despite the small number of subjects ($p < .05$).

These results tend to support the hypothesis that the response-time benefit measure may be more sensitive than the intelligibility benefit measure to the effects of frequency response. On the other hand, intelligibility benefit was more sensitive than response-time benefit to the effects of listening environment.

Figure 3 portrays the effects of visual speech cues on the two measures of benefit. The upper panel shows mean intelligibility benefit for audio-only and audiovisual speech presentation modes in each environment. There were no significant differences between the two modes in any environment. The lower panel gives the corresponding response-time benefit data for the two speech presentation modes. Although there are some fairly large mean

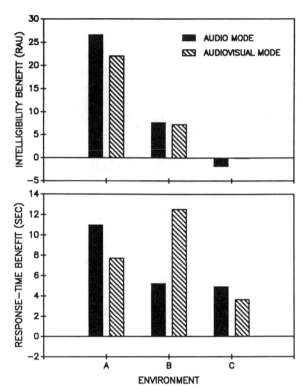

Figure 3. Mean intelligibility benefit measured in raus (upper panel) and mean response-time benefit measured in seconds (lower panel) for subjects listening to speech presented with (audiovisual mode) and without (audio mode) visual cues. Data are given for three listening environments. (Adapted in part from Cox and Alexander [1991a], with permission from *Ear and Hearing*.)

differences, especially in Environment B, these differences were, again, not statistically significant.

Relationship Between Hearing Loss and Benefit

Figure 4 depicts the relationship between speech reception threshold (SRT) and mean benefit for each subject. The upper panel illustrates intelligibility benefit, and the lower panel gives response-time benefit. Subjects listening in Environment A are represented with filled circles, Environment B with open triangles, and Environment C with open squares. The regression lines are shown for Environment A data. These regression lines illustrate that, in Environment A, there was a positive relationship between SRT and intelligibility benefit; that is, subjects with more hearing loss (higher SRT) obtained more benefit by both measures. For intelligibility data, the correlation between benefit and SRT was significant ($r = .76, p < .01$). However, the correlation coefficient for response-time data in Environment A ($r = .72$) was not statistically signifi-

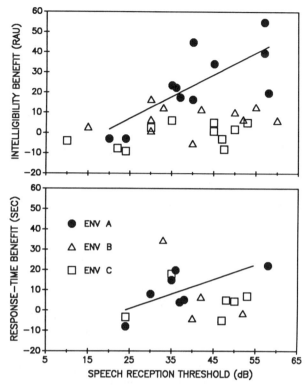

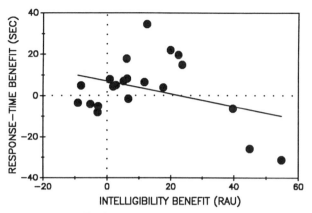

Figure 5. Intelligibility benefit data (raus) and response-time benefit data (seconds) for 21 hearing-impaired listeners. Each symbol depicts the pair of scores for one subject. The regression line is shown.

Figure 4. Mean hearing aid benefit in raus (upper panel) and seconds (lower panel) as a function of speech reception threshold (SRT) in dB re: ANSI (1969). Data are given for subjects serving in three listening environ ments. The regression lines are shown for Environment A data. (Adapted in part from Cox and Alexander [1991a], with permission from *Ear and Hearing*.)

cant, perhaps because of the small number of subjects. In Environments B and C there was no systematic relationship between benefit and hearing loss in spite of a fairly wide range of SRTs.

Relationship Between Objective Benefit Measures

It was of considerable practical and theoretical interest to determine whether the two measures of benefit quantify different aspects of hearing aid advantage. If intelligibility and response-time benefits are closely related, there is no reason to measure both. Conversely, if each type of data provides unique information about improvements in speech communication resulting from hearing aid use, an appropriate combination of the two may permit more accurate objective quantification of hearing aid benefit. Figure 5 reveals the relationship between intelligibility benefit and response-time benefit in this investigation. Each symbol gives the data for one subject averaged across all conditions. The regression line for these data is shown and suggests an

inverse relationship in which subjects with more intelligibility benefit had less response-time benefit. However, further inspection suggested that several subjects had provided misleading data for the response-time benefit measure. These subjects understood very little in the unaided condition. As a result, their response-time scores were unusually low: for many sentences, the response time was only long enough to indicate that they could not repeat any words. In the aided condition, on the other hand, they understood much more speech and required some processing time to formulate their responses. Thus, their response-time scores in the aided condition were greater than in the unaided condition. Consequently, response-time benefit was negative. Logic indicates that this was not a valid measure of the improvement in speech communication provided by the hearing aid for these subjects.

To address this problem, all subjects with mean unaided intelligibility scores less than 25 rau were eliminated from the analysis. Figure 6 displays the result after four subjects with very low unaided scores were eliminated. It is now clear that there was a significant positive relationship between intelligibility and response-time benefit ($r = .67, p < .01$). These data indicate that about 45% of the variance in response-time benefit scores can be attributed to the variance in intelligibility benefit scores. The source of the remaining 55% of the variance in response-time benefit scores remains unknown. Some is undoubtedly due to measurement error, and some presumably incorporates a contribution from factors relevant to speech communication that are independent of intelligibility benefit. More data are needed to separate these components.

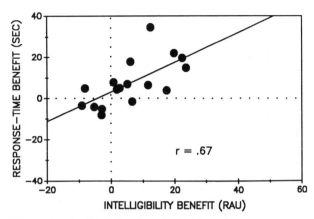

Figure 6. Intelligibility benefit data (raus) and response-time benefit data (seconds) for 17 hearing-impaired listeners with unaided intelligibility scores >25 raus. Each symbol depicts the pair of scores for one subject. The regression line is shown.

Summary

These results were consistent with the following conclusions about objectively measured hearing aid benefit.

First, intelligibility and response-time measures of benefit sometimes yielded different results: intelligibility benefit data revealed a significant difference in benefit across typical listening environments, whereas this was not seen with response-time benefit. However, intelligibility benefit did not distinguish among three moderately different frequency responses, whereas response-time benefit did, in a "cocktail party" type of listening environment.

Second, the intelligibility benefit data were consistent with the hypothesis that the frequency response differences produced by typical hearing aid prescriptive procedures do not produce different benefits in daily life. This is largely because volume control adjustments are used to compensate for the differences (Cox and Alexander 1991a). This outcome is at variance with some laboratory comparisons of prescriptive procedures (e.g., Byrne 1986; Humes 1986), but is consistent with several studies conducted in real-world types of settings (e.g., Stroud and Hamill 1989; Lynn and Lesner 1990).

Third, both benefit measures indicated that hearing aid benefit is not significantly affected by the presence or absence of visual cues to speech. This suggests that hearing aid benefit in the elderly can be measured validly using speech stimuli without visual cues.

Fourth, both benefit measures agreed that hearing aid benefit is significantly related to hear-

ing sensitivity loss only in the relatively favorable listening environment typified by one-to-one conversation in a home living room. In more difficult listening environments, benefit cannot be predicted from the audiogram.

Finally, when unaided performance was extremely poor, response-time measures, as used in this study, were not an appropriate approach to the quantification of hearing aid benefit.

Self-Assessment of Performance and/or Benefit in Daily Life

The opinion of the hearing aid wearer about the help provided by the instrument in the workaday world is both important and interesting. In the long run, the verdict of the hearing aid consumer determines whether or not the amplification strategy has been successful. The utility of laboratory measures of hearing aid benefit is very questionable if the laboratories give results that are at variance with the assessment made by the hearing aid wearer.

The literature contains many reports of investigations that have measured hearing aid benefit using questionnaires completed by hearing aid wearers themselves. For the most part, each investigation has produced a questionnaire that is customized to address the issues of interest in that study, and the resulting questionnaire has had limited application in other research. It is well known that the data yielded by attitude-measurement tools is often significantly influenced by the wording of items and other aspects of the inventory itself. Thus, self-assessed hearing aid benefit indicated by one questionnaire cannot be assumed to be equivalent to analogous data produced by another questionnaire. Because of this, standardized methods are needed to measure self-assessed benefit. Relatively few efforts have been reported to develop general-purpose questionnaires for quantification of self-assessed hearing aid benefit. A notable exception is the Hearing Aid Performance Inventory developed by Walden, Demorest, and Helper (1984).

The Profile of Hearing Aid Performance

To quantify daily life experience with hearing aids using a self-assessment approach, we developed a questionnaire called the Profile of Hearing Aid Performance, or PHAP (Cox and Gilmore 1990). The design objectives for the questionnaire were as follows: (1) benefit would be assessed using a profile of four scale scores, one for speech communication in each of our three listening environments and one measuring reactions to environmental sounds;[2] (2) each scale would be partitioned into subscales if the data suggested that this would be appropriate; (3) a relatively large number of response categories would be provided to maximize sensitivity; and (4) data produced by the inventory would be in terms of absolute performance. The last feature would allow direct comparison of different hearing aid conditions and comparison of subjective and objective performance data. In addition, benefit could be assessed by comparing responses to items for "with amplification" and "without amplification."

Figure 7 illustrates a typical item from the PHAP. There are seven response categories, each consisting of a descriptive word and an associated percentage. The instructions direct the subject to choose the response that comes closest to his or her everyday experience. The stem "When I wear my hearing aid:" appears before the first item and at the top of each new page. Table I provides an outline of the questionnaire. There are seven subscales and four scales. The Familiar Talkers (FT) and Ease of Communication (EC) subscales can be combined to form the Environment A scale (SA). The Reverberation (RV) and Reduced Cues (RC) subscales can be combined for the Environment B scale (SB). There are no subscales for the Environment C scale which is also referred to as the Background Noise (BN)

Table I. Summary of the Profile of Hearing Aid Performance (PHAP)

		Number Items
Subscales		
FT:	Familiar talkers	7
EC:	Ease of communication	7
RV:	Reverberation	9
RC:	Reduced cues	9
BN:	Background noise	16
AV:	Aversiveness of sounds	12
DS:	Distortion of sounds	6
Scales		
SA:	Speech, env A (FT + EC)	14
SB:	Speech, env B (RV + RC)	18
SC:	Speech, env C (BN)	16
ES:	Environmental sounds (AV + DS)	18

subscale. The Aversiveness of Sounds (AV) and Distortion of Sounds (DS) subscales combine for the Environmental Sound scale (ES). There are 66 items altogether. Coefficient alpha ranges from .70 to .90 for the scales and subscales.

An individual's responses to the PHAP questionnaire are evaluated using a computer graphic that is illustrated in figure 8. Note the seven-score and four-score profiles shown in the upper left. The profile shown with the filled circles is for the individual being tested. Two comparison profiles are provided: the heavy solid line depicts the mean profile for successful hearing aid wearers, and the dotted line shows the 85th percentile of scores for successful hearing aid wearers. The pie chart in the upper right depicts the number of times that each response alternative was used by this subject in completing the questionnaire. The line graph across the bottom tracks the pattern of responses through the questionnaire. These displays are used

[2]The literature contains numerous reports establishing that a negative response to the level or disruptive character of background sounds is a dominant factor in the failure of many hearing aid fittings. Thus, hearing aid benefit may be partially or completely cancelled by adverse reactions to amplified environmental sounds. Because of this, the PHAP was designed to evaluate both speech communication problems and reactions to environmental sounds.

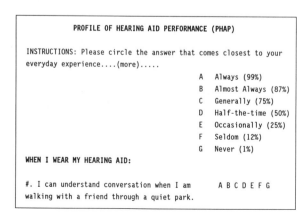

Figure 7. Typical item from the Profile of Hearing Aid Performance (PHAP).

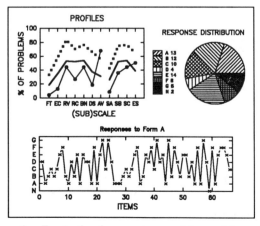

Figure 8. Facsimile of computer graphic used to evaluate responses to the PHAP questionnaire.

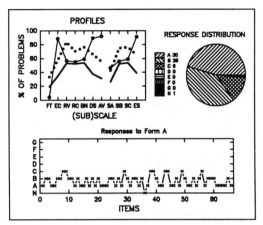

Figure 9.   Example of an invalid response to the PHAP questionnaire.

to evaluate the validity of the responses as well as the shape of the profiles. In our experience, five to ten percent of elderly hearing aid wearers do not complete the questionnaire in a valid manner.

Figures 9 and 10 give examples of invalid results. In figure 9 the invalid outcome was probably due to lack of question comprehension. The pie chart reveals that only three of the seven response alternatives have been used. This is judged to be invalid because PHAP items are written so that, to produce a consistent set of responses, it is necessary to use alternatives at both ends of the response continuum. In figure 10 the invalid outcome was probably due to fatigue. The pie chart shows a wide distribution of response categories, but the tracking graph at the bottom indicates that the subject apparently tired after 20 items and, thereafter, completed the inventory in a manner that is clearly fallacious.

Mean PHAP profiles for groups of normal hearers and successful hearing aid users are shown

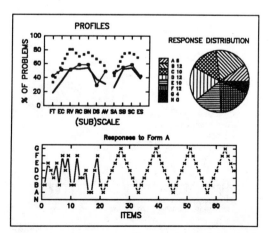

Figure 10.   Example of an invalid response to the PHAP questionnaire.

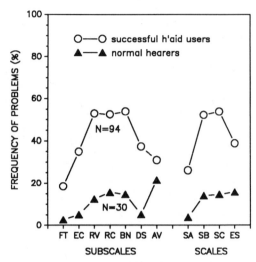

Figure 11.   Mean PHAP profiles for normal hearers and successful hearing aid wearers.

in figure 11. Standard errors of the means were too small to be seen on the figure. Responses are scored in terms of frequency of problems. Thus, a higher percentage is indicative of more problems. Successful hearing aid users were defined as current hearing aid wearers who reported that they had worn amplification more than seven hours/day for more than one year. The normal hearers completed a version of the questionnaire in which the stem "When I wear my hearing aid:" had been deleted. Note that even successful hearing aid wearers report many more problems in daily life than do normal hearers. Moreover, the biggest differences between the two groups are for the more difficult communication situations represented by Environments B and C (subscales RV, RC, and BN, and scales SB and SC).

Mean PHAP profiles for groups of successful and unsuccessful hearing aid users are compared in figure 12. For these data, unsuccessful users were individuals who indicated that they use their instruments one hour/day or less or have stopped using their hearing aids altogether. These profiles also show the standard errors of the means for the unsuccessful hearing aid users. There is a clear pattern across all scales and subscales for unsuccessful users to report more daily problems than do successful users. Individual t-tests revealed that many of the scale and subscale mean differences reached statistical significance. Asterisks above the X-axis labels indicate the instances where the difference between successful-user and unsuccessful-user means was significant ($p = < .05$).

The data of figure 12 have a noteworthy feature: significant differences between successful and unsuccessful users were seen for the subscales assess-

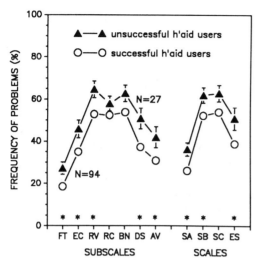

Figure 12. Mean PHAP profiles for successful and un-successful hearing aid wearers. Error bars depict ±1 standard error of the means. Asterisks denote subscales having significant mean differences.

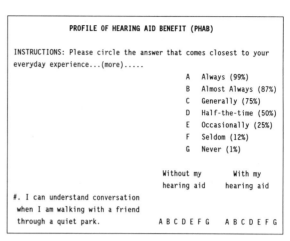

Figure 13. Excerpt from the Profile of Hearing Aid Benefit (PHAB).

ing speech communication performance in relatively easy listening situations (FT and EC) and for subscales quantifying reactions to amplified environmental sounds (DS and AV). Of the three subscales assessing speech communication in difficult listening situations (RV, RC, and BN), only RV produced a significant difference. The implication of this outcome is that speech communication in noisy situations, although clearly the most problematic issue for hearing-impaired listeners, is not the main factor that separates successful and unsuccessful hearing aid users. Instead, failure to realize adequate performance in relatively quiet, traditionally easy listening tasks may be a major component leading to rejection or underutilization of a hearing aid fitting. In addition, the observation that unsuccessful users report significantly more negative responses to amplified environmental sounds supports the proposal often advanced that this factor makes an important contribution to hearing aid rejection.

Comparison of Questionnaires to Measure Benefit

The PHAP quantifies user performance with a hearing aid in absolute terms. It does not produce a measure of hearing aid benefit as we have defined it, in terms of a difference between aided and unaided performance. However, two inventories to measure hearing aid benefit have been developed based on the PHAP.

The first benefit questionnaire is a direct derivative of the PHAP, called the Profile of Hearing Aid

Benefit, or PHAB. Figure 13 shows an excerpt from the PHAB. The instructions, items, and response alternatives are identical to those of the PHAP. However, to measure benefit using the PHAB, the subject responds twice to each item, once for "without my hearing aid" and once for "with my hearing aid." The difference between the two responses is the measure of benefit.

The second benefit questionnaire is called the Intelligibility Rating Improvement Scale, or IRIS. In the IRIS, there are no items assessing reactions to environmental sounds. This questionnaire is focussed entirely on speech communication in daily life and the items are slightly reworded versions of the speech communication items of the PHAP. The major difference between the two benefit questionnaires is in the response format. Figure 14 gives an excerpt showing the response format for the IRIS. For each item, the subject is provided with a scale from zero to one hundred, with the ends described as "no words understood" and "all words understood." They are asked to mark the scale twice,

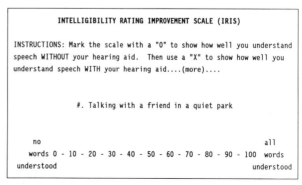

Figure 14. Excerpt from the Intelligibility Rating Improvement Scale (IRIS).

once for their understanding with amplification and again for their understanding without it. The difference is the measure of benefit.

We were interested in this response format because it has been useful for subjective estimation of speech intelligibility in both laboratory and clinical work (Speaks et al. 1972; Cox and McDaniel 1984, 1989). Thus, we wanted to assess its potential for use in a benefit questionnaire as well.

Cox, Gilmore, and Alexander (1991) administered both the PHAB and the IRIS to a group of 42 experienced hearing aid users. Some questions of interest were:

1. Is self-assessed hearing aid benefit equivalent for the two questionnaires? In other words, is estimated proportion of speech intelligibility improvement functionally equivalent to estimated proportion of situations in which intelligibility is improved?
2. Does self-assessed hearing aid benefit vary in the different types of listening environments addressed by the questionnaires? If so, is either questionnaire more sensitive to these situational differences?

To compare the results obtained with the two benefit questionnaires, mean benefit for each speech communication subscale was computed for PHAB and IRIS data. The results are shown in figure 15. Benefit for the PHAB represents a change in the percent of problem situations, whereas benefit for the IRIS represents a change in the percent of speech understanding.

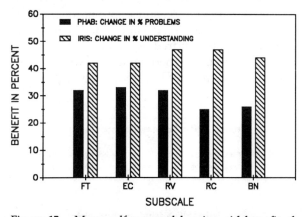

Figure 15. Mean self-assessed hearing aid benefit obtained using the PHAB and IRIS questionnaires. Data are given for the five speech communication subscales that are common to both questionnaires. (Adapted from Cox, Gilmore, and Alexander [1991], with permission from the *Journal of the American Academy of Audiology*.)

The figure reveals that neither questionnaire produced large benefit differences across the speech communication subscales. The range of mean benefit for the PHAB was about nine percent, and the range of mean benefit for the IRIS was about six percent. Thus, the PHAB produced a somewhat greater range of mean benefit scores, but neither questionnaire resulted in a range of self-assessed benefit as great as seen with our objective measure of intelligibility benefit.

The only subscale with a fairly high correlation across the two questionnaires was FT, which had a correlation coefficient of .76 ($p < .01$). The correlation for subscale BN was .54, which was also statistically significant ($p < .01$) but not especially high. This means that, generally, an individual's score for one subscale on the IRIS was not necessarily predictive of the score for the same subscale on the PHAB, and vice versa.

Finally, and most importantly, the pattern of self-assessed benefit for the PHAB data was different from that for the IRIS data. The IRIS yielded its greatest benefit for subscales RC, BN, and RV—the three subscales that produced the poorest self-assessed performance for the unaided condition. Results for the PHAB agreed with those for the IRIS in awarding relatively large benefit scores in the RV subscale. However, the PHAB also produced superior benefit scores for subscales FT and EC, the two subscales where unaided performance was reported to be the best. In other words, the IRIS benefit data suggested that hearing aids yield their greatest benefit in difficult listening conditions, whereas the PHAB benefit data indicated that hearing aid benefit is maximized in easy listening conditions.

Why did the two questionnaires produce different benefit patterns? In an attempt to understand this, we compared the aided and unaided data from each questionnaire, as shown in figure 16. To make the two sets of data comparable, it was necessary to reverse the PHAB data so that responses are in terms of percent of situations *without* problems. Examination of these data indicates that in the unaided condition, both inventories produced about the same result. That is, reported proportion of situations without speech communication problems was about equal to estimated proportion of speech intelligibility. However, in the aided condition, results diverged for the two inventories. For most of the subscales, estimated ability to understand speech was much greater than proportion of daily life situations without speech communication problems. Perhaps this outcome indicates that, despite consid-

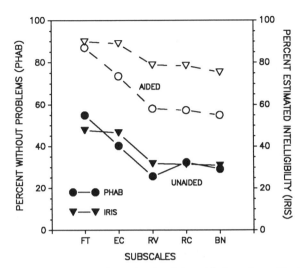

Figure 16. Mean data obtained for aided and unaided conditions using the PHAB and IRIS questionnaires. PHAB data are reversed for this comparison.

erable improvement in ability to understand speech when a hearing aid is worn, the typical hearing aid wearer still experiences many communication problems in daily life.

These data also provided the opportunity to examine the effect of questionnaire format on self-assessment of aided performance. Self-assessed aided performance data obtained using the PHAB questionnaire were compared with self-assessed aided performance data obtained from 30 similar subjects using the PHAP questionnaire. In the lat-

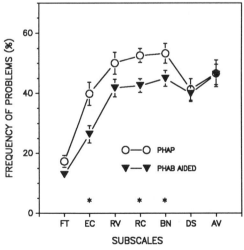

Figure 17. Mean aided performance data for seven subscales, obtained using the PHAB and PHAP questionnaires. Error bars depict ±1 standard error of the means. Asterisks denote subscales having significant mean differences.

ter questionnaire, subjects assessed their aided performance in an absolute sense, whereas, in the former case, they assessed their aided performance in relation to their unaided performance. Figure 17 shows mean aided subscale scores (plus/minus one standard error) measured using the PHAP compared with corresponding mean scores measured using the PHAB. Asterisks above the X-axis labels indicate the instances where t-tests revealed that the difference between PHAP- and PHAB-aided means was significant ($p < .05$). For the five speech understanding subscales, the reported frequency of problems was notably higher for the PHAP than for the PHAB. In other words, people evaluated their aided performance more favorably (i.e., with fewer problems) when they were making a direct comparison with unaided performance than when they were not simultaneously considering unaided performance. Note also that there was no difference at all in the aversiveness or distortion subscale scores (AV and DS). Apparently, direct comparison with unaided performance did not affect the responses to these items.

Summary

These data supported several observations about self-assessed hearing aid benefit:

1. Self-assessed benefit was affected by the types of listening environments assessed. However, with these questionnaires, the difference across types of environments was not as large as in our objective intelligibility measurements. The PHAB appeared somewhat more sensitive than the IRIS to situational differences.
2. Benefit measured by the two questionnaires was not equivalent. The PHAB tended to show the most benefit for subscales in which unaided performance was the best, whereas the IRIS tended to show the most benefit for subscales in which unaided performance was the worst.
3. Our comparisons of PHAP, PHAB, and IRIS data clearly demonstrated that self-assessed hearing aid benefit is strongly influenced by the precise format of the questionnaire used to measure it. Even two instruments as similar as the PHAP and the PHAB apparently do not produce equivalent data. We have yet to determine which of the three questionnaires produces results that are most in concert with the hearing aid wearer's daily life experiences.

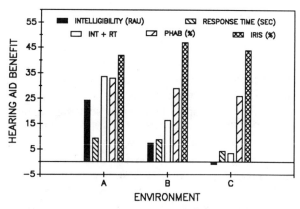

Figure 18. Comparison of self-assessed and objectively measured hearing aid benefit in three listening environments.

Comparison of Benefit Measures

Figure 18 presents a comparison of self-assessed benefit and objectively measured benefit. The figure shows mean benefit data measured in the three basic listening environments using intelligibility, response time, the PHAB, and the IRIS (for the PHAB and IRIS questionnaires, scales SA, SB, and SC are used). In addition, on the assumption that benefit in daily life incorporates both intelligibility and response-time improvements, these two types of objective data have been crudely combined by simply adding them, and the result is shown as the unfilled bars.

These data provide the opportunity to compare patterns of self-assessed and objective benefit measures across listening environments. The dominant pattern is for the most benefit to be seen in Environment A (the living room), and the least in Environment C (the cocktail party), the Environment B (the classroom lecture) somewhere in between. This result is quite consistent with many reports in the literature of self-assessed hearing aid benefit. The self-assessment results for the PHAB do show this pattern, but those for the IRIS do not. Because results for the PHAB are in substantial agreement with previous research on self-assessed benefit and because the PHAB questionnaire also allows us to measure reactions to amplified environmental sounds, our current hypothesis is that the PHAB is the more satisfactory instrument for self-assessment of hearing aid benefit.

It is important to note that the data described here were obtained on several different groups of subjects. In current work, we are obtaining both objective and self-assessed benefit measures on the same subjects. We are attempting to understand the bases of self-assessed benefit and to develop methods whereby it may be objectively quantified in the laboratory and, ultimately, in the clinic.

Software to score the Profile of Hearing Aid Performance was written by Robert Joyce.

References

ANSI 1969. ANSI S3.6-1969. American National Standard Specification for Audiometers (American National Standards Institute, New York).

Barcham, L.J., and Stephens, S.D.G. 1980. The use of an open-ended problems questionnaire in auditory rehabilitation. *British Journal of Audiology* 14:49–51.

Byrne, D. 1986. Effects of frequency response characteristics on speech discrimination and perceived intelligibility and pleasantness of speech for hearing-impaired listeners. *Journal of the Acoustical Society of America* 80:494–504.

Cox, R.M., Alexander, G.C., and Gilmore, C. 1987. Development of the Connected Speech Test (CST). *Ear and Hearing* 8(suppl):119S–126S.

Cox, R.M., Alexander, G.C., Gilmore, C., and Pusakulich, K.M. 1988. Use of the Connected Speech Test (CST) with Hearing-Impaired Listeners. *Ear and Hearing* 9:198–207.

Cox, R.M., Alexander, G.C., Gilmore, C., and Pusakulich, K.M. 1989. The Connected Speech Test Version 3: Audiovisual Administration. *Ear and Hearing* 10:29–32.

Cox, R.M., and Alexander, C.G. 1991a. Hearing aid benefit in everyday environments. *Ear and Hearing* 12:127–39.

Cox, R.M., and Alexander, C.G. 1991b. Preferred hearing aid gain in everyday environments. *Ear and Hearing* 12:123–26.

Cox, R.M., and Gilmore, C. 1990. Development of the Profile of Hearing Aid Performance (PHAP). *Journal of Speech and Hearing Research* 33:343–57.

Cox, R.M., and McDaniel, D.M. 1984. Intelligibility ratings of continuous discourse: Application to hearing aid selection. *Journal of the Acoustical Society of America* 76:758–66.

Cox, R.M., and McDaniel, D.M. 1989. Development of the Speech Intelligibility Rating (SIR) Test for Hearing Aid Comparisons. *Journal of Speech and Hearing Research* 32:347–52.

Cox, R.M., Gilmore, C., and Alexander, G.C. 1991. Comparison of two questionnaires for patient-assessed hearing aid benefit. *Journal of the American Academy of Audiology* 2:in press.

Gatehouse, S., and Gordon, J. 1990. Response times to speech stimuli as measures of benefit from amplification. *British Journal of Audiology* 24:63–68.

Golabek, W., Nowakowska, M., Siwiec, H., and Stephens, S.D.G. 1988. Self-reported benefits of hearing aids by the hearing impaired. *British Journal of Audiology* 22:183–86.

Hagerman, B., and Gabrielsson, A. 1984. Questionnaires

on desirable properties of hearing aids. *Karolinska Inst. Report* TA109.

Haggard, M.P., Foster, J.R., and Iredale, F.E. 1981. Use and benefit of postaural aids in sensory hearing loss. *Scandinavian Audiology* 10:45–52.

Hecker, M.H., Stevens, K.N., and Williams, C.E. 1966. Measurements of reaction time in intelligibility tests. *Journal of the Acoustical Society of America* 39:1188–1189.

Humes, L.E. 1986. An evaluation of several rationales for selecting hearing aid gain. *Journal of Speech and Hearing Disorders* 51:272–81.

Hutton, C.L. 1983. Hearing aid wear times for planning and intervention in aural rehabilitation. *Journal of the Academy of Rehabilitative Audiology* 16:182–201.

Hutton, C.L., and Canahl, J.A. 1985. Scaling patient reports of hearing aid benefit. *Journal of Auditory Research* 25:255–69.

Kapteyn, T.S. 1977. Satisfaction with fitted hearing aids. *Scandinavian Audiology* 6:171–77.

Lynn, J.M., and Lesner, S.A. 1990. Comparison of hearing aid prescriptions: Use, benefit and satisfaction. *Audiology Today* 2(2):33.

Pratt, R.L. 1981. On the use of reaction time as a measure of intelligibility. *British Journal of Audiology* 15:253–55.

Speaks, C., Parker, B., Harris, C., and Kuhl, P. 1972. Intelligibility of connected discourse. *Journal of Speech and Hearing Research* 15:590–602.

Stroud, D.J., and Hamill, T.A. 1989. A multidimensional evaluation of three hearing aid prescription formulae. *ASHA* 31(10):60.

Studebaker, G.A. 1985. A "rationalized" arcsine transform. *Journal of Speech and Hearing Research* 28:455–62.

Walden, B.E., Demorest, M.E., and Hepler, E.L. 1984. Self-report approach to assessing benefit derived from amplification. *Journal of Speech and Hearing Research* 27:49–56.

Wright, R., Spanner, M., and Martin, M. 1981. Pilot experiments with a reaction time audiometer. *British Journal of Audiology* 15:275–81.

CHAPTER 18

Clinical Observations of Self-Report and Global Measures of Hearing Aid Benefit

Patricia McCarthy

At the first Vanderbilt Conference on Amplification, workshop participants were asked to identify the most pressing needs in hearing aid research. Validation of hearing aid success was identified as the most urgent need (Bess 1982). Nine years later, I am very pleased to discuss some of the progress that has been made in this area through the development of self-report and global measures of hearing aid benefit. The chapter by Dr. Robyn Cox provides an excellent description of her work in developing tools to measure hearing aid benefit. The purpose of this presentation is to discuss some of the additional work that has been done in the subjective measurement of hearing aid success with a focus on the clinical utility of these measures.

Interest in self-report measures of hearing aid benefit seems to have evolved for at least two reasons. First, while psychophysical and electroacoustical measures used in traditional hearing aid evaluations can quantify many aspects of hearing aid performance, these measures fall short in the area of predictive validity. Hearing aid evaluation techniques are insufficient in predicting success with amplification, and results obtained in the clinic typically cannot be generalized to everyday communication. Walden (1982) has suggested that a prerequisite to the evaluation of predictive validity is the development of relevant criterion measures. Consequently, some research efforts have focused on the development of self-report methods as criterion measures because they reflect performance in everyday communication.

The second reason for the growing interest in self-report measures of hearing aid benefit appears to be the increased emphasis on documentation of rehabilitative outcome in health care. Because hearing aids act as the nucleus of most aural rehabilitation plans, documentation of the benefits of amplification can serve as one indicator of the success of aural rehabilitation. Furthermore, the information obtained from these self-reports allows modification of the hearing aid, thus possibly enhancing the overall success of aural rehabilitation.

Research efforts in the use of self-report methodology have taken two different avenues. Some researchers have attempted to design new tools to measure benefit from hearing aids subjectively, while others have examined the use of existing inventories to measure hearing aid success.

Innovative Measures of Hearing Aid Benefit

One of the earliest attempts to predict success with amplification was developed by Rupp, Higgins, and Maurer (1977) for use with older hearing-impaired patients. The Feasibility Scale for Predicting Hearing Aid Use (FSPHAU) consists of 11 prognostic indicators of hearing handicap that purportedly predict success with amplification. The indicators include motivation, self-assessment of communication difficulties, "fault" for communicative difficulties, magnitude of hearing loss, informal verbalizations during the hearing aid evaluation, flexibility and adaptability, age, manual dexterity, visual ability, financial resources, and the presence of a significant other. Each of these factors is weighted according to its potential contribution to success with amplification, with motivation assigned the greatest weighted value. Percentage scores are calculated using a six-point scale for each factor. Patients with high scores (76–100%) are considered likely to be more successful with hearing aids than those with low scores (0–40%). Examination of the FSPHAU reveals some strengths but several weaknesses undermining its clinical utility. Obviously, it represents an innovative attempt to examine formally many of the factors that ultimately contribute to hearing aid acceptance and success. However, scoring of this scale is subjective and requires value judgments on the part of the audiologist. Clearly, there is room for misjudgment. An additional strength of the FSPHAU is that it was the initial attempt to predict hearing aid success. However, although the authors supplied anecdotal reports of its use, no data describing the reliability or predictive or criterion validity were reported.

Recently, Chermak and Miller (1988) examined both the test-retest reliability and the criterion validity of a revised form of the FSPHAU. The Hearing Handicap Inventory for the Elderly (Ventry and Weinstein 1982) served as the criterion measure of hearing aid success as predicted by the FSPHAU. Unfortunately, Chermak and Miller found the test-retest reliability of the revised FSPHAU was inadequate as indicated by significant changes in scores between administrations. Although discussion of validity in the absence of reliability is irrelevant, results of this study did not support the criterion validity of the FSPHAU for predicting hearing aid success. Therefore, while the FSPHAU would seem to be a clinically useful predictive measure, psychometric data do not support its use. Chermak and Miller report they are looking at further modifications of the FSPHAU that might improve its reliability and validity.

Prompted by an interest in the compounding factors that create difficulties for the elderly in adjusting to amplification, the Bill Wilkerson Hearing and Speech Center has developed four abbreviated self-appraisal questionnaires for use with elderly hearing aid patients (Lazenby et al. 1986). Questionnaire 1 focuses on the patient's attitude toward hearing loss and hearing aids, while Questionnaire 2 examines the patient's ability to manipulate and care for a hearing aid. Questionnaire 3 was designed to evaluate hearing aid success, while Questionnaire 4 probes the patient's perception of services.

Although no psychometric data have been published, Lazenby et al. (1986) report that these questionnaires have been helpful in assessing hearing aid success under a variety of listening conditions. Interestingly, the majority of their patients agreed that their hearing aids were worth their financial investment, while only 10% were uncertain about their investment. Questioning the financial value of the hearing aid appears to be a novel, highly pragmatic way of measuring hearing aid benefit with a strong consumer emphasis. The authors suggest that these questionnaires have been useful in providing direction for counseling as well as modification of electroacoustic characteristics of the hearing aid. Furthermore, these questionnaires appear to be useful tools for documenting rehabilitative outcome.

Perhaps the best designed self-report approach to assessing benefit derived from amplification is the Hearing Aid Performance Inventory (HAPI) (Walden, Demorest, and Hepler 1984). This 64-item questionnaire utilizes a 5-point rating scale ranging from "Very Helpful" to "Hinders Performance."

Walden, Demorest, and Hepler (1984) used the HAPI to assess the potential of a self-report instrument as a criterion measure for studying the predictive validity of hearing aid selection procedures. They found excellent internal consistency reliability ($\alpha = .96$), suggesting that individual differences in perceived benefit from amplification can be assessed reliably using the HAPI. Furthermore, factor analysis led to the identification of four types of situations that could be used as criterion measures: (a) noisy situations, (b) quiet situations with the speaker in proximity, (c) situations with reduced signal information, and (d) situations with nonspeech stimuli. These results suggest that hearing aid benefit for an individual patient in quiet may not be predicted well from his or her performance in noise. In fact, patients in this study generally reported significantly more benefit from their aid in quiet than in noise. This is consistent with the findings of Scherr, Schwartz, and Montgomery (1983), whose survey results showed consistently higher hearing aid ratings in quiet than in noisy conditions. Walden, Demorest, and Hepler (1984) suggest it may be useful to assess benefit from amplification separately for noisy and quiet listening conditions. The authors concluded that self-report methodology for measuring hearing aid success in daily life appears promising as a criterion measure for future predictive validation studies.

From a clinical standpoint, modifications of the HAPI may be necessary before it can be used routinely in most hearing aid dispensing programs. The 64-item length appears to be the greatest deterrent. However, Walden, Demorest, and Hepler (1984) report that the high value of the reliability coefficient alpha (.96) implies that the questionnaire could be reduced in length considerably without greatly affecting reliability. They suggest that estimated reliability of a 32-item questionnaire would still be .92 while further reduction to a 16-item measure would lower alpha to .86. In addition to its length, many of the HAPI items are not applicable to the elderly population, thus possibly limiting its clinical use. However, given the strength of its psychometric properties, one hopes that future research efforts will focus on modifying it for clinical use.

Use of Existing Inventories

Several researchers have attempted to demonstrate the utility of existing hearing handicap inventories in assessing hearing aid benefit. Tannahill (1979) reported on use of the Hearing Handicap Scale (HHS) (High, Fairbanks, and Glorig 1964) as a measure of hearing aid benefit by comparing responses obtained prior to hearing aid use with that obtained following hearing aid use. Subjects ranging from 56 to 91 years of age demonstrated a significant reduction in handicap following four weeks of hearing aid use. Tannahill concluded that the HHS is useful for assessing hearing aid benefit and supplementing audiometric results.

The results of Tannahill's study coupled with the reliability of the HHS suggest it is a viable measure of hearing aid benefit. However, the scope of the HHS is so narrow that it limits its ability to reflect everyday communication difficulties validly. Consequently, its clinical value in assessing hearing aid benefit remains limited.

Dempsey (1986) investigated the effectiveness of the Hearing Performance Inventory (HPI) (Giolas et al. 1979) in measuring hearing aid benefit. After a six-week interval, he found a significant reduction in hearing handicap for the Understanding Speech and Intensity sections of the HPI. However, the ability to generalize these results is somewhat limited because the sample size was only 10. Given the broad scope of the HPI, further investigation may support its use in measuring hearing aid benefit. From a clinical perspective, the length of the scale (90 items) and the complexity of some of the items have been considered problematic. Consequently, many hearing aid dispensers may find it cumbersome to use on a pre- and post-evaluation basis.

Hutton (1980) investigated use of the Hearing Problem Inventory to measure hearing aid benefit. The HPI was administered to 329 patients prior to a hearing aid evaluation and again six weeks after the hearing aid had been fitted. Comparisons of pre- and post-data showed reductions in problems reported and increases in hearing aid wear time. Interestingly, Hutton reported larger systematic reductions in self-assessed problems in new hearing aid users than in those patients being seen for re-

placement hearing aids. Hutton's ongoing study of hearing aid benefit as measured by the HPI focuses on hours per day the aid is worn, its benefit in various situations, and degree of satisfaction (Hutton and Canahl 1985). The length of this inventory (84 items) precludes its routine use for many clinics. The HPI appears to be a research oriented tool at this point.

Measurement of hearing aid benefit in the elderly as measured by the Hearing Handicap Inventory for the Elderly (HHIE) (Ventry and Weinstein 1982) has been studied recently by Weinstein and her colleagues. Newman and Weinstein (1988) administered the HHIE to a group of elderly hearing-impaired adult males prior to and following one year of hearing aid use. Their findings showed a significant reduction in the perceived emotional and social effects of hearing impairment as measured by the HHIE. Ongoing interest in the optimal time interval necessary to measure hearing aid benefit prompted Malinoff and Weinstein (1989a) to administer the HHIE to a group of 45 new hearing aid users prior to and following three weeks of hearing aid use. A statistically significant reduction in perceived handicap was found again. In order to monitor reaction to the benefits of amplification over a one year period, Malinoff and Weinstein (1989b) administered the HHIE to 25 older adults at three weeks, at three months, and at one year after initial hearing aid fitting. Again, a significant reduction in perceived handicap was found after three weeks of hearing aid use. However, a significant increase in perceived handicap was observed during the interval between three weeks and three months, with a stabilization occurring between three months and one year. The authors suggested that a three-month interval is probably more realistic than three weeks. The greater reduction handicap noted after the shorter interval may have been influenced by the initial enthusiasm and positive feelings about amplification. The authors suggest that the three month interval is more likely to be realistic because it allows hearing aid users more time to evaluate the limitations of amplification. However, Demorest and Erdman (1988) caution that lengthening the test-retest interval increases the likelihood that the true test score will change due to personal and environmental factors rather than as a result of hearing aid use. Clearly, more research is needed to determine the optimal time interval(s) to assess hearing aid benefit using self-report methods.

Given the validity and reliability of the HHIE, its use as a clinical tool to measure hearing aid outcome with the elderly population is promising. To date, the work of Weinstein and colleagues in this area has been with the full-length version of the HHIE. The abbreviated length of the screening form (HHIE-S) makes it an attractive clinical tool for assessing hearing aid benefit in the elderly population. Because the validity and reliability of the screening version of the HHIE-S have been documented, future efforts should focus on its use in measuring hearing aid success.

Conclusions

The initial work in the use of self-report methodology to assess hearing aid benefit is encouraging. Self-report tools appear to have potential as clinical measures of hearing aid outcome and as criterion measures for examining the predictive validity of hearing aid evaluation procedures. However, the work done to date is only the beginning. Some of the points on which future research needs in this area might focus are the following:

1. Because self-report methodology seems viable as a criterion measure, predictive validation studies of hearing aid evaluation procedures should be initiated.

2. Traditional hearing aid evaluation procedures typically produce better results in noise than in quiet, whereas self-report measures appear to show just the opposite (Walden, Demorest, and Hepler 1984; Scherr, Schwartz, and Montgomery 1983). Research should continue to focus on the issue of quiet versus noisy listening conditions as two separate criterion measures in assessing hearing aid benefit. Clearly, this is important information for effective hearing aid counseling.

3. Many audiologists feel self-assessment inventories yield much data, but they are unsure how to translate this information into effective audiologic rehabilitation (McCarthy, Montgomery, and Mueller 1990). Further study is needed to investigate how self-report data can be used in rehabilitation planning and hearing aid counseling.

4. The feasibility of using personal computers for administration and scoring of self-report inventories should be investigated. Humes (1988) has developed a software program (HI-5) that is a collection of five existing hearing inventories: HHS, HHIE, HHIE-S, HPI, and HAPI. Software of this type should be evaluated for its clinical utility in measuring hearing aid benefit, particularly with elderly hearing aid patients.

5. From a clinical perspective, the issue of administration time cannot be ignored. Despite the apparent utility of several self-report inventories in documenting hearing aid benefit, self-report tools will continue to be underused if hearing aid dispensers deem them to be too time consuming (McCarthy, Montgomery, and Mueller 1990). Research efforts should focus on development and/or refinement of reliable, valid, and time-efficient self-report methods.

There are many unanswered questions surrounding self-report and global methods of assessing hearing aid benefit. Clearly, continued research in this area will benefit us as hearing aid dispensers. But perhaps the greatest benefit of this type of research is that it focuses our attention on what the patient is telling us rather than what our audiometric results suggest. Ultimately, this should result in improved hearing aid service delivery to the consumer.

References

Bess, F.H. 1982. Amplification for the hearing impaired: Research priorities. In *The Vanderbilt Hearing Aid Report: State of the Art–Research Needs,* eds. G.A. Studebaker and F.H. Bess. Monographs in Contemporary Audiology. Upper Darby, PA: E.R. Libby.

Chermak, G.D., and Miller, M.C. 1988. Shortcomings of a revised feasibility scale for predicting hearing aid use with older adults. *British Journal of Audiology* 22:187–94.

Demorest, M.E., and Erdman, S.A. 1988. Retest stability of the communication profile for the hearing impaired. *Ear and Hearing* 9:237–42.

Dempsey, J.J. 1986. The hearing performance inventory as a tool in fitting hearing aids. *Journal of the Academy of Rehabilitative Audiology* 19:116–25.

Giolas, T., Owens, E., Lamb, H., and Schubert, E. 1979. Hearing performance inventory. *Journal of Speech and Hearing Disorders* 44:169–95.

High, W.S., Fairbanks, G., and Glorig, A. 1964. Scale for self-assessment of hearing handicap. *Journal of Speech and Hearing Disorders* 29:215–30.

Humes, L. 1988. HI-5, Version 1.1. Bloomington, IN: Venture 4th.

Hutton, C.L. 1980. Responses to a hearing problem inventory. *Journal of the Academy of Rehabilitative Audiology* 13:133–54.

Hutton, C.L., and Canahl, J. 1985. Scaling patient reports of hearing aid benefit. *Journal of Auditory Research* 25:255–65.

Lazenby, B.B., Logan, S.A., Ahlstrom, J., and Bess, F.H. 1986. Self-assessment questionnaire for the elderly: Hearing aid dispensary use. *The Hearing Journal* 39: 18–21.

Malinoff, R.L., and Weinstein, B.E. 1989a. Measurement of hearing aid benefit in the elderly. *Ear and Hearing* 10:354–56.

Malinoff, R.L., and Weinstein, B.E. 1989b. Changes in self-assessment of hearing handicap over the first year of hearing aid use by older adults. *Journal of the Academy of Rehabilitative Audiology* 22:54–60.

McCarthy, P.A., Montgomery, A.A., and Mueller, H.G. 1990. Decision making in rehabilitative audiology. *Journal of the American Academy of Audiology* 1:23–30.

Newman, C.W., and Weinstein, B.E. 1988. The hearing handicap inventory for the elderly as a measure of hearing aid benefit. *Ear and Hearing* 9:81–85.

Rupp, R., Higgins, J., and Maurer, J. 1977. A feasibility scale for predicting hearing aid use (FSPHAU) with older individuals. *Journal of the Academy of Rehabilitative Audiology* 10:81–104.

Scherr, C.K., Schwartz, D.M., and Montgomery, A.A. 1983. Follow-up survey of new hearing aid users. *Journal of the Academy of Rehabilitative Audiology* 16:202–209.

Tannahill, J.C. 1979. The hearing handicap scale as a measure of hearing aid benefit. *Journal of Speech and Hearing Disorders* 44:91–99.

Ventry, I., and Weinstein, B.E. 1982. The hearing handicap inventory for the elderly: A new tool. *Ear and Hearing* 3:128–34.

Walden, B.E. 1982. Validating measures for hearing aid success. In *The Vanderbilt Hearing Aid Report: State of the Art–Research Needs*, eds. G.A. Studebaker and F.H. Bess. Monographs in Contemporary Audiology. Upper Darby, PA: E.R. Libby.

Walden, B.E., Demorest, M., and Hepler, E.L. 1984. Self-report approach to assessing benefit derived from amplification. *Journal of Speech and Hearing Research* 27:49–56.

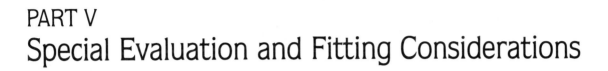

PART V
Special Evaluation and Fitting Considerations

CHAPTER 19

Aural Rehabilitation
Review and Preview

Allen A. Montgomery

In this chapter, I examine several issues and developments under the general heading of hearing aids and aural rehabilitation. I begin by discussing the role of aural rehabilitation in hearing aid fitting. Then I introduce five overall goals of the aural rehabilitation process and illustrate in some detail two of them (auditory-visual integration and cognitive processing). These two processes seem to be especially amenable to progress in the next decade. Following this, a briefer review of several promising clinical and technological topics is presented. Finally, an appeal is made for audiologists to accept responsibility for the overall management of the hearing-impaired adult and to view the aural rehabilitation group meeting as the ideal mechanism for implementing that responsibility.

Role of Hearing Aids in Rehabilitation

It is most appropriate to ask the question, "What is the role of the hearing aid in the overall management and rehabilitation of the hearing-impaired adult with acquired hearing loss?" However, the focus of this book is on hearing aids, and to a large extent, hearing aid technology, so I will rephrase the question to read, "What is the role of aural rehabilitation in the fitting and dispensing of hearing aids?" There are at least four relatively distinct ways in which aural rehabilitation can assist the process of hearing aid fitting.

Insurance

The most important function of aural rehabilitation is that it insures (as much as currently possible) that the patient will actually use the aid! It is nonsense for members of a profession to spend large amounts of money, time, and research efforts to provide the ideal frequency/gain characteristics in an aid and then do little to insure that the aid is worn. It is like giving a person a new computer and saying, "I'll show you how to turn it on and where to get it repaired, but it's up to you to learn how to use it." Aural rehabilitation, especially in the form of the aural rehabilitation group that serves as the analogous "users' group," provides support and guidance during the initial adjustment and acceptance period (Binnie and Hession 1990). I return to this point later, when considering some efficient ways for the audiologist to conduct aural rehabilitation.

Auditory-Visual Integration

Aural rehabilitation stresses the importance of speechreading in communication and, more importantly, the use of speechreading in combination with amplified auditory speech. It is safe to say that all patients with reasonable vision will benefit from integration of the auditory and visual components of speech. Auditory-visual integration (AVI), however, is a skill to be acquired, and many patients perform at a suboptimal level. Indeed, as we see in a subsequent section, the exact specifications of optimal AVI are not well understood or easily measured.

User Education

Aural rehabilitation strives to produce an informed user who can understand and use hearing aid technology and assistive listening devices to the extent needed for his or her particular circumstances. This aspect of aural rehabilitation will be especially important in the next few years as hearing aid technology evolves more options for the user and more ways for the aid to adapt to changing acoustic environments. The most successful systems will be those that allow meaningful on-line user selection of various options, rather than those that are completely automatic. Let the intelligence reside in the human being, not in the microprocessor. In fact, as a general principle, it is probably true that the more control the user has over an instrument, the more likely he or she is to use it.

Hearing Aid Failure

For patients with moderate or worse losses, hearing aids typically do not restore speech understanding to its previous level. Because the hearing loss is not a simple filter function (as erroneously implied by the audiogram), the patient has difficulty using the aid, especially in noisy environments. One of the specific goals of aural rehabilitation is to produce an assertive communicator who can actively reduce or avoid noisy circumstances ("Let's not go to Charlie's for lunch, it's too noisy there"). This produces a person who can compensate and adjust those circumstances where the hearing aid is not particularly effective, not just serve as a passive listener who either "gets" something or does not. That is, in the process of aural rehabilitation, the patient gets to know the weaknesses and failures of the aid as well as its strengths, and how to deal with them.

The Five Maximizations

I have focused so far on four specific areas where aural rehabilitation has a direct impact on hearing aid use. Now I consider the broader, overall goals of aural rehabilitation. These are cast in the form of trying to maximize five hierarchically arranged processes, depending on a particular patient's abilities and needs. Table I shows the goals that provide direction for our adult group and individual rehabilitation services. They proceed from supplying the best possible visual and amplified audio input (goal 1) to integrating those sources of information (goal 2) and applying knowledge of the world, the current situation, and the language to the task of reducing the ambiguity of the incomplete sensory signal (goal 3). Finally, specific problems in the work and home environments are addressed (goal 4), and an assertive/interactive way of communicating and repairing communication breakdown (Erber 1988) is promoted (goal 5). We have chosen two

Table I. Goals in Adult Aural Rehabilitation

1. Maximize Sensory Input
2. Maximize Sensory Integration
3. Maximize Cognitive Processing
4. Maximize Family/Work Communication
5. Maximize Interactive Communication

of them, sensory integration and cognitive processing, for elaboration.

Auditory-Visual Integration (AVI)

It is obviously important for the hearing-impaired individual to combine the amplified auditory speech information with the visible signal available through speechreading. Numerous studies have demonstrated the tremendous benefit derived from adding speechreading to an auditory speech recognition task (Sumby and Pollack 1954; Binnie, Montgomery, and Jackson 1974). Surprisingly enough, many patients need to be convinced of this benefit before they will consciously incorporate speechreading into daily use. The data shown in figure 1 are derived from a classic study by Sumby and Pollack (1954) and illustrate the effects of combining the auditory and visual speech signals. Obviously, at lower auditory-only performance levels, substantial benefit is derived.

Optimal AVI

It is often said that at the phoneme level, for example, the visual information is used to select from among audibly similar candidates (Walden, Prosek, and Worthington 1975). For example, /p/, /t/, and /k/ may sound alike to an impaired individual, but are usually distinct visually; /p/, /b/, and /m/ look alike, but are audibly different. Thus, an optimal com-

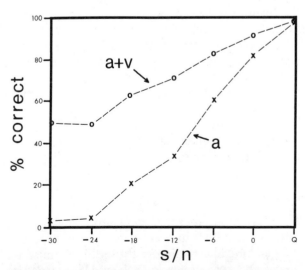

Figure 1. Auditory and auditory-visual speech recognition data for the mean of 64- and 128-word sets, taken with permission from Sumby and Pollack (1954).

bination of these two categorizations would result in the recognition of /p/ when it is presented.

In reality, however, the process is rarely that simple. The distinction between the /p, t, k/ auditory cluster and other phonemes is not complete, but has a certain probability associated with it (as do the visual clusters). The patient may also favor one modality over the other. Thus, if the auditory signal (wrongly) sounds somewhat like /t/ but looks like /p/, the patient may override the correct visual input and perceive /t/ because of his or her auditory bias. It becomes a complex matter of probabilities, biases, weights, and decisions in the face of uncertainty and conflicting information. There is no reason at all to assume that the integration process is optimal in a given patient. This is illustrated in table II, which shows a confusion matrix drawn from Walden et al. (1987). In this study, hearing-impaired subjects were presented with consonant-vowel (CV) nonsense syllables for recognition under three conditions: unamplified-auditory only (UNAMP), amplified auditory-only through their hearing aids (AMP), and amplified audio plus speechreading (AMP + VIS). The /p, b, m/ part of a larger matrix is shown for the UNAMP condition. Thus, when /m/ was presented, /b/ was perceived 13 times out of a total of 240 trials, /m/ was correctly recognized 181 times, and responses to 42 other consonants were made. The /m/ stimulus rows from the AMP and the AMP + VIS matrices are added at the bottom for comparison. When the signal is amplified, some of the errors on the other consonants are resolved to the main diagonal, as would be expected. However, when vision is added, not only do the other errors go wrongly to /b/ (41 entries instead of 13), but the number of correct /m/ responses only increases from 191 to 198. Thus, for these subjects, vision does

not improve recognition of /m/. When the 34 other consonant errors (35−1=34) are distributed in a more optimal way (based on audition, which is one of several ways to define optimal, such that the proportion of /b/ and /m/ responses remains at 13:191), the correct recognition of /m/ jumps to 223, or 92.9% correct. These patients are obviously not performing optimally in their auditory-visual integration. Unfortunately, as mentioned above, calculating optimal auditory-visual (AV) from auditory and visual performance is not simple, and at the moment no acceptable method is available. Some promising models are being developed however (Braida 1988; Massaro 1987), and some techniques may emerge that will permit assessment of a patient's auditory-visual performance relative to his or her theoretical maximum. At that point, but not before, quantitative evaluation of the effect of AV training becomes feasible and should be the focus of clinical research.

Auditory-Visual Articulation Index (AV-AI)

Another aspect of AV integration that merits audiologists' attention is the possibility of developing an auditory-visual version of the Articulation Index (AV-AI). Of course, the ANSI AI standard (1969, pg. 22) has a function that relates calculated AI to effective AI with visual cues. The amount added to the auditory AI for speech-reading ranges from 15% in the lower AI range to 5–6% in the higher range, tapering to zero at AI = 1.0. This conversion, however, assumes that the visual contribution to intelligibility is a function strictly of the overall AI, not of the individual frequency bands. Audiologists currently devote a great deal of time to determining the exact amount of gain needed by a patient at each point in the frequency/gain (F/G) function to maximize auditory speech recognition. I propose that the question audiologists should be addressing instead is, "What is the F/G function that will produce the maximum AV intelligibility?" It is reasonable to assume that most hearing aid use takes place where the talker is visible to the user (especially if one considers the large amounts of time spent watching TV), and the best possible AV speech recognition is therefore an obvious goal. (Ideally the best solution is to have three or four F/G settings: one of which is the best auditory-only configuration, and the others, the best AV settings for various noise environments. This calls for an informed user—one of the goals assigned to aural rehabilitation.)

Conventional wisdom suggests that the lower

Table II. Confusion Matrix from Unamplified, Auditory-Only Conditions (UNAMP) (Taken from Walden et al. (1987) showing responses to /p/, /b/, and /m/.) Responses to /m/ from amplified (AMP), amplified with vision (AMP + VIS), and a theoretical optimal response are added for comparison.

	Responses				
	P	B	M	Etc.	
Stimuli					
P	144	4	1	91	
B	13	110	1	116	
M	4	13	181	42	Unamp
M	1	13	191	35	Amp
M	0	41	198	1	Amp + Vis
M	1	15	223	1	Optimal

frequencies, where the invisible voicing and nasality cues are most prominent, would be more heavily weighted in the AV-AI. However, this expectation is based on CV nonsense-syllable recognition (Miller and Nicely 1955; Binnie, Montgomery, and Jackson 1974), and should not necessarily hold for AV sentence recognition where the performance-intensity (PI) functions are extremely steep and top-down processing is heavily involved. The role of temporal processing of sentence-length material is also important. The amplitude envelope of the speech wave form, which is generally distributed in frequency, contains much information on stress, timing, word and syllable boundaries, and phoneme onset characteristics; in combination with speechreading, it contributes strongly to sentence recognition. Breeuwer and Plomp (1984), for example, showed that time/amplitude information alone in a one-octave band centered at 500 Hz raised AV sentence intelligibility from 22% (V only) to 66%. Similar results are obtained by adding fundamental frequency information (Rosen, Fourcin, and Moore 1981).

This proposal to maximize AV intelligibility raises some interesting possibilities. First, we may find a need to trade off some possible upward spread of masking for increased temporal information in the low frequencies, especially for patients with flat losses and poor temporal speechreading skills. (The low frequencies, of course, may contribute to sound quality and thus to user acceptance as well.) Second, it would be necessary to develop efficient AV testing procedures. The AV connected speech test (CST) material developed by Cox and her colleagues (1989) may be very valuable in this regard. Also, the continuous discourse/perceived intelligibility procedure developed by Hawkins et al. (1988) may be useful as well. In this task a subject is seated in a moderately reverberant room with noise from three loudspeakers at 90°, 180°, and 270° and continuous discourse from a TV monitor and loudspeaker at 0° azimuth. The subject makes repeated estimations of percent intelligibility (similar to the procedure of Cox and McDaniel 1984) as the examiner varies the noise level to create a range of signal-to-noise (S/N) ratios. The procedure is done under auditory-only and auditory-visual conditions. Figure 2 shows a smoothed example of the PI functions obtained from a hearing subject. It can be seen that the slopes are quite steep, as would be expected from continuous discourse. In this case the opportunity to speechread provides approximately 9 dB resistance to noise. The results are in dB S/N and are comparable to those of Middelweerd and Plomp (1987), who used sentences presented in A

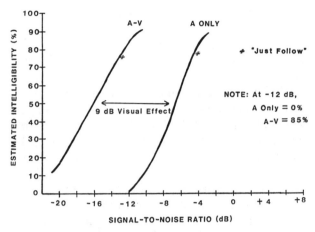

Figure 2. Performance intensity functions from one normal-hearing subject. Performance is based on subject's estimates of intelligibility of connected discourse. Procedure is based on Hawkins et al. (1988).

and AV formats. As noted, at a particular S/N (−12 dB), adding vision raises estimated intelligibility from zero to approximately 85% intelligibility, which is sufficient to allow the subject generally to follow the monologue.

Grant (1987, 1988) has begun to investigate the AV-AI. To date, his results on sentence processing are consistent with a large role of temporal visual processing (and thus not a lot of differences in the AV band weights). However, given the large differences in talker visual intelligibility (Kricos and Lesner 1982) and the even larger range of speechreading skills (Montgomery and Sylvester 1984), it is very unlikely that the best auditory-only F/G function will also be the best AV setting for individual patients. The AV-AI needs to be explored fully, and if its value for even a modest percentage of patients (such as the good speechreaders) can be demonstrated, then it should be incorporated into our fitting procedures to better prepare the hearing aid user for the auditory-visual world.

The advent of specific models of AVI, even though presently only at the CV monosyllable level, and the availability of lower cost videodisc recorders as well as players, indicate that the next decade will yield significant improvements in the assessment and training of the hearing impaired adult's most important skill, auditory-visual integration.

Sentence Understanding

Now let us turn our attention to another topic that shows equal promise for advancement and benefit for the hearing-impaired population. The last 20 years have seen the "cognitive revolution" in psychology in which behaviorism has been replaced by an understanding of human beings as highly sophisticated "pre-wired" processors of information (Osherson and Lasnik 1990, offers a good introduction to this subject). It is appropriate that aural rehabilitation draws upon whatever concepts and insights arise from cognitive psychology. One of the areas where it may be helpful to aural rehabilitation is in the attempts by cognitive psychologists to study word recognition and sentence understanding. Neither of these cognitive activities is well understood yet, but word recognition is currently the subject of considerable activity (Frauenfelder and Tyler 1987; Marslen-Wilson 1989). Normal sentence understanding is also receiving attention (see Garrett 1990). Our concern, however, is with sentence (and eventually continuous discourse) processing by the hearing-impaired adult. The following is a demonstration of one initial attempt to deduce some of the cognitive processes that underlie the errors made while speechreading sentences. The procedure has been called the Repeated Sentence Task (RST).

Repeated Sentence Task

In the RST, a hearing-impaired person is asked to speechread repeatedly a videodisc presentation of a sentence produced by a talker. No sound is included. After each presentation, the subject writes down what he or she perceived, guessing where possible. The sentence typically is presented up to 12 times or until the sentence is perceived correctly, whichever comes first; that number can be increased if the subject seems to be close to a correct response. The goal is to get a sequence of responses to the same sentence that shows a progression of understanding from zero or a few words or fragments to a correct rendering of the sentence. This sequence is then studied in a deductive, nonquantitative way to determine, if possible, the perceptual and cognitive processes apparent in the resolution of errors and false starts that characterize the sequence. Table III shows examples of RST sequences obtained from two subjects under a visual-only speech recognition condition. In the first example the subject responds initially with some erroneous but visually reasonable words. Nothing changes until the fourth response, however, when he sees "brush," and by the next repetition he has

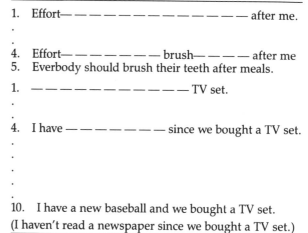

Table III. Responses from Two Hearing-Impaired Subjects on a Sentence Recognition Test. (Sentences were presented repeatedly in a visual-only mode.)

1. Effort— — — — — — — — — — — — after me.
.
.
4. Effort— — — — — — — brush— — — — after me
5. Everbody should brush their teeth after meals.
1. — — — — — — — — — — — TV set.
.
4. I have — — — — — — since we bought a TV set.
.
.
.
10. I have a new baseball and we bought a TV set.
(I haven't read a newspaper since we bought a TV set.)

figured it out. He was thus able to abandon his earlier guesses both preceding and following the correct word and fill in appropriately. The subject in the second example is not so successful. He gets "TV set" correct immediately, and gets the entire last phrase by the fourth exposure to the sentence. However, he is unable to move backward through the presentation and find any meaning in the first half that logically leads to the correctly received second phrase. In fact, by repetition ten, he has even abandoned his correct "since" to make his "baseball" guess more sensible, and he has decided on two sentences joined by "and."

These examples illustrate only a few of the many patterns of response progression (or failure!) that may arise from the RST. Some of the more common patterns I have seen lead to interpretations as follows:

1. The subject fixates rigidly on a wrong choice and will not experiment and change it, even when it is obviously wrong.
2. The subject must get the initial few words before any later word. He is unable to work backward toward the beginning of the sentence.
3. When faced with difficulty, the subject resorts to a series of simple conjoined sentences rather than the correct, more complex one.
4. The subject does not detect brief visual units such as the end of contractions, function words, and unstressed syllables. This person appears to be a candidate for structured speechreading training.
5. The subject cannot detect many word boundaries, misses syllable stress indicators, and gets the wrong number of syllables by more than

two. This pattern suggests a lack of time domain information, and the person presumably would show improvement with even a minimal auditory supplement.

6. The subject misses many content words, and so, gets few reliable words from which to build a sentence. This person, presumably, is a poor speechreader at the single word level.

7. The subject gets words or phrases correct, then later abandons them. The person either lacks confidence or is unable to confirm his or her responses upon repetition.

In this procedure we have substantially removed memory from the task in order to examine the processes underlying the errors in visual sentence recognition and, in effect, to get a slow motion look at his or her thinking. In my experience, much more insight into the nature of the subjects' difficulties is available from looking at several repetitions of a few sentences than from looking at single responses to many different sentences. The RST tells you *what* the problems are to some extent, whereas the first attempt only tells you whether or not they exist. One doesn't see the time domain problems, the rigidity, or the lack of confidence without examining the sequence of repetitions. While this technique is still under development it seems to be helpful for problem cases and for structuring individual aural rehabilitation procedures.

Clinical and Research Developments

In this section I consider several developments, both real and potential, which may affect the way aural rehabilitation is conducted in the future. The list is quite selective and makes no attempt to be complete. Tactile aids and cochlear implants are omitted completely, for example. Also, the important topics of AV test battery development and self-assessment procedures have been treated recently and are not included here (Montgomery and Demorest 1988).

AV Asynchronization

It is only a matter of time before various advanced forms of speech signal processing (SSP) are incorporated into hearing aids and cochlear implants. (See Levitt, this volume, Chapter 8, for more information.) The SSP algorithms face a clear limit, however, on the amount of time they have for process-

ing before the audio signal is sufficiently delayed behind the speechreading signal to be noticeable and interfere with AV integration. Several studies have addressed this issue (McGrath and Summerfield 1985; Pandey, Kunov, and Abel 1986; Dixon and Spitz 1980). The best estimate seems to be about 80 ms (McGrath and Summerfield 1985), but little is known about continuous discourse processing, and no study to date has determined the amount to which tolerable AV asynchrony may be increased through training. This question must be addressed before complex SSP techniques can be implemented in wearable units.

Automatic Speech Recognition (ASR)

It is commercially and humanistically desirable to be able to recognize speech with a computer. Considerable progress has been made in this very difficult engineering problem (Lee 1989), and it now appears to be possible to identify continuous speech with an ASR system under certain circumstances. When this capability is developed fully, it will have tremendous implications for the deaf and hearing-impaired population. Ideally, at a large conference a screen would display speech orthographically a few seconds after it was produced! ASR systems, however are very prone to errors and sensitive to noise. It may be necessary, again, to let some of the intelligence reside in the viewer, that is, to let the individual have some idea of the possibilities considered by the computer and to choose the correct meaning from the possible ones. Figure 3 shows a possible output from an ASR system processing the sentence (referring to golf) "I'll bet you can't find out if she parred it or not." The path selected by the computer is shown by the asterisks and the correct path is shown by the dotted line. The exact error rates and the size of the word-candidate pool that can be tolerated by deaf viewers is unknown. In fact, the whole human factor issue of how best to display error-prone information to the deaf is largely unexplored. This will certainly become a

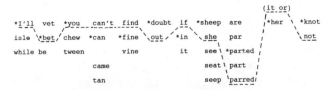

Figure 3. Illustration of hypothetical sentence path as produced by an automatic speech recognition system. Dotted lines indicate correct response, asterisks mark words selected by computer from pool of candidates.

useful area for research as the exact nature and quality of ASR output becomes known.

An interesting example of human factor research in visual displays is seen in the ongoing development of the autocuer (Research Triangle Institute 1984; Cornett and Beadles 1989). This device processes speech in near real time and displays speech features available in cued speech, such as voicing and nasality, as a series of small vertical and horizontal bars. These bars are located on the surface of the user's glasses and light up when the particular feature is present. Field trials are apparently underway to determine if this type of processing and display will supplement speechreading in the same successful manner as does manually cued speech.

Sign Systems for the Elderly

On a much less technical level, Marcia Montgomery and I are pursuing the use of a modified sign language system for use by an elderly couple where one spouse has acquired a profound hearing loss and the other has relatively normal hearing. Results to date are promising, as our test couple uses signs and fingerspelling to resolve serious communication breakdowns, but are not yet using signing in all situations where it might be helpful. This approach would appear to be an alternative to be considered in special cases, although further refinement of the teaching procedures is needed.

Tinnitus Rehabilitation

No audiologist can avoid the question, "What about the ringing in my ears?" At present, there is no optimistic answer to this frequent query (Tyler, Stouffer, and Schum 1989), but research on the psychoacoustic properties of tinnitus in its wide variety of forms and masking patterns is proceeding (Penner 1988). At some time in the future it may be possible to develop a tinnitus "site of lesion" battery to assist us in the treatment and rehabilitation process. It is hoped that, as remediation of tinnitus begins to be possible in more cases, audiologists will assert their rightful role in the differential diagnosis and management of this distressing audiologic problem.

Interactive Videodiscs

One of the main technological breakthroughs in the past few years has been the low-cost availability of the interactive videodisc. The hardware and soft-

ware allow us to present audio-visual stimuli without the frustrating time constraints of the videotape medium. Thus, it permits great freedom in the development of testing materials and computer-aided instruction (Mahshie 1987). The materials mentioned earlier by Cox, Alexander, and Pusakulich (1989) that may be obtained on videodisc are one of several examples of AV materials that are available. (See Sims [1988] for a more complete list.) By far the most useful development, however, is the availability of videodisc recorders for under $15,000. With these units one can easily make videodiscs for research and clinical purposes without the complicated process previously required. Speech and hearing laboratories at CUNY and Walter Reed have the Panasonic version of the "portable" videodisc recorder, for example. Unfortunately the discs produced are not compatible with the standard disc players, but improvements in price and compatibility are to be expected.

Fiberoptic Telephone/Video Lines

Fiberoptic lines for the transmission of high quality data are rapidly becoming available. This technology has several implications for hearing-impaired persons. First, it will be possible to have a true high-fidelity speech signal available through the telephone, which may assist many mild and moderately impaired individuals. Second, it will become possible to receive a synchronized video image of the talker with acceptable image quality. This would enable hearing-impaired users to receive sign language and speechreading information with the audio signal. The equipment and lines will be expensive, but with enough demand and perhaps assistance from the Americans with Disabilities Act of 1990, costs may come down.

We are hopeful that the 1990s will produce breakthroughs in both hardware and "skinware" (human innovations) that will promote and improve the services available for the rehabilitation of the hearing-impaired adult.

Clinical Suggestions

Aural rehabilitation ensures that the client will be wearing the aid six months from now. The risk is 20% (perhaps 30%) that a client will not be wearing the aid. This is equivalent to building a $300,000 house and then not insuring it, knowing that it has a 30% chance of burning down in six months! From a professional point-of-view, a resources management point-of-view, a quality assurance point of view, and a human happiness point-of-view, it is simply unacceptable to omit or cut short aural rehabilitation following a hearing aid fitting. So what should an audiologist do?

I believe that the most efficient way to conduct aural rehabilitation is through an adult aural rehabilitation group where clients with spouses and/or other close associates attend a regular meeting, perhaps two hours, once a week for six weeks. Now, this is *not* a traditional lipreading group, although we work hard on speechreading strategies; it is more a problem-solving and support group. The advantages of the group include the following:

1. First, it is not hard to do. With a little organization and material support, the group almost runs itself.
2. For the client, it provides support during the initial adjustment period.
3. Clients develop realistic expectations based on others' experiences.
4. Including spouses allows you to solve many problems that you otherwise could not solve or would not even know about.
5. Most importantly, it gives the client an opportunity for weekly contact with you to solve the many problems that occur. ("How do you use the telephone?," "The earmold hurts my ear," "It's too loud," "It sounds funny," . . .). These are the problems that they might not make an appointment to see you about, but which eventually contribute to their decision not to wear the aid. It's just common sense that the more support they get, the more contact with you, the more reassurance, the more likely the clients are to wear the aid.

Finally, I'm concerned that our profession, in its clear ongoing success at incorporating technology and miniaturizing hearing aids, has led us to be technicians, not professionals. If all you are doing is pure tone testing, making an earmold for an ITE, sending it off, waiting for it to come back, putting it on the client, doing a little hearing aid orientation and sending the client away, *hoping he or she will not be back*, then you're acting like a technician. On the other hand, if you make aural rehabilitation a part of the hearing aid fitting process, if you arrange it so you are sure that you will see the client on an ongoing basis through an adult aural rehabilitation group, you are a professional, taking responsibility for the management of the client. So that is one test—do you hope your clients never come back?

Or do you ensure that you will see them again? Another test is, what do you do with the hearing-impaired *non*hearing aid wearer? Throw up your hands? These people are prime candidates for the aural rehabilitation group—even if they refuse to wear an aid, there are a lot of things we can do to help!

So, in conclusion:

. . . if you are showing some of these technician symptoms,
. . . if you want to increase the chances that your client will use the aid,
. . . if you want to reach the nonhearing aid wearer,
. . . if you are *bored with your work,*

try a little aural rehabilitation in the form of an adult aural rehabilitation group. You will find it rewarding and, frankly, fun. As the television commercial says: JUST DO IT!

References

American National Standards Institute 1969. American national standard method for the calculation of the articulation index. New York: ANSI.

Binnie, C.A., Montgomery, A.A., and Jackson, P.L. 1974. Auditory and visual contributions to the perception of consonants. *Journal of Speech and Hearing Research* 17:619–30.

Binnie, C.A., and Hession, C. 1990. A four-week communication skillbuilding program. *ADA Feedback* Winter:37–41.

Braida, L.P. 1988. Development of a decision model for multidimensional identification experiments. Paper presented at ASA 116th meeting, November 1988, Honolulu, HI.

Breeuwer, M., and Plomp, R. 1984. Speechreading supplemented with frequency-selective sound-pressure information. *Journal of the Acoustical Society of America* 77:686–91.

Cornett, D., and Beadles, R. 1989. The autocuer and the use of cued speech. Paper presented at the International Conference on Artificial Intelligence, August 1988, Detroit, MI.

Cox, R.M., Alexander, G.C., and Pusakulich, K.M. 1989. The Connected Speech Test Version 3: Audiovisual Administration. *Ear and Hearing* 10(1):29–32.

Cox, R., and McDaniel, M. 1984. Intelligibility rating of continuous discourse: Application to hearing aid selection. *Journal of the Acoustical Society of America* 76:758–66.

Dixon, N.F. and Spitz, L. 1980. The detection of auditory visual desynchrony. *Perception* 9:719–21.

Erber, N.P. 1988. *Communication Therapy for Hearing-Impaired Adults.* Abbotsford, Australia: Clavis Publishing.

Frauenfelder, U.H., and Tyler, L.K. 1987. *Spoken Word Recognition.* Cambridge, MA: The MIT Press.

Garrett, M.F. 1990. Sentence processing. In *Language: An*

Invitation to Cognitive Science, Vol. I, eds. D.N. Osherson and H. Lasnik. Cambridge, MA: The MIT Press.

Grant, K.W. 1987. Evaluating the Articulation Index for auditory-visual input. *Journal of the Acoustical Society of America* 82:S4.

Grant, K.W. 1988. Further studies on the auditory-visual Articulation Index. *Journal of the Acoustical Society of America* 83:S86.

Hawkins, D.B., Montgomery, A.A., Mueller, H.G., and Sedge, R.K. 1988. Assessment of speech intelligibility by hearing-impaired listeners. In *Noise as a Public Health Problem,* Vol. II, eds. B. Berglund, U. Berglund, J. Karlsson, and T. Lindvall. Stockholm: Swedish Council for Building Research.

Kricos, P.B., and Lesner, S.A. 1982. Differences in visual intelligibilty across talkers. *The Volta Review* 84:219–25.

Lee, K.F. 1989. ASR: *The Development of the Sphinx System.* Kluwer Academic Publications.

McGrath, M., and Summerfield, Q. 1985. Intermodal timing relations and audio-visual speech recognition by normal-hearing adults. *Journal of the Acoustical Society of America* 77:678–85.

Mahshie, J.J. 1987. A primer on interactive video. *Journal for Computer Users in Speech and Hearing* 3:39–57.

Marslen-Wilson, W. 1989. Access and integration: Projecting sound onto meaning. In *Lexical Representation and Process* ed. W. Marslen-Wilson. Cambridge, MA: The MIT Press.

Massaro, D.W. 1987. *Speech Perception by Ear and Eye: A Paradigm for Psychological Inquiry.* Hillsdale, NJ: Lawrence Earlbaum Associates.

Middelweerd, M.J., and Plomp, R. 1987. The effect of speechreading on the speech-reception threshold of sentences in noise. *Journal of the Acoustical Society of America* 82:2145–2147.

Miller, G.A., and Nicely, P.E. 1955. An analysis of perceptual confusions among some English consonants. *Journal of the Acoustical Society of America* 27:338–52.

Montgomery, A.A., and Demorest, M.E. 1988. Issues and developments in the evaluation of speechreading. *The Volta Review* 90:193–214.

Montgomery, A., and Sylvester, S. 1984. Streamlining the aural rehabilitation process. *Hearing Instruments* 35:46–48.

Osherson, D.N., and Lasnik, H. 1990. *Language.* Vol. I. Cambridge, MA: The MIT Press.

Pandey, P.C., Kunov, H., and Abel, S.M. 1986. Disruptive effects of auditory signal delay on speech perception with lipreading. *The Journal of Auditory Research* 26:27–41.

Penner, M.J. 1988. Masking of tinnitus and central masking. *Journal of Speech and Hearing Research* 30:147–52.

Research Triangle Institute 1984. Autocuer field tests begin. *Hypotenuse* September/October:2–5.

Rosen, S.M., Fourcin, A.J., and Moore, B.C.J. 1981. Voice pitch as an aid to lipreading. *Nature* 291:150–51.

Sims, D. 1988. Video methods for speechreading instruction. *The Volta Review,* 90:273–88.

Sumby, W.H., and Pollack, I. 1954. Visual contribution to speech intelligibity in noise. *Journal of the Acoustical Society of America* 26:212–15.

Tyler, R.S., Stouffer, J.L., and Schum, R. 1989. Audiological Rehabilitation of the tinnitus client. *Journal of the Academy of Rehabilitative Audiology* 22:30–42.

Walden, B.E., Cord, M.T., Demorest, M.E., and Montgomery, A.A. 1987. Effects of amplification and visual cues on consonant recognition. Paper presented at a meeting of the Military Audiology and Speech Pathology Society, 1987, Baltimore, MD.

Walden, B.E., Prosek, R.A., and Worthington, D.W. 1975. Auditory and audiovisual feature transmission in hearing-impaired adults. *Journal of Speech and Hearing Research* 18:272–80.

CHAPTER 20

New Perspectives in Audiological Rehabilitation

Carl Binnie

My comments are directed toward new perspectives in audiological rehabilitation as I see them from my position as an audiology educator and practitioner. As I see it, there are several reasons the audiological rehabilitation process has changed during the past few years and reasons adults with hearing impairment can expect better quality services from audiologists in the future. First, since June of 1978 there has been a significant change in the hearing aid delivery system so that audiologists now are selecting, evaluating, fitting, and validating hearing instruments within their own hospitals, clinics, or private practices. Prior to this audiologists had to "refer out" to hearing aid dealers and were expected to handle problem cases by providing postfitting communication training. Currently, the hearing aid is the focal point of the audiological rehabilitation process. We have come a long way since audiology was born in military aural rehabilitation programs following World War II. We recognize the experiences and philosophies of these programs, especially the leadership provided by the Department of Veterans Affairs as evidenced by their joint sponsorship of this conference.

A second change in the audiological rehabilitation process is related to improvements in hearing aid technology, especially "speech enhancement" designs or techniques that attempt to improve the quality of the amplified signal and the hearing instrument's performance in a noise background. We know more about our patients and what they want. We understand their communication complaints better. Research and development are consumer driven and hearing aid manufacturers are working diligently to address consumer concerns. The potential of digital signal processing to improve the intelligibility of speech for hearing-impaired persons has never been greater. In addition, there is a strong interpersonal component to speech enhancement as evidenced by research that shows that "speaking clearly" to a hearing-impaired person can make a difference in what the listener understands. There also is evidence that individual and group com-munication training programs can reduce the communication deficit.

Third, legislative efforts designed to assist hearing-impaired people in telephone communication, television communication, and communication access have become more evident and successful and have increased audiologists' interest and attention to assistive listening devices and systems (ALDS). Compton (1989, 1990) has taken the lead by highlighting assistive technology with its numerous and varied applications to hearing-impaired consumers. In addition, recent legislative efforts have increased the visibility and availability of these various sensory devices. For example, Public Law 97-410 legislation, effective August 16, 1989, mandates that new telephones must be compatible with hearing aids or be labeled incompatible if they are not. This legislation also requires hotels and motels to provide 10% of their rooms with compatible telephones. Many hotels now provide closed-caption decoders and special wake-up alarms for their hearing-impaired guests. The Americans with Disabilities Act (ADA) was signed by President Bush in July 1990 and guarantees an estimated 43 million disabled Americans access to employment, transportation, public accommodations, and telecommunications services (Bebout 1990). The ADA mandates that telephone handset amplifiers, telephones compatible with hearing aids, TDD devices, and signed langue or oral interpreters be provided to hearing-impaired persons. Hotels, motels, restaurants, churches, cinemas, theaters, auditoria, stadia, convention centers, retail establishments, hospitals, health-care facilities, museums, libraries, and zoos fall under the public accommodations provision of this Act.

The impact will be significant for the assistive devices market because every hearing-impaired person has a right to enter a public place and be able to hear in that situation. On April 12, 1991, the Federal Communications Commission adopted standards for closed caption decoding and display as directed by The Television Decoder Circuitry Act of 1990. This law required closed caption decoding capability to be a built-in feature of all television sets that are 13" or larger imported or manufactured in the United States after July 1, 1993. There is a 24-hour nationwide toll free number for TDD Directory Assistance (800-855-1155) and TDD relays are becoming more evident in some of the larger metropolitan areas with 17 states having some type of limited relay system.

Fourth, significant, positive changes in audiological rehabilitation programming have emerged from the testing/training protocol available for cochlear implant patients. There are new testing and training materials and there have been several reports that support the contention that short-term skill building can reduce the communication deficit for adult patients (Binnie 1976; Danz and Binnie 1983; DeFilippo and Scott 1978; Hutchinson 1990; Montgomery et al. 1984; Rubinstein 1985; Rubinstein and Boothroyd 1987; Walden et al. 1977; Walden et al. 1981). As a result of these recent advances many audiologists are declaring that audiological rehabilitation has "returned" (Ross 1987) and that attention to communication training efforts can make a difference in the lives of the adult hearing-impaired persons they serve. These rehabilitative efforts take into consideration several changes in our knowledge of speech perception theory, especially auditory-visual integration, word and sentence intelligibility, and those various cognitive strategies that hearing-impaired adult patients use to sort out message identification, especially when the signal is attenuated or filtered as is the case with high-frequency hearing impairment. Montgomery has addressed some of these in his chapter.

Finally, in order to provide a sufficient number of audiologists who are well-educated and skillful there will need to be changes in audiology curricula in university training programs. There are a number of significant responsibilities that graduating audiologists must assume. Schwartz (1990) called for increased attention to "audiologic history" by increasing graduate students' knowledge of where we've been in order to understand where we are going and to demand the respect required to function as a hearing health-care professional.

Similarly, Kileny (1990) calls for audiologists to assemble a patient's history, audiologic and vestibular results to formulate a coherent audiologic diagnosis. There is a call for a new curriculum in audiology and a new degree designation so that educated and skilled audiologists can serve hearing-impaired persons. Our scope of practice also includes the di-agnosis of communication deficits. Audiologists of the future must be able to determine the communication status of patients seen in audiology clinics and to make appropriate recommendations for selection and evaluation of sensory aids with accompanying communication training efforts. McCarthy (1990) does an excellent job of reminding audiology practitioners about their responsibilities regarding aural rehabilitation.

Audiological rehabilitation has been defined as a series of nonmedical therapeutic techniques designed to reduce the communication deficit secondary to a hearing impairment. The audiological (aural) rehabilitation process refers to services and procedures for facilitating both receptive and expressive communication. The sequences and content of the audiological rehabilitation process are described in a well-developed audiological management model (Binnie 1990). As stated by ASHA (1984) these services include (1) identification and evaluation of sensory capabilities (auditory, visual, and tactile-kinesthetic); (2) interpretation of results, counseling, and referral; (3) intervention through skill building efforts to reduce communication deficits; (4) reevaluation of the patient's status; and (5) evaluation and modification of the intervention program.

Speech Enhancement

The effectiveness of hearing aid design has improved considerably during the past five years with special attention to noise reduction circuitry. The goal of most hearing aid designs is to provide improved sound quality and speech enhancement. However, several major problems still exist. First of all, approximately 80% of those with hearing impairment do not own hearing aids (Goldstein 1984). For those who do own hearing aids many find that present-day hearing instruments are not able to deal with difficult message/competition environments (groups, restaurants, cocktail parties, theaters, churches, etc.). Hearing Industries Association's data (1984) presented statistics indicating approximately 14% of the four million hearing aid owners do not wear their hearing aids, with noise being cited as the major reason. Suter (1985) has documented the decrement in speech intelligibility among hearing-impaired persons, including even those with mild impairments. Hearing-impaired persons typically require a greater signal-to-noise ratio for good speech intelligibility than do normally hearing persons. In addition, there is a progressive decrease in speech intelligibility for hearing-impaired persons above 50 years of age. Certainly the hearing instrument should not be expected to compensate for these age-related speech intelligibility decrements.

Preves (1990) reported that persons with sensorineural hearing loss typically are sensitive to an upward spread of masking on the basilar membrane as a result of low-frequency environmental noise, as well as to masking from distortion components produced by the hearing aid itself in high noise level background environments. According to Preves, these distortion components are the result of insufficient "headroom" (a condition resulting from low SSPL [SSPL90] combined with high gain causing clipping at high input levels. Distortion components produced by hearing aids with inadequate headroom are thought to cause subjective judgments of poor sound quality and poor speech clarity by hearing aid users. Simply providing audible acoustic cues of speech and presenting them at a comfortable level through the hearing aid may not result in optimal intelligibility. This is especially true when the speech and the noise are similar spectrally as is the case in many adverse listening environments.

Montgomery (1984) and Williamson and Punch (1990) reviewed speech enhancement techniques that sought to increase the intelligibility for hearing-impaired adults. Most hearing-impaired persons wear hearing aids to reduce the communication deficit. They want to improve their understanding of speech. Speech enhancement techniques are thought to include those that improve intelligibility through signal manipulation in both time and frequency domains. Montgomery presented a rationale for speech enhancement based on three distinct but interdependent components. The first is referred to as the filtering component or the effects of threshold hearing loss. The filtering component can be compensated very well by using selective amplification. It is likely, though, that speech recognition performance may still be low, suggesting that other components may be operating. The second component is the effect of reduced signal resolution caused by the impaired cochlea. This includes reduced frequency resolution, reduced temporal resolution, and impairment of speech feature detectors. The third effect is the behavior of the impaired cochlea processing a speech signal in noise. Plomp and Duquesnoy (1982) have suggested an excellent way to measure the attenuation and distortion components of a speech signal in a noise background. Their data support the fact that most hearing-impaired patients are handicapped in a noisy environment, more so with steeply sloping losses, and that hearing aids do not give much help in noisy conditions.

If the term speech enhancement refers to the alteration or exaggeration of specific cues or segments, or environmental properties, as suggested by Montgomery (1984), then there are some non-instrumental (rehabilitative) approaches that may have an impact on improved speech intelligibility. Summers and colleagues (1988) addressed the effects of noise on speech production and found clear and consistent differences in the acoustic-phonetic patterns for speech produced in quiet versus noise environments. When persons were asked to speak in high noise levels, utterances were found to be more intelligible than those produced in quiet. This finding appeared even though the talkers were not told or asked to change their speaking patterns. This has some striking applications to audiological rehabilitation for adult hearing-impaired patients.

In another example of speech enhancement, Picheny et al. completed a series of studies (1985, 1986, 1989) concerned with enhancing speech by speaking clearly. He found a 17% average improvement in speech intelligibility in clearly spoken speech as compared to the same stimuli spoken in a typical conversational manner. Because hearing-impaired persons often accuse talkers of mumbling, it is prudent to examine whether the talker can make his or her speech clearer by using good articulation when talking to hearing-impaired persons. Summers et al. (1988) suggested that it may be possible to train talkers to improve their performance when speaking to others, especially in noise. This is a particularly effective audiological rehabilitation approach within the family when both the hearing-impaired person (typically a new hearing instrument user) and normally hearing spouse or other family member talk to one another.

When we deliberately speak clearly we emphasize certain cues in the speech signal and this improves the intelligibility of what we say. What do we do when we try to speak more clearly?

1. We tend to speak louder
2. We change the way we articulate words
3. We are careful not to omit words
4. We speak more slowly
5. We pronounce vowels more precisely
6. We release stop consonants more carefully.

Bess (1982) identified the validation of hearing aid selection procedures as the most urgent need. Audiologists now use several of these techniques to validate the hearing aid fitting, including word recognition testing, subjective ratings of intelligibility and quality, measures of real-ear aided responses or theoretical application of the Articulation Index. Walden (1984) stated that the ultimate goal of these validation procedures is to predict successful use of amplification in daily listening and communication environments. This can be accomplished only in an individualized audiological rehabilitation approach.

Consumer Considerations

Counseling is the cornerstone of any audiologic rehabilitation effort, especially as related to hearing aid acceptance, adjustment, and speech enhancement. It has been demonstrated that the shaping of attitudes, increasing motivation, modifying the level of expectations, and developing a better understanding of the communication process leads to a more positive hearing aid adjustment (Binnie 1977, 1990; Brooks 1979; Erdman, Crowley, and Gillespie 1984).

Erdman, Crowley, and Gillespie (1984) reported that improvements in hearing aid technology and "state of the art" fitting procedures will not be sufficient if a patient questions the need for amplification, has obvious concerns about the cosmetics of the instrument, or has had previous unsatisfactory experiences with hearing instruments. Frankel (1981) reported that psychological and social variables were more closely related to adjustment strategies than to the presence of hearing impairment. She did not find any clear-cut trends for psychological problems among hearing-impaired adults but did conclude that some patients simply do not adjust to their hearing impairment as well as others. Frankel reported that approximately two-thirds of her patients wanted to talk to someone about their hearing impairment and wanted to find ways to reduce communication deficit. The most commonly cited reasons included: (1) wanting information, 74%, (2) difficulty at home, 49%, (3) difficulty at work, 43%, (4) interpersonal problems related to the hearing impairment, 32%, and (5) wanting hearing aid information, 20%.

Erdman, Crowley, and Gillespie (1984) discussed some common considerations regarding audiological rehabilitation needs of 300 hearing-impaired (HI) adult patients who responded to items from the Communication Profile for the Hearing Impaired (CPHI). They found that approximately one-third of their patients identified feelings of stress, frustration, anger, and embarrassment. These reactions seem to be situation-based because patient reactions differed substantially from one environment to another. For example, feelings of stress, incompetency, stupidity, and embarrassment were more common in work and social settings. A feeling of isolation, being left out, was most common in social situations, and feelings of anger or irritation were most common in home environments.

Audiologists must recognize that their patients exhibit a wide variety of behavioral traits and find ways to talk to them, to understand the impact of a hearing impairment and a hearing aid on the communication deficit. Howard E. "Rocky" Stone (1990), Executive Director of Self Help for Hard of Hearing People stressed the importance of the consumer in the hearing health-care system. This means being aware of the needs of the whole person and not just the technological advances of hearing instruments. He stated that counseling may well be the most effective service we can give to our hearing-impaired patients—they are looking for well-educated and skillful practitioners who will respect them as well as treat them.

Thomas (1984) stated that knowledge of each individual hearing-impaired person has four main aspects: (1) understanding the causes, onset and progression of the hearing impairment; (2) developing the realization that communication demands vary from one situation to another, especially at home, at work, and socially, with the understanding that information and solution for one situation may not work in the other; (3) increasing our knowledge about how individuals cope with hearing impairment and how others with whom they are in regular contact are also affected; and (4) realizing that adjustment to a hearing impairment is a psychological process in which the individual's self esteem, personality, temperament, and attitude toward the impairment may override the hearing aid and the communication training program. New models of speech perception are important but may not be very helpful in reducing the psychological stress associated with the impairment. Detailed and comprehensive hearing handicap scales may do little to capture the variety of ways in which hearing impairment affects people and those they live with if the unique social and psychological factors associated with each individual's life are not taken into account.

Group Communication Skills Program

Audiologists have a number of evaluation and training procedures available to treat a person with an acquired hearing impairment. The focal point of audiological rehabilitation is the hearing aid selection, fitting, evaluation, validation, and orientation process. Many individuals respond positively to these rehabilitative approaches. However, there are several other evaluation and training procedures. These include speech perception testing (auditory versus auditory-visual), counseling, visual speech communication, telephone communication training, and hearing tactics.

In this section, I discuss group and individual audiological rehabilitation in the Audiology Clinic at Purdue University. Our facility is a full-service clinic offering all aspects of audiological diagnosis and rehabilitation, including the dispensing of hearing aids. There is a group adult rehabilitation program available every month for persons who are undecided about amplification, persons who have just been fitted with hearing instruments, persons who desire a "refresher" on communication tactics, and persons who have relatively normal hearing but who report communication problems in certain situations such as groups and noise environments. Referral is not reserved for the "problem case," but is made available to all who want to take part. The cost is built into the hearing aid evaluation and hearing aid consultation components of the program. Referrals are accepted from other audiological facilities in the community.

The Communication Skills Program is offered every month (once in the afternoon and once in the evening) and consists of four one and one-half hour sessions each week for a total of six hours. The ideal group size is 8 to 10 people with equal numbers of hearing-impaired and normally hearing family members. It is our philosophy that participation in the group program provides an opportunity to talk, to convey thoughts and concerns, and to learn speech enhancement techniques. The fundamental goal of our audiological rehabilitation program is to facilitate the communication functioning of the hearing-impaired person in various real life situations. The program is held in a specially designed home-like environment that facilitates counseling and communication training in situations like those experienced outside of the clinic. The communication training environment is arranged in a living room format with ceiling-mounted loudspeakers in each corner and an audio-mixer that permits the

generation of a variety of noise types and signal-to-noise ratios. There is an audio loop, infrared, FM, and direct audio input for television listening. A switchboard controls five different telephones and a variety of doorbell and telephone ring signalers are part of the assistive devices alternatives.

The program is based on several premises:

PREMISE 1: Most hearing-impaired persons, even those who wear hearing aids, continue to experience situation-based communication problems in groups and noise environments.

PREMISE 2: Hearing impairment acceptance and hearing aid adjustment can be facilitated in a short-term group audiological rehabilitation program of approximately six hours.

PREMISE 3: Counseling strategies can be implemented in a group setting using several hearing-impaired persons and significant others.

PREMISE 4: Speech enhancement can be facilitated by managing the communication environment and learning how to talk clearly to people with hearing impairment.

PREMISE 5: Patients understand that assertiveness is the learned ability to express feelings and preferences without infringing on the rights of others. Assertiveness can help bring about positive changes in communication behavior by telling others how to help.

PREMISE 6: The short-term group audiological rehabilitation program will provide a referral pool for those who can benefit from assistive devices, telephone communication training, listening training, or visual communication training.

The program content and sequence have been reported by Binnie and Hession (1990) and will only be summarized here:

I. SESSION 1/Communication Strategies
   A. Orientation to Program Format
   B. Group Discussion of Communication Problems
   C. Speech Enhancement Techniques
      1. Basic Suggestions for Effective Communication
      2. Assertiveness Options
      3. Listening Strategies
      4. Speaking Clearly
   D. Practice and Role Playing
II. SESSION 2/Hearing Loss and Audiogram Interpretation
   A. Anatomy of the Ear
   B. Causes of Hearing Loss
   C. Hearing Conservation

A brief comment should be made about the evaluation of the program. Our observation is that the majority of those who attend the first session continue on through the four-week sequence. Evaluation of our program by participants demonstrate that most report a sense of personal benefit related to communication performance. Some patients have emerged from the Communication Skills Program purchasing assistive listening devices and others have been referred for more intensive, short-term individual skill building efforts.

Individual Skill Building

Montgomery and Demorest (1988) addressed issues and developments regarding the evaluation of speechreading. They claim that speechreading is vital to the practice of audiological rehabilitation in order (1) to determine the patient's current level of performance, (2) to form some impression of the potential for improvement, and (3) to monitor progress as the skill building efforts proceed. Most models of audiological rehabilitation evaluation stress the importance of examining communication function. Binnie (1976, 1990), Sedge and Scherr (1979), Goldstein and Stephens (1981), and Garstecki (1981) all advocate auditory-visual (AV) testing as part of a battery designed to obtain information related to speech understanding. Erber (1975, 1988) suggested that auditory-visual assessment should be a routine procedure in the evaluation of communication performance. Auditory-visual testing can give the audiologist a valid estimate of the patient's ability to communicate person-to-person. AV test results may help convince patients with low motivation that hearing aids are beneficial and may be helpful in selecting hearing instruments. Comparing AV scores with A-only scores may demonstrate to the patient that he or she does have some speechreading ability and can benefit from hearing aid use. Auditory-visual testing may provide descriptions of auditory and auditory-visual errors in speech recognition. These descriptions may help the audiologist analyze ways in which the patient uses the two types of sensory information to complement one another. The test results may suggest whether the patient should receive rehabilitation emphasis with the auditory or visual modality.

Auditory-Visual Interaction

It is generally accepted that information received through one sensory mode can affect the way in which one perceives that available from another mode. In everyday face-to-face communication, auditory-visual cues are typically available. These cues help people to develop acceptable communication styles, to establish eye contact and to gain from visible articulatory gestures, including facial and postural gestures available from the speaker.

Some of the literature suggests the possibility of correlated auditory-visual systems (Shipley 1954; Gebhardt and Mowbray 1959; Etlinger 1967; Brown and Hopkins 1968; Sanders 1982). In these studies, it is posited that the brain processes the products of sensory information so that when information from two different sensory channels is complementary, the integration of sensory data reduces the dependency on either single channel.

The reception of speech is essentially an auditory process although a number of variables may affect differentially the way a listener understands speech. Correct speech recognition depends upon the intensity at which the materials are presented, the context of the speech materials, the acoustic spectrum available to the listener's ear, and those cognitive strategies that a listener uses to understand it. The speech signal can be degraded in many ways (attenuated, amplified, compressed, masked, or filtered) yet intelligibility may remain quite good. When the auditory signal is altered sufficiently in terms of frequency distortion and attenuation, such as seen with high-frequency hearing impairment, speech intelligibility will decrease.

Several researchers have demonstrated the importance of the integration of the auditory-visual signals to speech perception (Erber 1969; Sumby and Pollack 1954; Sanders and Goodrich 1971); Binnie (1973) plotted bisensory articulation functions and demonstrated that maximum intelligibility was achieved at 16 dB SL for auditory-visual presentations as compared to 24 dB SL for auditory-only. It was concluded that a pair of eyes is worth about 8 dB. In 1978, Steele, Binnie, and Cooper used an adaptive procedure to adjust the S/N ratio until a preselected percentage of correct answers were obtained for auditory-only and auditory-visual presentations. They found that the addition of vision to a hearing-only condition was worth about 13 to 14 dB and this improvement is equivalent to a 50% increase in the intelligibility of speech.

There have been several studies examining auditory (Miller and Nicely 1955; Owens, Benedict, and Schubert 1971; Bilger and Wang 1976), visual (Woodward and Barber 1964; Fisher 1968; Binnie, Jackson, and Montgomery 1976; Walden, Prosek, and Scherr 1974), and auditory-visual (Erber 1972; Binnie, Montgomery, and Jackson 1974; Walden, Prosek, and Worthington 1974) distinctive feature identification. Walden, Prosek, and Worthington described a procedure to predict auditory-visual consonant recognition for hearing-impaired adults. It was speculated that if the visual recognition of consonant sounds did not vary greatly across observers, then variations in auditory-visual consonant recognition would reflect subtle differences in auditory recognition performance. From their results, Walden, Prosek, and Worthington (1974) developed the redundancy hypothesis, which states that "for simple consonant stimuli, the improvement in recognition that a hearing-impaired observer obtains from the addition of visual cues is determined by the degree of redundancy between the auditory and visual confusions among consonants" (p. 273). Walden, Prosek, and Worthington (1974) found an orderly, predictable negative relation between the percentage of auditory information transmitted for the visibility feature and the superiority of auditory-visual consonant recognition over auditory-only recognition. These data support the hypothesis that the degree of redundancy between a hearing-impaired person's auditory and visual consonant confusions strongly determines the benefit available to him or her from visual cues. The

dominant variable in the audiovisual recognition of consonants is the pattern of auditory confusions produced by the hearing-impaired patient. This finding is an extremely important one in that it stresses to audiologists the need to examine each person's auditory and auditory-visual error patterns in order to plan effective audiological rehabilitation. Computer applications to auditory and auditory-visual confusion matrices will enhance audiologists' use of this testing procedure.

Montgomery's suggestion to develop an auditory-visual Articulation Index with the goal of selecting various gain and frequency response characteristics of hearing instruments is a good one. Pavlovic (1989) examined Articulation Index predictions of speech intelligibility in hearing aid evaluations. The Articulation Index has been incorporated into hearing aid prescriptive formulas such as the CID Phase IV. Humes, Dirks, and Bell (1986) developed a speech-transmission index-based procedure and related it to the SHAPE software program with attempts to predict NST scores from the aided audiogram. Berger (1990) employed a modified Articulation Index to compare POGO (McCandless and Lyregaard 1983), the Berger Method, and the NAL Method (Byrne and Dillon 1986). Montgomery's suggestion in the previous chapter that the relationship between auditory and visual speech perception may help audiologists alter the various frequency bands of speech energy through manipulation of the hearing instrument has some interesting clinical applications.

Word and Sentence Recognition

There is no single, satisfactory index of everyday speech communication performance. It is unlikely that suprathreshold tests of monosyllabic stimuli can be used as a criterion measure to predict hearing aid use. To be sure, PB word lists "do not sample the domain of all speech" and "polysyllables, sentences and continuous discourse introduce a greater variety of speech syntax and morphology for speech recognition tests" (Elkins 1984, p. 77). The California Consonant Test (Owens and Schubert 1977) has some clinical applications to hearing aid evaluations (Tecca and Binnie 1984) especially to evaluate the high-frequency spectral components. Dubno and Dirks (1981) and Dubno, Dirks, and Langhofer (1981) reported on the Nonsense Syllable Test (NST). They found that it is highly repeatable, the CV or

VC structure tends to produce minimal learning effects, the test utilizes both male and female talkers and is recorded in both quiet and noisy environments. Both the CCT and the NST allow for the opportunity to produce a pattern of consonant confusions, unique to each observer. The Revised SPIN test (Bilger et al. 1984) has high face validity by virtue of ease of administration, low predictability (acoustic-phonetic) versus high predictability (linguistic-contextual) scoring, and presentations of stimuli in a multispeaker babble. Last, recognition and comprehension of contextual material can be evaluated using the speech tracking method advocated by DeFilippo and Scott (1978) and discussed by DeFilippo (1988).

One of the interesting applications to audiological rehabilitation is the determination of which approach to communication training actually makes a difference. Some audiologists disagree about the value of formal auditory training (or speechreading training). Instead, they recommend a counseling-oriented approach that attempts to shape attitudes and behavior change by discussion rather than drill (Fleming 1973). Others advocate formal skill building efforts, but disagree about the form it should take. Some advocate an analytic approach (Sedge and Scherr 1979; Walden et al. 1977; Hutchinson 1990), while others hold out for a synthetic format (Davis and Hardick 1981; Sanders 1982). Still others feel that in addition to synthetic training there is some value to including both analytic and synthetic approaches (Owens 1978; Smith and Karp 1978; Tye-Murray et al. 1990). Interestingly, there have been several studies that have demonstrated that training in one approach generalizes to the other (Danz and Binnie 1983; Montgomery et al. 1984; Rubinstein and Boothroyd 1987). An interesting and encouraging finding from the Rubinstein and Boothroyd research is that the gains achieved during the formal communication training program were not lost in the month following the termination of training. These findings suggest that the benefits of auditory training occurred as a result of an increased use of sentence context as an aid to word recognition. Walden et al. (1981) found that hearing-impaired subjects improved their recognition of an auditory-visual sentence task following either auditory training or speechreading training. In addition, there was a significant increase in consonant recognition performance demonstrating that both analytic auditory and speechreading training was effective. Danz and Binnie (1983) found that training in the auditory-visual tracking of connected speech resulted in an improved ability in speech tracking over a span of several training sessions. Furthermore, the results indicated a significant improvement on post-training tests of syllable recognition and intelligibility judgment (IJ) of connected discourse. The IJ seems to be a powerful clinical tool because speech does seem to be as intelligible as a listener says it is (Cox, Alexander, and Gilmore 1987; Cox et al. 1988).

Another interesting application to the adult audiological rehabilitation process is to study how hearing-impaired people learn. What strategies do they find helpful to resolve the communication deficit? Are there individual differences in their approach to problem solving? Erber and Greer (1973) observed the repair strategies used by classroom teachers during their instruction at an oral school for the deaf. They identified four basic response patterns (repetition, emphasis, structural change, and supplementary information) used by teachers when hearing-impaired children fail to understand the spoken message. Others advocate the use of providing key words, signing, writing, fingerspelling, and requesting confirmation or clarification (Kaplan, Bally, and Garretson 1987).

Repair strategies, coping strategies, or cognitive strategies have been the target of research in continuous discourse tracking for both hearing aid and cochlear implant users. Owens and Telleen (1981) studied "coping strategies" of hearing-impaired adult patients to resolve "communication blockages." They found that the majority of patients preferred to have the sender/talker repeat a portion of the phrase (63%), followed by repetition of the whole phrase (20%), spell the word (6%), and repeat one word (5%). Tye-Murray and Tyler (1988) recommended that both the sender and receiver obtain training in the speech tracking procedures and then the sender's "repair strategies" should be limited to an orderly and sequenced number of alternatives. DeFilippo (1988) reported on the use of several "fail safe" strategies designed to resolve the communication breakdown. Gagne and Wyllie (1989) studied the effectiveness of three repair strategies: (1) repetitions, (2) synonyms, and (3) paraphrases for a group of adults who viewed experimental videotapes. The results indicated that providing an exact repetition of a misidentified stimulus did not constitute an effective repair strategy. A significant improvement in performance was seen when the observers were provided with a substitute stimulus (i.e., a synonym or a paraphrase), with paraphrases being a more effective repair strategy. Gagne and Wyllie suggested that the most appropriate repair strategy for a given situation depends upon several factors, including: (1) the cause and the extent of the communication breakdown, (2) the kind of relevant linguistic and contextual cues available, (3) the appropriateness of using a substitute stimulus, (4) the ability of the sender to apply repair strategies, and (5) the cognitive and linguistic competencies of the sender as well as the receiver.

It should be clear, then, that learning to use and to request appropriate repair strategies should be incorporated into communication training programs. Trychin and Boone (1985) developed a communication training program entitled "Did I Do That?" which is designed to serve as a guide to improve relationships between hearing-impaired persons and family, friends, and co-workers. Tye-Murray et al. (1988) described a computerized laser videodisc program to train assertive communication behaviors. This approach holds considerable promise in the application of technology to speech perception testing and training as suggested by Boothroyd et al. (1988). Tye-Murray and Tyler (1988) suggested that future research should focus on the development of a test that reflects a natural communication interaction such as one that engages the hearing-impaired person in a conversational style of listening. It is likely that this approach may best be studied through the use of an interactive video that records the style of learning and those various repair strategies which help resolve daily communication deficits.

In summary, there is a growing interest in the rehabilitative aspects of audiology, especially with regard to the selection, fitting, and evaluation of hearing instruments. Other audiological rehabilitative interests have emerged from the recent explosion of technological advancements in the field, especially digital signal processing hearing aids, assistive listening devices, cochlear implants, sophisticated real ear measures, laser videodisc applications, and other noninstrumental speech enhancement techniques.

References

Definition of and competencies for aural rehabilitation. 1984. *American Speech-Language Hearing Association* 26:37–41.

Bebout, J.M. 1990. The Americans with Disabilities Act: American dream achieved for the hearing impaired? *The Hearing Journal* 43:11–13, 16–19.

Berger, K.W. 1990. The use of an articulation index to compare three hearing aid prescriptive methods. *Audecibel* 16–19.

Bess, F. 1982. Amplification for the hearing impaired: Research priorities. In *The Vanderbilt Hearing-Aid Report,* eds. G.A. Studebaker and F.H. Bess. Upper Darby, PA: Monographs in Contemporary Audiology.

Bilger, R.C., and Wang, M.D. 1976. Consonant confusions in patients with sensorineural hearing loss. *Journal of Speech and Hearing Research* 19:718–40.

Bilger, R.C., Nuetzel, J.M., Rabinowitz, W.M., and Rzeczkowski, C. 1984. Standardization of a test of speech perception in noise. *Journal of Speech and Hearing Research* 27:32–48.

Binnie, C.A. 1973. Bi-sensory articulation functions for normal hearing and sensori-neural hearing loss patients. *Journal of the Academy of Rehabilitative Audiology* 3:43–52.

Binnie, C.A. 1976. Relevant aural rehabilitation. In *Hearing Disorders,* ed. J.L. Northern. Boston, MA: Little, Brown and Co.

Binnie, C.A. 1977. Attitude changes following speechreading training. *Scandinavian Audiology* 6:13–19.

Binnie, C.A. 1990. Communication training through amplification. Unpublished manuscript, Purdue University.

Binnie, C.A., and Hession, C.M. 1990. A four-week communication training program. *Academy of Dispensing Audiologists, ADA Feedback* Winter 1990:37–41.

Binnie, C.A., Jackson, P.L., and Montgomery, A.A. 1976. Visual intelligibility of consonants: A lipreading screening test with implications for aural rehabilitation. *Journal of Speech and Hearing Disorders* 41:530–39.

Binnie, C.A., Montgomery, A.A., and Jackson, P.L. 1974. Auditory and visual contributions to the perception of consonants. *Journal of Speech and Hearing Research* 17:619–30.

Boothroyd, A., Yeung, E., Hanin, L., Hnath-Chisolm, T., Kishon-Rabin, L., Medwetsky, L., Broecker, B., Eran, O., and Plant, N. 1988. Application of interactive video laserdisc technology to speech perception testing and training. A scientific exhibit at the 1988 Convention of the American Speech-Language-Hearing Association, Boston, MA.

Brooks, D.N. 1979. Hearing aid candidates—some relevant features. *British Journal of Audiology* 13:81–84.

Brown, A.E., and Hopkins, H.K. 1968. Interaction of the auditory and visual sensory modalities. *Journal of the Acoustical Society of America* 41:1–6.

Byrne, D., and Dillon, H. 1986. New procedure for selection gain and frequency response of a hearing aid. The National Acoustic Laboratories (NAL). *Ear and Hearing* 7:257–65.

Compton, C.L. 1989. Assistive devices. *Seminars in Hearing.* Vol. 10, No. 1. NY: Thieme Medical Publishers.

Compton, C.L., 1990. Assistive devices: An overview. *ADA Feedback* Winter 1990:19–29.

Cox, R.M., Alexander, G.C., and Gilmore, C. 1987. Intelligibility of average talkers in typical listening environments. *Journal of the Acoustical Society of America* 81:1598–1608.

Cox, R.M., Alexander, G.C., Gilmore, C., and Pusakulich, K.M. 1988. Use of the Connected Speech Test (CST) with hearing impaired listeners. *Ear and Hearing* 9:198–207.

Danz, A.D., and Binnie, C.A. 1983. Quantification of the effects of training the auditory-visual reception of connected speech. *Ear and Hearing* 4:146–51.

Davis, J.M., and Hardick, E.J. 1981. *Rehabilitative Audiol-*

ogy for Children and Adults. New York: John Wiley and Sons.

DeFilippo, C.L. 1988. Tracking for speechreading training. In *New Reflections on Speechreading*, Vol. 90, No. 5, eds. C. L. DeFilippo and D. G. Sims. Washington, D.C.: The Volta Review.

DeFilippo, C.L., and Scott, B.L. 1978. A method for training and evaluating the reception of ongoing speech. *Journal of the Acoustical Society of America* 63:1186–1192.

Dubno, J.R., and Dirks, D.D. 1981. Evaluation of hearing-impaired listeners using a nonsense syllable test. I. Test reliability. *Journal of Speech and Hearing Research* 25:135–41.

Dubno, J.R., Dirks, D.D., and Langhofer, L.R. 1981. Evaluation of hearing-impaired listeners using a nonsense syllable test. II. Syllable recognition and consonant confusion patterns. *Journal of Speech and Hearing Research* 25:141–48.

Elkins, E. 1984. Recommendations for speech recognition research. In *ASHA Reports No. 14: Speech Recognition by the Hearing Impaired*, 77–79.

Erber, N.P. 1969. Interaction of audition and vision in the recognition of oral speech stimuli. *Journal of Speech and Hearing Research* 12:423–25.

Erber, N.P. 1972. Auditory, visual and auditory-visual recognition of consonants by children with normal and impaired hearing. *Journal of Speech and Hearing Research* 15:413–22.

Erber, N.P. 1975. Auditory-visual perception of speech. *Journal of Speech and Hearing Disorders* 40:481–92.

Erber, N.P. 1988. *Communicaiton Therapy for Hearing-Impaired Adults*. Abbotsford, Victoria, Australia: Clavis Publishing.

Erber, N.P., and Greer, C.W. 1973. Communication strategies used by teachers at an oral school for the deaf. *The Volta Review* 75:480–85.

Erdman, S., Crowley, J., and Gillespie, G. 1984. Considerations in counseling the hearing impaired. *Hearing Instruments* 35:50–58.

Ettlinger, G. 1967. Analysis of cross modal effects and their relationship to language. In *Brain Mechanisms Underlying Speech and Language*, ed. F.L. Darley. New York: Grune and Stratton, Inc.

Fleming, M. 1972. A total approach to communication therapy. *Journal of the Academy of Rehabilitative Audiology* 5:28–31.

Fisher, C.G. 1968. Confusions among visually perceived consonants. *Journal of Speech and Hearing Research* 11:796–804.

Frankel, B.J. 1981. Adult onset hearing impairment: Social and psychological correlates of adjustment. Doctoral Dissertation. The University of Western Ontario, London, Ontario.

Gebhardt, J.W., and Mowbray, G.H. 1959. On discriminating the rate of visual flicker and auditory flutter. *American Journal of Psychology* 72:521–29.

Gagne, J., and Wyllie, K.A. 1989. Relative effectiveness of three repair strategies on the visual-identification of misperceived words. *Ear and Hearing* 10:368–74.

Garstecki, D.D. 1981. Auditory-visual training paradigm for hearing impaired adults. *Journal of the Academy of Rehabilitative Audiology* 14:223–38.

Goldstein, D.P. 1984. Hearing impairment, hearing aids and audiology. *ASHA* 25:24–38.

Goldstein, D.P., and Stephens, S.D.G. 1981. Audiological rehabilitation: Management model I. *Royal National Throat, Nose, Ear Hospital Technical Memo* 3.

Hearing Industries Association (HIA) Market Survey. 1984. A *Summary of Findings and Business Implications for the US Hearing Aid Industry*. Washington, D.C.: HIA.

Humes, L.E., Dirks, D.D., and Bell, T.S. 1986. Application of the Articulation Index and the Speech Transmission Index to the recognition of speech by normal-hearing and hearing-impaired listeners. *Journal of Speech and Hearing Research* 29:447–62.

Hutchinson, K. 1990. An analytic distinctive feature approach to auditory training. *The Volta Review* 92:5–7.

Kaplan, H., Bally, S.J., and Garretson, C. 1987. *Speechreading: A Way to Improve Understanding*, 2nd Ed. Washington, D.C.: Gallaudet University Press.

Kileny, P. 1990. *Diagnostic Audiology* January/February:2, 25.

McCarthy, P. 1990. Aural rehabilitation. *Audiology Today* January/February:25.

McCandless, G.A., and Lyregaard, P.E. 1983. Prescription of gain/output (POGO) for hearing aids. *Hearing Instruments* 34:16–20.

Miller, G.A., and Nicely, P.A. 1955. An analysis of perceptual confusions among some English consonants. *Journal of the Acoustical Society of America* 27:338–52.

Montgomery, A.A. 1984. A review of speech signal enhancement for the hearing impaired. In *Symposium on Hearing Technology: Its Present and Future*. Washington, D.C.: Gallaudet University Press.

Montgomery, A.A., and Demorest, M. 1988. Issues and developments in the evaluation of speechreading. In *New Reflections on Speechreading*, Vol. 90, No. 5, eds. C.L. DeFilippo and D.G. Sims. Washington, D.C.: The Volta Review.

Montgomery, A.A., Walden, B.E., Schwartz, D.M., and Prosek, R.A. 1984. Training auditory-visual speech recognition in adults with moderate sensorineural hearing loss. *Ear and Hearing* 5:30–36.

Owens, E. 1978. Consonant errors and remediation in sensorineural hearing loss. *Journal of Speech and Hearing Disorders* 43:331–47.

Owens, E., and Schubert, E. 1977. Development of the California Consonant Test. *Journal of Speech and Hearing Research* 20:463–74.

Owens, E., Benedict, M., and Schubert, E.D. 1971. Consonant phonemic errors associated with pure-tone configurations and certain kinds of hearing impairment. *Journal of Speech and Hearing Research* 15:308–322.

Owens, E., and Telleen, C.C. 1981. Tracking as an aural rehabilitative process. *Journal of the Academy of Rehabilitative Audiology* 14:259–73.

Pavlovic, C.V. 1989. Speech spectrum considerations and speech intelligibility predictions in hearing aid evaluations. *Journal of Speech and Hearing Disorders* 54:3–8.

Picheny, M.A., Durlach, N.I., and Braida, L.D. 1985. Speaking clearly for the hard of hearing. I: Intelligibility differences between clear and conversational speech. *Journal of Speech and Hearing Research* 28:96–103.

Picheny, M.A., Durlach, N.I., and Braida, L.D. 1986. Speaking clearly for the hard of hearing. II: Acoustic characteristics of clear and conversational speech. *Journal of Speech and Hearing Research* 29:434–46.

Picheny, M.A., Durlach, N.I., and Braida, J.D. 1989. Speaking clearly for the hard of hearing. III: An attempt to determine the contribution of speaking rate to differences in intelligibility between clear and conversational speech. *Journal of Speech and Hearing Research* 32: 600–603.

Plomp, R., and Duquesnoy, A.J. 1982. A model for the speech reception threshold in noise without and with a hearing aid. *Scandinavian Audiology* Suppl. 15:1–17.

Preves, D.A. 1990. Approaches to noise reduction in analog, digital and hybrid hearing aids. *Seminars in Hearing* 11:39–67.

Ross, M. 1987. Aural rehabilitation revisited. *Journal of the Academy of Rehabilitative Audiology* 20:13–23.

Rubinstein, A. 1985. The effect of a synthetic only versus synthetic plus analytic approach to auditory training with adventitiously hearing-impaired adults. Unpublished doctoral dissertation. Graduate School of the City University of New York, New York.

Rubinstein, A., and Boothroyd, A. 1987. Effect of two approaches to auditory training on speech recognition by hearing impaired adults. *Journal of Speech and Hearing Research* 30:153–160.

Sanders, D.A. 1982. *Aural Rehabilitation: A Management Model (2nd Ed.).* Englewood Cliffs, N.J.: Prentice Hall.

Sanders, D.A., and Goodrich, S.J. 1971. The relative contribution of visual and auditory components of speech to speech intelligibility as a function of three conditions of frequency distortion. *Journal of Speech and Hearing Research* 14:154–59.

Schwartz, D.M. 1990. Clinical perspectives: What ever happened to those bygone days? *Audiology Today* 2:26–27.

Sedge, R.K., and Scherr, C. 1979. Aural rehabilitation for individuals with high frequency hearing loss. *Journal of the Academy of Rehabilitative Audiology* 12:47–61.

Shipley, T. 1954. Auditory flutter-driving of visual flicker. *Science* 145:1328–1330.

Smith, C.R., and Karp, A. 1978. *A Workbook in Auditory Training for Adults.* Springfield, IL: Charles C Thomas.

Steele, J.A., Binnie, C.A., and Cooper, W.A. 1978. Combining auditory and visual stimuli in the adaptive testing of speech discrimination. *Journal of Speech and Hearing Disorders* 43:115–22.

Stone, H.E. 1990. Hearing health care in the 1990s. *Audiology Today* July/August:14–17.

Sumby, W.H., and Pollack, I. 1954. Visual contributions to speech intelligibility in noise. *Journal of the Acoustical Society of America* 26:212–15.

Summers, W. Van., Pisoni, D.B., Bernacki, R.H., Pedlow, R.I., and Stokes, M.A. 1988. Effects of noise on speech production: Acoustical and perceptual analyses. *Journal of the Acoustical Society of America* 84:917–28.

Suter, A.H. 1985. Legal status of the hearing conservation amendment and its effects on the C.Q. *Sound and Vibration* December 1985.

Tecca, J.E., and Binnie, C.A. 1984. The application of an adaptive procedure to the California Consonant Test for hearing aid evaluation. *Ear and Hearing* 3:72–76.

Thomas, A.J. 1984. *Acquired Hearing Loss: Psychological and Psychosocial Implications.* Academic Press, London.

Tye-Murray, N., and Tyler, R.S. 1988. A critique of continuous discourse tracking as a test procedure. *Journal of Speech and Hearing Disorders* 53:226–31.

Tye-Murray, N., Tyler, R.S., Bong, B., and Nares, T. 1988. Computerized laser videodisc programs for training speechreading and assertive communication behaviors. *Journal of the Academy of Rehabilitative Audiology* 21:129–42.

Tye-Murray, N., Tyler, R., Lansing, C., and Bertschy, M. 1990. Evaluating the effectiveness of auditory training stimuli using a computerized program. *The Volta Review* 25–30.

Trychin, S., and Boone, M. 1985. *Communication Rules for Hard of Hearing People: A Workbook for Wrong/Right Ways for Effective Communication.* Washington, D.C.: Gallaudet University Press.

Walden, B.E. 1984. Speech perception of the hearing-impaired. In *Hearing Disorders in Adults,* ed. J. Jerger. San Diego: College-Hill.

Walden, B.E., Erdman, S.A., Montgomery, A.A., Schwartz, D.M., and Prosek, R.A. 1981. Some effects of training on speech recognition by hearing-impaired adults. *Journal of Speech and Hearing Research* 24:207–216.

Walden, B.E., Prosek, R.A., and Scheer, C.K. 1974. Dimensions of visual consonant perception by hearing impaired observers. Paper presented at the annual convention of the American Speech and Hearing Association, Las Vegas, NV.

Walden, B.E., Prosek, R.A., and Worthington, D.W. 1974. Predicting audiovisual consonant recognition performance of hearing-impaired adults. *Journal of Speech and Hearing Research* 17:270–78.

Walden, B.E., Prosek, R.A., Montgomery, A.A., Scherr, C.K., and Jones, C.J. 1977. Effects of training on the visual recognition of consonants. *Journal of Speech and Hearing Research* 20:130–45.

Williamson, M.J., and Punch, J.L. 1990. Speech enhancement in digital hearing aids. *Seminars in Hearing* 11: 68–78.

Woodward, M.F., and Barber, C.G. 1964. Phoneme perception in lipreading. *Journal of Speech and Hearing Research* 3:212–22.

CHAPTER 21
Special Amplification Considerations for Elderly Individuals

Sandra Gordon-Salant

A small percentage of hearing-impaired elderly individuals use hearing aids successfully. In 1990, there were approximately 9.9 million hearing-impaired people aged 65 years and older, representing 39% of the elderly population (Hotchkiss 1989). Among this hearing-impaired group, approximately 20% own hearing aids (Ries 1982). Surveys indicate that between 53% and 72% of elderly hearing aid owners use their hearing aids constantly (Upfold and Wilson 1983; Salomon, Vesterager, and Jagd 1988). These data suggest that a large percentage of elderly individuals with hearing loss reject the use of amplification.

Some of the most prominent reasons for rejecting hearing aids by older people are shown in table I (Franks and Beckmann 1985). Among the major concerns are cost, appearance, and amplification of noise. Alternatively, a number of studies have examined perceived hearing aid benefit by older users. Table II presents some of the benefits of hearing aids as perceived by elderly subjects, as reported in four studies. Essentially, elderly listeners report or exhibit improved communication function, social function, emotional function, and cognitive function, with the use of hearing aids. Thus, a number of benefits can be realized by elderly hearing-impaired individuals with hearing aid use. For some elderly individuals, however, the negative aspects of hearing aids outweigh possible benefits.

This chapter examines the factors that potentially limit hearing aid acceptance and satisfaction by elderly hearing-impaired individuals and furnishes suggestions for optimizing hearing aid use among this population. A series of recommendations is included for future research directed at improving our understanding of the unique problems experienced by elderly individuals and improving hearing aid technology to meet these specific needs. Elderly individuals composed approximately 60% of the clients of hearing aid dispensers in 1989 (Cranmer 1990); hence, the amplification re-

quirements of this group should be a high priority to those involved in designing and evaluating hearing aids.

Age-related Changes in Auditory Function

Numerous anatomical and physiological changes in the auditory system are thought to occur with the passage of time. Deterioration has been observed at every site of the auditory system in elderly subjects (Kirikae 1969; Hansen and Reski-Nielson 1965). As a consequence, an elderly individual may exhibit a peripheral hearing loss or evidence of central auditory nervous system dysfunction. In addition, certain cognitive abilities are known to decline with age. Peripheral, central, and cognitive factors potentially affect performance with hearing aids.

Peripheral Hearing Loss

Pure-tone Audiogram Average audiograms of individuals of different ages usually show that pure-tone thresholds deteriorate with increasing age and that men exhibit poorer thresholds than women of comparable age (Corso 1963; Moscicki et al. 1985; Kryter 1983). Figure 1 exemplifies these findings (Moscicki et al. 1985). The "typical" presbycusic loss is mild-to-moderately severe in degree, sensorineural, and gradually sloping in configuration for women and sharply sloping for men.

A recent longitudinal study examined rate of aging in pure-tone air conduction thresholds in men over a 20 year period (Brant and Fozard 1990). The results (figure 2) indicate a steady increase in threshold of about 1 dB per year at 8000 Hz, with an accelerated increase in thresholds at 500, 1000, and 2000 Hz at 60 years and older. Significant individual variability in the magnitude of threshold shifts with age was also reported. These data underscore the

Table I. Survey Items Ranked by Mean Rating. Percent Agreement and Disagreement for All Respondents. N = 100. (Adapted from Franks and Beckmann 1985.)

	Survey Item by Overall Rank	Mean Rating	% Agree	% Disagree
1	Cost too much	2.9	72	27
2	Call attention to handicap	3.1	72	25
3	Dealers use deceptive practices	3.6	57	39
4	Amplify noise	3.6	55	43
5	Inconvenient to wear	3.7	53	39
5A	Dealers use high pressure	3.7	49	32
6	Difficulty manipulating	3.7	45	49
7	Dealers' interest only in money	3.7	40	46
8	Would not know where to buy	3.7	48	48
9	Make sounds too loud	3.8	49	42
10	Dealers not trained	3.8	43	45
11	Uncomfortable to wear	3.9	36	45
11A	Questionable help from aid	3.9	46	48
12	For most severe problems	3.9	41	47
13	Fear of wrong choice	3.9	55	41
14	Not instructed in use	3.9	45	47
15	Sounds unnatural	4.1	40	56
16	Poor experience of others	4.1	35	48
17	Can't afford	4.1	41	56
18	Words unclear	4.2	34	60
19	No transportation	4.2	43	54
19A	Unattractive	4.2	40	60

fact that individuals age at different rates and that an elderly person may exhibit auditory thresholds that do not conform with averaged data. Selection of appropriate hearing aids for elderly people should accommodate individual patterns of hearing sensitivity and potential age-related shifts in auditory thresholds.

Suprathreshold Peripheral Distortions Peripheral hearing loss often affects a listener's ability to perform suprathreshold auditory processing tasks with simple stimuli (Humes 1983). A few studies have shown that elderly listeners also are impaired on some of these tasks, although abnormal performance may be associated with the sensitivity loss.

Table II. Reported and Perceived Benefits of Hearing Aids by Older Users

Benefit	Scale	# S's	Age (Yrs)	Study
Improved communication in quiet situations	Hearing Aid Performance Inventory	24	62–87	Kricos, Lesner, Sandridge, Yanke (1987)
Improved reception of nonspeech signals				
Improved communication in situations with reduced signal information				
Higher self-concept	Tennessee Self-Concept Scale	86	60+	Harless and McConnell (1982)
Improved communication efficiency	Speech Intelligibility Questionnaire			
Improved emotional function	Hearing Handicap for the Elderly	45	55–90	Malinoff and Weinstein (1989)
Improved social function				
Improved emotional function	Hearing Handicap for the Elderly	95	64+	Mulrow et al. (1990)
Improved social function				
Improved communication function	Quantified Denver Scale			
Improved cognition	Short Portable Mental Status Questionnaire			
Improved affect	Geriatric Depression Scale			

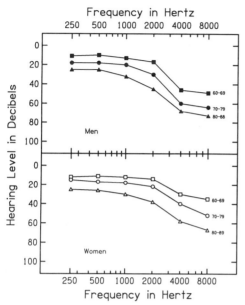

Figure 1. Mean pure-tone thresholds in the better ear of men and women as a function of frequency and age (Total *N* = 2293). (Adapted from Moscicki et al. 1985.)

For example, Patterson and colleagues (1982) found that the frequency selectivity of the auditory filter deteriorated progressively with increasing age in listeners over the age of 55 years. Klein and co-workers (1990) found that most elderly hearing-impaired subjects exhibited excessive upward-masked thresholds. However, the performance of the elderly hearing-impaired subjects was not significantly different from that of younger subjects with hearing loss.

Deficits in suprathreshold auditory processing that occur with sensitivity loss have implications for hearing aid use. First, some measures of supra-

threshold processing with simple acoustic signals are related to speech recognition in noise (Tyler et al. 1982; Irwin and McCauley 1987; Klein, Mills, and Adkins 1990; Dreschler and Plomp 1980, 1985). Second, one of the major problems experienced by elderly listeners is speech recognition in noise (CHABA 1988). Third, as noted earlier, elderly listeners report limited benefit from hearing aids in understanding speech in noise. Although not yet shown empirically, limited benefit with amplification may be related to deficits in suprathreshold auditory processing. Because a hearing aid enables a listener to receive an acoustic signal at suprathreshold levels, performance with amplification may be less than optimal because of the underlying distortions in peripheral processing. There is a need, then, to evaluate systematically the independent effects of age and hearing loss on processing of signals in the temporal, spectral, and intensive domains, and to examine the relationship of such effects to speech recognition performance in noise with and without hearing aids.

Speech Recognition Performance Elderly listeners usually do not exhibit significant deficits in speech recognition performance in quiet conditions at high presentation levels (Gordon-Salant 1987a). However, in less-than-ideal acoustic situations, performance of elderly listeners may be excessively poor. Degraded acoustic environments encountered in daily situations include noise, reverberation, and fast talkers.

Age-related performance differences have been observed in noise backgrounds and relatively difficult conditions (Dubno, Dirks, and Morgan 1984; Gordon-Salant 1987a). For example, Gordon-Salant (1987a) assessed the signal-to-babble (S/B) ratio required for 50% criterion performance by young and elderly normal and hearing-impaired subjects on items from the Modified Rhyme Test (Kruel et al. 1968) and Northwestern University Test No. 6 (NU6) (Tillman and Carhart 1966). The results, shown in figure 3, demonstrated a significant age effect for all measures. Thus, combining the presence of noise with the adaptive S/B ratio procedure created added stimulus and task complexity. Combinations of complex conditions may be particularly difficult for elderly listeners and may reveal deficits that exceed peripheral hearing loss effects.

Speech recognition performance by elderly individuals is reduced in reverberant environments. Nabelek and Robinson (1982) tested recognition performance for speech presented at three reverberation times, by subjects between 10 and 72 years. As

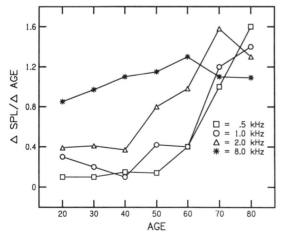

Figure 2. Rates of change in pure-tone threshold for four frequencies over seven age groups. (Redrawn from Brant and Fozard 1990.)

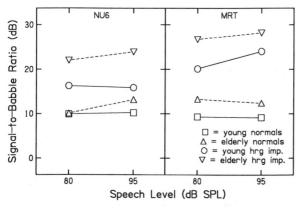

Figure 3. Recognition of NU6 and MRT in noise, expressed as S/B ratio for 50% criterion performance, by four subject groups at two signal levels.

shown in figure 4, subjects aged 64 years and older exhibited significantly greater deficits than the younger subjects at the longer reverberation times. However, mild high-frequency loss was present in the older subjects, which could have contributed to the reduced speech intelligibility in the reverberant conditions (Nabelek and Mason 1981). Recently, Helfer and Wilber (1990) assessed recognition of nonsense syllables distorted by reverberation and noise by young and elderly subjects with minimal hearing loss and with hearing impairment. The older subjects showed marked difficulty identifying the nonsense syllables in noise and reverberation, even when the effects of hearing loss were controlled statistically. Thus, performance-based studies verify that elderly hearing-impaired listeners experience difficulty understanding speech in everyday listening situations that include reverberation and noise. Moreover, elderly listeners experience excessive deficits in environments that combine reverberation and noise.

Conversational speech is sometimes rapid and is characterized by a reduction in the duration of phonetic segments and the duration of interword pauses (Picheny, Durlach, and Braida 1986). Several cognitive theories of aging propose a generalized slowing of mental perceptual processing (Birren, Woods, and Williams 1980), or diminished speed of perceptual processing (Salthouse 1980) with increasing age. As a consequence, elderly listeners may experience particular difficulty recognizing rapidly presented speech.

Methods used for studying the effects of speeded speech without introducing spectral distortions include natural rate alterations and time compression. Elderly subjects usually perform more poorly than younger subjects on time-compressed speech tests (Konkle, Beasley, and Bess 1977; Schmitt 1983; Schon 1970; Sticht and Gray 1969) and on naturally speeded speech tests (Schmitt and Carroll 1985). Figure 5 shows the shifts in recognition of time-compressed speech that occur with age. The age-related decrement could be associated with differences in high-frequency sensitivity between young and older subjects, because high-frequency hearing loss is known to affect recognition of time-compressed speech (Grimes, Mueller, and Williams 1984; Harris, Haines, and Myers 1963). As shown in figure 6, when young and elderly listeners are matched for pure-tone sensitivity, they perform comparably on time-compressed speech tasks (Otto and McCandless 1982). These results suggest that elderly hearing-impaired listeners may not be at a significant disadvantage for listening to rapid speech, compared to younger hearing-impaired listeners, when simple linguistic materials are presented in quiet. However, elderly listeners may experience exaggerated difficulty for

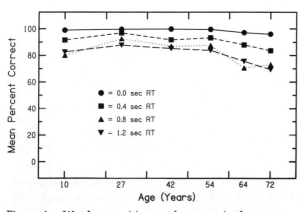

Figure 4. Word recognition performance in three reverberant conditions and one anechoic condition, as a function of age. (Adapted from Nabelek and Robinson 1982.)

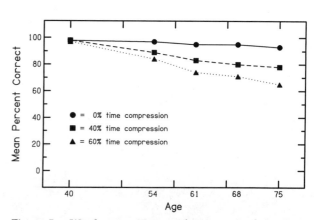

Figure 5. Word recognition performance in three time compression conditions, as a function of age. (Adapted from Konkle, Beasley, and Bess 1977.)

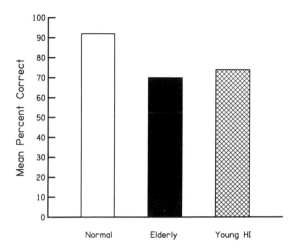

Figure 6. Word recognition for time-compressed speech, by young normal listeners, elderly listeners with sensorineural hearing loss, and young listeners with sensorineural hearing loss. (Redrawn from Otto and McCandless 1982.)

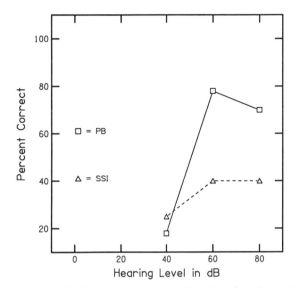

Figure 7. Performance-intensity function for phonetically balanced words (PB) and the Synthetic Sentence Identification test (SSI), demonstrating the "central aging effect."

rapid speech when stimulus and task demands increase (Wingfield et al. 1985).

Central Auditory Processing Disorder

A central auditory processing disorder (CAPD) is defined operationally as a deficit in speech understanding that cannot be explained on the basis of the peripheral sensitivity loss (Jerger et al. 1989). Presumably, it results from deterioration of one or more of the nuclei composing the central auditory nervous system. Jerger and Hayes (1977) and others (Davidson and Wall 1988; Rodriguez, DiSarno, and Hardiman 1990) have shown that CAPDs characterize the performance of many elderly individuals, and that such disorders may limit an older person's success with amplification. The following methods have been used to identify CAPDs in elderly individuals: comparison of PI-PB versus PI-SSI functions, masking-level differences, and dichotic speech tests. The relationship of the "central aging effect" to performance with hearing aids must be examined carefully to avoid the confounding influence of peripheral hearing loss. Nevertheless, clear evidence of a CAPD in an elderly person implies that distinctive hearing aid selection strategies and counseling goals may be warranted.

PI-PB Versus PI-SSI Functions   Jerger and Hayes (1977) compared performance-intensity (PI) functions for phonetically balanced words (PB) and the Synthetic Sentence Identification test (SSI) (Speaks and Jerger 1965) among subjects with known auditory system lesions. They identified a central pat-

tern, presented in figure 7, in which the PI-SSI function was poorer than the PI-PB function in the presence of normal hearing sensitivity. This PB-SSI discrepancy was also observed in elderly subjects and was termed the "central aging effect." Younger individuals with peripheral low-frequency hearing loss also exhibited this pattern. Thus, the finding of the PB-SSI discrepancy in older listeners with low frequency hearing loss is equivocal.

The relationship of central findings to performance with hearing aids was examined in a follow-up study (Hayes and Jerger 1979). Subjects over the age of 60 years were classified into three groups: primarily central component (PB-max score > SSI-max score by more than 20%), primarily peripheral hearing loss (SSI-max score ≥ PB-max score), and mixed peripheral-central components (PB-max > SSI-max by 20% or less). Monaural aided performance on the SSI presented at decreasing message-to-competition ratios (MCRs) was compared among groups. The results are shown in figure 8. At −10 dB MCR, the peripheral group performed best whereas the central group performed poorest. Hayes and Jerger concluded that as the central component increased, aided performance decreased systematically. They suggested that a hearing aid may not be warranted in cases of mild hearing loss and CAPD, and recommended that elderly clients with CAPD be counselled to expect very limited benefit of hearing aids in background noise. Davidson and Wall (1988) further suggested that if an interaural asymmetry in the PB-SSI central aging ef-

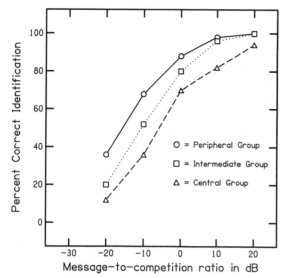

Figure 8. Aided performance in the sound field for elderly subjects classified with primarily central component, primarily peripheral component, and mixed peripheral-central components. (Redrawn from Hayes and Jerger 1979.)

fect exists, then the ear without the central aging effect should receive amplification.

In contrast, perceived hearing aid benefit among elderly listeners does not seem to be affected by the presence of CAPD. Kricos and colleagues (1987) compared scores on the Hearing Aid Performance Inventory (Walden, Demorest, and Hepler 1984) between elderly subjects with peripheral hearing loss and elderly subjects with a central component (as defined by the PI-SSI comparison). The results, shown in figure 9, reveal that there was no relationship between perceived hearing aid benefit and central auditory functions.

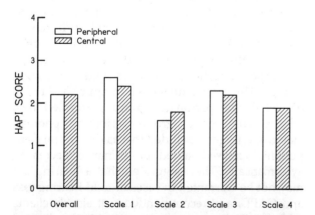

Figure 9. Comparison of scores on the Hearing Aid Performance Inventory (HAPI) for elderly subjects classified with central hearing loss and peripheral hearing loss. (Adapted from Kricos et al. 1987.)

The presence of CAPD as defined by the PB-SSI abnormality does not have an effect on elderly listener's binaural performance. In one study, Kaplan and Pickett (1981) compared performances of an elderly central group and an elderly peripheral loss group on recognition of speech in noise presented in monotic, dichotic, and diotic modes. Both groups showed significant improvement in speech recognition in the dichotic and diotic modes compared to the monotic mode; there were no significant differences between the groups. In a second study, Stach (1990) examined the influence of central auditory processing status, age, and hearing loss on the aided binaural advantage. Hearing-impaired subjects, ranging in age from 24 to 93 years (mean = 68 years), were tested with the SSI at varying MCRs in unaided, monaural-right, monaural-left, and binaural conditions. Subjects of all ages showed the binaural advantage, as did subjects with CAPD (as defined by the PB-SSI discrepancy). The binaural advantage was reduced, however, as the degree of hearing loss increased.

The source of the discrepant findings reported by Hayes and Jerger (1979) and others (Kricos et al. 1987; Kaplan and Pickett 1981; Stach 1990) may be differences in the measurement of hearing aid benefit: self-report on a questionnaire versus aided monaural speech discrimination scores versus binaural speech discrimination scores. A second source suggested by Kricos and colleagues (1987) is the method for defining central auditory deficit. Other measures for identifying central auditory dysfunction are available. Because the sensitivity and specificity of the PI-SSI pattern for identifying central aging effects are unknown at present, corroborating evidence from more than one test is desirable for identification of CAPD.

Masking Level Difference A second measure of central auditory function is the Masking Level Difference (MLD). Normal-hearing listeners exhibit improved thresholds for binaural signals in binaural noise when the signals are presented out-of-phase rather than in-phase and when the signals are low in frequency (Hirsh 1948). Jeffress (1972) has shown that the MLD is mediated by correlational processes in the central auditory nervous system (CANS). Other researchers (Olsen, Noffsinger, and Carhart 1976) have shown that the MLD is abnormally reduced in subjects with lesions of the auditory brainstem. The MLD also is reduced by interaural threshold asymmetry and significant peripheral hearing loss (Jerger, Brown, and Smith 1984; Hall, Tyler, and Fernandes 1984). As a measure of central auditory function, it is applied most judiciously in cases of normal hearing or bilateral symmetrical high-frequency hearing loss.

The MLD is reduced in elderly listeners with hearing loss (Olsen, Noffsinger, and Carhart 1976), but not in elderly listeners with normal hearing (Jerger, Brown, and Smith 1984). Jerger and coworkers (1984) developed correction factors to MLDs for people with high-frequency sensorineural loss and minimal low-frequency loss. Application of the correction factors should permit a determination of the significance of reduced MLDs in elderly individuals with primarily high-frequency hearing loss.

If applied appropriately, the measure of MLDs could prove useful in hearing aid selection. A large MLD indicates that a listener can perform a binaural signal analysis that improves signal reception in noise. With binaural amplification, this listener should be able to capitalize on binaural cues and improve speech recognition in noise. Elderly listeners who exhibit reduced MLDs might not benefit from binaural amplification for improving speech understanding in noise.

A related procedure for assessing binaural signal processing in noise was described by Warren and coworkers (1978). Suprathreshold speech recognition in noise by young and elderly normal hearing listeners was compared for diotic and dichotic signal presentations. The expected improvement in intelligibility in the dichotic condition, observed for younger subjects, was reduced in the elderly subjects. Warren and colleagues suggested that a hearing aid that increases interaural differences prior to reception might improve speech intelligibility in noise for hearing-impaired elderly listeners. These hypotheses need to be examined empirically.

Dichotic Speech Tests   Dichotic tests require recognition of two different signals, one presented to each ear, and are sensitive to lesions of the auditory cortex (Milner, Taylor, and Sperry 1968). Dichotic procedures may be useful for detecting cortical dysfunction in elderly people resulting from possible deterioration of cortical fibers (Hansen and Reski-Nielson 1965). For this application, dichotic tests that control for the effects of peripheral hearing loss should be selected. These tests include the SSW, DSI, and dichotic digits.

The Staggered Spondaic Word Test (SSW) (Katz 1962) presents one spondee to each ear, with one syllable of each spondee overlapping in time. A correction factor is applied to raw SSW scores to reduce the effect of peripheral distortion. Figure 10 shows that corrected SSW (C-SSW) error scores increase with age, beyond 70 years, in subjects with bilateral, symmetrical sloping sensorineural hearing

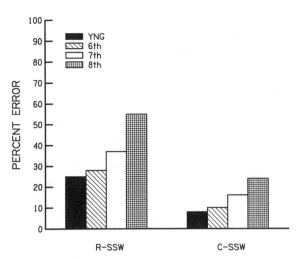

Figure 10.   Mean raw-SSW (R-SSW) scores and corrected-SSW (C-SSW) scores from young normal-hearing listeners and elderly listeners in the 6th, 7th, and 8th age decades. (Adapted from Arnst 1982.)

losses (Arnst 1982). However, subjects with pure-tone-averages (PTAs) exceeding 40 dB HL exhibit significantly poorer C-SSW scores than subjects with more mild hearing losses, at all ages. The SSW test, then, appears to be useful for detecting a central effect in older listeners up to age 70 years, with PTAs less than 40 dB HL.

A second dichotic measure that provides clinical norms for listeners with peripheral hearing loss is the Dichotic Sentence Identification Test (DSI) (Fifer et al. 1983). In this test, two sentences from the SSI are presented dichotically. The listener is required to identify the two sentences presented from a closed set of choices. Normal cutoff values are available for subjects with PTAs ranging from 0 to 50 dB HL. Jerger and colleagues (1989) used the DSI as one of three tests to determine the presence of CAPD in 130 elderly subjects. Of the subjects identified with CAPD (N = 65), approximately 50% showed abnormal performance on the DSI alone or in combination with another measure.

Dichotic signals that are brief in time and carefully aligned in onset and offset are considered the stimuli of choice for detecting cortical lesions (Noffsinger and Kurdziel 1979). Dichotic digits and consonant-vowel stimuli (CVs) meet these criteria, although dichotic digits are much less affected by the presence of peripheral hearing loss (Speaks, Niccum, and Van Tasell 1985). Elderly subjects with minimal hearing loss exhibit the expected right ear advantage for dichotic digits (Rodriguez, DiSarno, and Hardiman 1990). Among a sample of 25 elderly subjects with minimal hearing loss, 40% exhibited abnormally reduced scores on the dichotic digits test, 60% showed significant SSI rollover, and none showed abnormal SSW scores (Rodriguez, Di-Sarno, and Hardiman 1990). Comparing the two dichotic procedures, it appears that the dichotic digits test may be more sensitive to subtle central auditory aging effects than the SSW.

Dichotic procedures may serve to complement other measures of central auditory disorder. Elderly subjects do exhibit performance deficits on these measures, even when the effects of hearing loss are controlled. The relationship of performance on the SSW, DSI, and dichotic digits test to performance with hearing aids by elderly subjects is unknown at present.

Cognitive Dysfunction

Cognitive processing skills are related to speech understanding ability (CHABA 1988). Moreover, decline in certain cognitive skills is known to occur with aging. In some elderly individuals, deterioration of cognitive function may be associated with speech understanding difficulty and limited benefit of hearing aids.

Cognitive skills that seem to be most relevant to speech understanding include memory (dynamic working memory, secondary episodic memory, semantic memory), selective attention, and semantic processing (Cohen 1987). Studies have shown that age differences exist in each of these skills, favoring younger subjects (see CHABA 1988; Cohen 1987). In addition, several cognitive theories of aging propose that there is a generalized slowing of mental perceptual processing (Salthouse 1980; Birren, Woods, and Williams 1980). The rate of perceptual processing becomes noticeably poorer as the number of mental operations increases, as in cases of increased stimulus or task complexity (Wingfield et al. 1985). This factor may be the source of the excessively poor performance exhibited by elderly subjects in conditions that combine multiple distortions.

The correspondence between cognitive abilities and audiologic performance among elderly subjects has been examined recently by Jerger and colleagues (1989). Subjects were categorized as having a cognitive deficit if they showed abnormal performance on a neuropsychological battery. CAPD was identified on the basis of abnormal performance on the PB-SSI, DSI, or Revised Speech Perception in Noise test (R-SPIN) (Bilger et al. 1984). The classification of the 130 elderly subjects is presented in figure 11. Normal cognitive status without a significant speech recognition deficit was observed in 36%

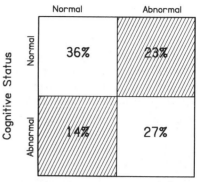

Figure 11. Prevalence of normal and abnormal function on measures of central auditory processing and cognition among 130 elderly persons. (From Jerger et al. 1989.)

of the subjects, whereas cognitive deficits and abnormal speech recognition performance were seen in 27% of the subjects. This congruence in cognitive status and speech recognition performance, however, does not establish a cause-and-effect relationship.

Reports on cognition and aging indicate that elderly people can overcome cognitive limitations through practice (CHABA 1988). Fozard (1980) suggests that elderly people can be trained successfully with approaches that incorporate self-pacing, repetition, and familiarization. These findings imply that when cognitive factors limit hearing aid adjustment and use, a carefully constructed training program may be advantageous. The effects of specific cognitive deficits on unaided and aided audiological performance in elderly listeners need to be evaluated systematically. In the interim, awareness of cognitive effects in this population should guide selection of hearing aids, evaluation of hearing aid performance, orientation to hearing aids, and design of new hearing aids. These issues will be considered in the succeeding sections.

In summary, age-related changes in peripheral, central, and cognitive function may be present in elderly individuals. The hearing loss itself probably limits suprathreshold auditory processing and understanding of speech distorted by noise, reverberation, and fast talkers. Difficulties in speech understanding that seem to be uniquely related to aging are evident when multiple speech distortions are presented or when signal distortion and task complexity are combined. These aging effects may be the result of CAPDs or cognitive deficits. Listening to amplified speech in real-world situations represents a condition of multiple distortions and complexities. Elderly people with CAPD or cognitive deficits may not be able to realize a significant benefit from amplification, unless hearing aids are selected to minimize the influence of multiple distortions. Moreover, training with amplification is necessary to enable the elderly hearing aid user to overcome task complexities. The next section will review strategies that meet these goals.

Hearing Aid Strategies for Elderly Listeners

Hearing Aid Candidacy

Because many elderly hearing-impaired individuals are dissatisfied with their hearing aids, it may be useful to screen for hearing aid candidacy prior to hearing aid selection. Those people who do not appear to be good candidates should be counselled more carefully regarding benefits and limitations of amplification. Two measures have been suggested as predictors of hearing aid candidacy: expression of hearing handicap and improved speech recognition performance in noise at high signal levels.

Older people who report difficulty communicating in quiet and noise without visual cues may derive more benefit from amplification than those who do not report these problems. Salomon and coworkers (1988) compared three groups of elderly subjects on a number of measures, including pure-tone thresholds, speech discrimination in the sound field in quiet and noise with and without visual cues, health history, communication handicap, and hearing handicap. Results showed that the most effective indicator of the need for a hearing aid was hearing handicap. Need for hearing aids was defined on the basis of improvement experienced by the patient during discrimination tests in quiet and noise. Others have reported that elderly subjects who are satisfied with hearing aids tend to be more positive in their psychosocial attitudes than people who reject hearing aids (Franks and Beckmann 1985; Kapteyn 1977). Screening measures of hearing handicap or psychosocial status may therefore be useful in selecting hearing aid candidates.

Speech recognition performance in noise has also been recommended as a predictor of hearing aid candidacy. Dirks, Morgan, and Dubno (1982) described an adaptive procedure that measures the average S/B ratio required by a listener to achieve 50% recognition performance. Derived psychometric functions of S/B ratios versus signal presentation level were obtained for presbycusic listeners and young normal hearing listeners. Examples of performance by two elderly listeners are shown in figure 12. The listener who shows better performance (lower S/B ratios) at high intensity levels is predictably a good hearing aid candidate, whereas the listener who doesn't improve with increasing level is expected to derive more limited benefit from amplification in noise.

In a previous section, the relationships between central auditory processing and cognitive function to hearing aid use were discussed. The presence of CAPD or cognitive dysfunction does not obviate the use of a hearing aid, because results of studies to date are inconclusive.

Selection of Hearing Aid Characteristics

Hearing aid recommendations for elderly listeners require careful consideration of style, gain, mode (binaural/monaural), and noise suppression techniques. Fortunately, these issues have been addressed in the literature on aging.

Style The second highest ranked reason for rejecting hearing aids among elderly people is that they call attention to a handicap (Franks and Beckmann 1985). For this reason, in-the-ear (ITE) hearing aids are preferable to this population. Elderly hearing-impaired users demonstrate good-to-excellent speech discrimination scores in noise with ITE hearing aids and report that ITE hearing aids are beneficial (Clasen, Vesterager, and Parving 1987). Nevertheless, approximately 20% of elderly sub-

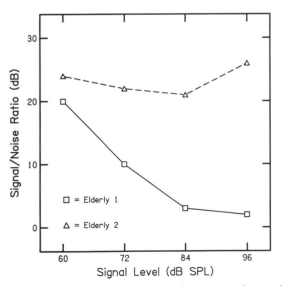

Figure 12. Performance-intensity functions of speech recognition in noise from two elderly hearing-impaired listeners.

jects from a sample size of 70 had difficulty handling the ITE hearing aids. Specific problems included volume control manipulation, hearing aid insertion, and battery replacement. In users with dexterity problems, BTE or body hearing aids with easily manipulated controls should be recommended.

Gain Several studies (Leijon, Eriksson-Mangold, and Bech-Karlsen 1984; Clasen, Vesterager, and Parving 1987; Humes and Kirn 1990) have reported that the average preferred gain of hearing aid users aged 60 years and older is considerably less than the amount recommended by various prescriptive formulae. Indeed, Leijon and colleagues (1984) found that the average preferred insertion gain was approximately 10 dB.

Some newer formulae prescribe somewhat less gain than the earlier formulae. The revised formula of the National Acoustic Laboratories (R-NAL) (Byrne and Dillon 1986) prescribes gain according to the ½-gain rule, but also compensates for differences in audiogram slope by a factor that is less than ⅓ the difference in the frequency response slope. A validation study (Byrne and Cotton 1988) of the R-NAL method tested 44 subjects aged 55 to 90 years (median = 72 years). There was excellent agreement between the three frequency average prescribed gain (16.2 dB) and three-frequency average gain (15.8 dB) preferred by listeners for providing the best speech intelligibility and most pleasant quality.

Preferred insertion gain values of elderly (> 75 years) and younger (< 60 years) subjects have been compared to gain values predicted by the POGO, R-NAL, Berger, and ⅓-gain formulae (Ryals and Auther 1990). An age effect for average insertion gain value was not observed. However, as shown in figure 13, there was a significant difference between prescribed gain and insertion gain which varied with the formula type. For the R-NAL and ⅓ gain methods, there were no significant differences between average predicted and preferred gain. However, for both the POGO and Berger methods, there was significantly more predicted gain than preferred gain. These results confirm one previous report (Berger and Hagberg 1982) that hearing aid gain does not vary specifically as a function of age. Moreover, these results suggest that formulae that predict relatively low gain values provide appropriate target insertion gain values for older adults.

Mode Binaural amplification is usually preferred over monaural amplification for individuals with bilateral hearing impairment. The theoretical

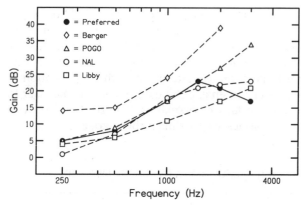

Figure 13. Average insertion gain measured at each frequency for young and elderly subjects combined (Preferred) compared with predicted gain using the Berger, POGO, NAL, and Libby prescriptive formulae. (Redrawn from Ryals and Auther 1990.)

advantages of binaural amplification are improved localization, improved speech recognition in noise, and binaural summation. Binaural amplification may not be warranted for some elderly hearing-impaired people, however, because of increased cost and difficulty with manipulating two aids.

As noted in an earlier section, binaural listening and binaural amplification do seem to improve speech recognition in degraded environments for elderly people, compared to monaural listening. Elderly people exhibit higher speech recognition scores in dichotic or diotic modes compared to monaural modes for listening to speech in noise (Kaplan and Pickett 1981), speech subjected to reverberation (Nabelek and Robinson 1982), and speech that has been time compressed (Antonelli 1978). These improvements in performance with binaural listening support the use of binaural hearing aids in theory for elderly people, especially in situations with reduced acoustic information. In addition, Stach (1990) reported that subjects aged 24 to 93 years (mean = 68 years) experienced an aided binaural advantage of 10% to 20% for speech recognition in noise (figure 14). Because a major complaint of elderly hearing-impaired people is difficulty understanding speech in degraded environments, binaural amplification should be considered when practical.

Noise Suppression Another strategy for improving speech understanding in noise is with noise suppression techniques. These methods include high-pass amplification, directional microphones, automatic low-frequency adjustment (automatic signal processing, or ASP), and adaptive filtering (e.g., Zeta circuitry). Hearing-impaired

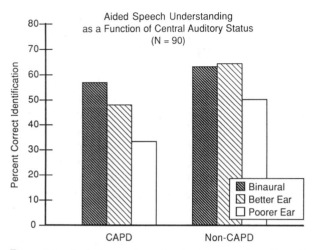

Figure 14. Aided speech understanding as a function of central auditory status (*N* = 90; mean age = 68 years). (From Stach 1990.)

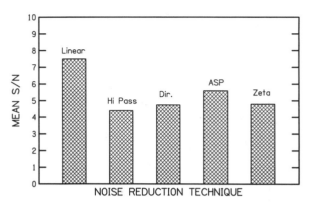

Figure 15. Mean S/N ratio required for 50% correct word recognition by elderly hearing-impaired listeners, obtained in linear, high-pass, directional microphone, automatic signal processing, and ZETA amplification modes. (From Schum 1990.)

subjects have shown improved speech recognition scores in noise with high-pass amplification (Gordon-Salant 1984) and directional microphones (Hawkins and Yacullo 1984), but minimal improvement with either ASP hearing aids (Tyler and Kuk 1989) or Zeta I circuitry (Van Tasell, Larsen, and Fabry 1988; Klein 1989; Tyler and Kuk 1989) in noise.

Elderly subjects do appear to benefit from these noise reduction methods, although this varies among individuals. Schum (1990) compared scores for word recognition in cafeteria noise by elderly subjects in five aided modes: linear amplification, high-pass amplification, directional microphone, ASP amplification, and Zeta II circuitry. Significantly poorer performance was obtained with linear amplification than with the noise reduction strategies (see figure 15), although differences between the noise reduction strategies were not significant. Individual rank ordering of performance with each device revealed large inter-subject variability, suggesting that any one noise suppression method is not optimal for all elderly listeners. Rather, the benefits of a variety of noise reduction techniques should be assessed for each elderly person.

Hearing Aid Adjustment and Training

Two models for rehabilitation of new hearing aid users have been used with elderly listeners. One method (Hardick and Gans 1982) is essentially an extended hearing aid trial period for elderly individuals who might have difficulty adjusting to amplification. The program attempts to overcome the common problems experienced by elderly hearing aid users. For example, time is devoted during each session to individual practice in assembling the hearing aid, placing it in the ear, and manipulating the controls. Information about hearing aids is presented repeatedly, because secondary memory and attention may be poor. These elements of the program are based on the suggestion that elderly people learn best under conditions using self-pacing, repetition, and familiarization (Fozard 1980).

Traditional auditory training methods also are successful with elderly listeners. Rubenstein and Boothroyd (1987) assigned elderly hearing aid users (56 to 79 years) to either a synthetic training program or a combined synthetic/analytic training program, and evaluated speech recognition with the Nonsense Syllable Test (NST) (Resnick et al. 1975), High Predictability (HP)-SPIN and Low Predictability (LP)-SPIN on two occasions prior to training and two occasions following training. As shown in figure 16, a performance increase of 10% was observed following training, and the amount of improvement was comparable with both training methods. In general, the greatest improvement was seen in HP-SPIN scores, and improvement continued after the training ended. Thus, the primary skill acquired with training was an improvement in the use of contextual cues, regardless of the type of training method (analytic versus synthetic).

Rehabilitative programs for promoting adjustment to hearing aids are essential for elderly people. These programs should be aimed at overcoming physical limitations that affect hearing aid use, fostering knowledge about hearing aids, and improving awareness of available contextual information in reduced acoustic environments.

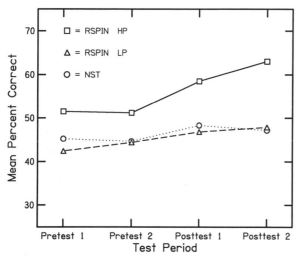

Figure 16. Mean test scores of 20 adults (56–79 years) for four test periods and three test types, for analytic + synthetic and synthetic training modes combined. (From Rubinstein and Boothroyd 1987.)

Research Needs

A number of cross-cutting issues for future research on amplification and the elderly are apparent from the foregoing discussion. Five broad areas for further research are presented. Collectively, the goal is to improve communication for elderly hearing-impaired people in realistic environments and thereby to promote hearing aid use.

The effects of peripheral, central, and cognitive factors on hearing aid success need to be specified. Toward this end, suprathreshold processing distortions among elderly listeners, which are related to hearing aid use, must be identified. In addition, efficient and valid clinical procedures that identify CAPD while controlling for peripheral hearing loss are needed. Cognitive measures that are sensitive to decline in auditory processing skills among elderly listeners need to be determined. Available measures of hearing aid success should be validated and compared to each other. For example, measures of hearing handicap, perceived hearing aid performance, hours of hearing aid use, speech recognition in noise, and pleasantness of speech quality have all been used to assess hearing aid success, but little is known about the cross-correlations among these measures.

Hearing aids designed to enhance speech intelligibility in noise must be evaluated specifically with elderly listeners, and new design techniques should be explored. An increasing number of

"Adaptive Frequency Response" (AFR) hearing aids that employ adaptive high-pass filtering or multichannel compression (Fabry and Walden 1990) are becoming available. However, these amplification devices have not yet been evaluated directly with elderly listeners. Moreover, other types of digital speech enhancement methods that attempt to improve speech intelligibility in noise have been described. For example, increasing consonant energy improves speech recognition performance in noise by elderly listeners (Gordon-Salant 1986, 1987b). Potential methodologies such as these should be considered for the development of digital hearing aids for the future.

New developments in adaptive filtering and digital technology should aim at improving speech recognition by elderly listeners in reverberation and with fast talkers. Reverberation smooths temporal fluctuations in the speech waveform and produces an effect that is comparable to low-pass filtering (Duquesnoy and Plomp 1980). A multiple microphone technique that filters uncorrelated signals may be one method that reduces the effects of reverberation (Levitt, Weiss, and Rabinowitz 1987; Levitt 1990). For improving recognition of fast speech, techiques that convert conversational speech to clear speech by increasing phonetic segments and interword pause time should be developed further (Gordon-Salant 1986, 1987b; Montgomery and Edge 1988; Picheny, Durlach, and Braida 1989).

Procedures for hearing aid selection and evaluation of aided performance for elderly listeners should be refined. Prescriptive fitting approaches should include methods for selecting compression variables for elderly listeners. Based on the complaint of elderly hearing-impaired listeners that their hearing aids are too loud (Franks and Beckmann 1985), the effect of age on SSPL requirements should be assessed. A protocol for evaluation of an elderly listener's performance with a hearing aid should be developed. Procedures included should be brief, reliable, and should reveal the special problems that might be encountered by an elderly person.

Numerous other factors that change with age potentially influence an elderly person's satisfaction with a hearing aid. Among these factors are personality attributes, perceived age, general health, and visual acuity. The effect of each of these variables on hearing aid benefit should be determined and, depending on the outcome, methods to minimize the negative impact of these factors should be devised.

Technological advances and applied research

need to keep pace with the special hearing aid requirements of elderly hearing-impaired individuals. The speech processing problems of this group are complex, and are affected by inherent changes in the individual as well as environmental conditions. Amplification devices and techniques for selection, evaluation, and training need to be constructed with an awareness of the special peripheral, central, and cognitive characteristics of elderly people that affect speech processing. Validation of new developments with elderly people with differing audiologic profiles should ensure that the individualized needs of this population are fulfilled.

References

Antonelli, A.R. 1978. Auditory processing disorders and problems with hearing-aid fitting in old age. *Audiology* 17:27–31.

Arnst, D.J. 1982. Staggered spondaic word test performance in a group of older adults: A preliminary report. *Ear and Hearing* 3:118–23.

Berger, K.W., and Hagberg, E.N. 1982. Gain usage based on hearing aid experience and subject age. *Ear and Hearing* 3:235–37.

Bilger, R.C., Nuetzel, J.M., Rabinowitz, W.M., and Rzeczkowski, C. 1984. Standardization of a test of speech perception in noise. *Journal of Speech and Hearing Research* 27:32–48.

Birren, J.E., Woods, A.M., and Williams, M.V. 1980. Behavioral slowing with age: Causes, organization, and consequences. In *Aging in the 1980's: Psychological Issues*, ed. L.W. Poon. Washington, D.C.: American Psychological Association.

Brant, L.J., and Fozard, J.L. 1990. Age changes in pure-tone hearing thresholds in a longitudinal study of normal human aging. *Journal of the Acoustical Society of America* 88:813–20.

Byrne, D., and Cotton, S. 1988. Evaluation of the National Acoustic Laboratories' new hearing aid selection procedure. *Journal of Speech and Hearing Research* 31:178–86.

Byrne, D., and Dillon, H. 1986. The National Acoustic Laboratories' (NAL) new procedure for selecting the gain and frequency response of a hearing aid. *Ear and Hearing* 7:257–65.

Committee on Hearing Bioacoustics and Biomechanics (CHABA). 1988. Speech understanding and aging. *Journal of the Acoustical Society of America* 83:859–95.

Clasen, T., Vesterager, V., and Parving, A. 1987. In-the-ear hearing aids. *Scandinavian Audiology* 16:195–200.

Corso, J. 1963. Age and sex differences in pure-tone thresholds. *Archives of Otolaryngology* 77:383–405.

Cohen, G. 1987. Speech comprehension in the elderly: The effects of cognitive changes. *British Journal of Audiology* 21:221–26.

Cranmer, K. 1990. Hearing instrument dispensing—1990. *Hearing Instruments* 41:4–12.

Davidson, S.A., and Wall, L.G. 1988. Hearing aid selection for the elderly: Consideration of central aging effects. *Folia Phoniatr* 40:270–76.

Dirks, D.D., Morgan, D.E., and Dubno, J.R. 1982. A procedure for quantifying the effects of noise on speech recognition. *Journal of Speech and Hearing Disorders* 47:114–22.

Dreschler, W.A., and Plomp, R. 1980. Relation between psychophysical data and speech perception for hearing-impaired subjects I. *Journal of the Acoustical Society of America* 68:1608–1616.

Dreschler, W.A., and Plomp, R. 1985. Relation between psychophysical data and speech perception for hearing-impaired subjects II. *Journal of the Acoustical Society of America* 78:1261–1270.

Dubno, J.R., Dirks, D.D., and Morgan, D.E. 1984. Effects of age and mild hearing loss on speech recognition in noise. *Journal of the Acoustical Society of America* 76:87–96.

Duquesnoy, A.J., and Plomp, R. 1980. Effect of reverberation and noise on the intelligibility of sentences in cases of presbycusis. *Journal of the Acoustical Society of America* 68:537–44.

Fabry, D.A., and Walden, B.F. 1990. Noise Reduction Hearing Aids. *ASHA* 32:48–51.

Fifer, R.C., Jerger, J.F., Berlin, C.I., Tobey, E.A., and Campbell, J.C. 1983. Development of a dichotic sentence identification test for hearing-impaired adults. *Ear and Hearing* 4:300–305.

Fozard, J.L. 1980. The time for remembering. In *Aging in the 1980's: Psychological Issue*, ed. L.W. Poon. Washington, D.C.: American Psychological Association.

Franks, J.R., and Beckmann, N.J. 1985. Rejection of hearing aids: Attitudes of a geriatric sample. *Ear and Hearing* 6:161–66.

Gordon-Salant, S. 1984. Effects of reducing low-frequency amplification on consonant perception in quiet and noise. *Journal of Speech and Hearing Research* 27:483–93.

Gordon-Salant, S. 1986. Recognition of natural and time/intensity altered CV's by young and elderly subjects with normal hearing. *Journal of the Acoustical Society of America* 80:1599–1607.

Gordon-Salant, S. 1987a. Age-related differences in speech recognition performance as a function of test format and paradigm. *Ear and Hearing* 8:277–82.

Gordon-Salant, S. 1987b. Effects of acoustic modification on consonant recognition by elderly hearing-impaired subjects. *Journal of the Acoustical Society of America* 81:1199–1202.

Grimes, A., Mueller, G., and Williams, D.L. 1984. Clinical considerations in the use of time-compressed speech. *Ear and Hearing* 5:114–17.

Hall, J.W., Tyler, R.S., and Fernandes, M.A. 1984. Factors influencing the masking level difference in cochlear hearing-impaired and normal hearing listeners. *Journal of Speech and Hearing Research* 27:145–54.

Hansen, C.C., and Reski-Nielsen, E. 1965. Pathological studies in presbycusis. *Archives of Otolaryngology* 82:115–32.

Hardick, E.J., and Gans, R.E. 1982. An approach to rehabilitation with amplification. *Ear and Hearing* 3:178–82.

Harris, J.D., Haines, H.L., and Myers, C.K. 1963. The importance of hearing at 3Kc for understanding speeded speech. *Laryngoscope* 70:131–46.

Hayes, D., and Jerger, J. 1979. Aging and the use of hearing aids. *Scandinavian Audiology* 8:33–40.

Hawkins, D.B., and Yacullo, W.S. 1984. Signal-to-noise

ratio advantage of binaural hearing aids and directional microphones under different levels of reverberation. *Journal of Speech and Hearing Disorders* 49:278–86.

Helfer, K.S., and Wilber, L.A. 1990. Hearing loss, aging and speech perception in reverberation and noise. *Journal of Speech and Hearing Research* 33:149–55.

Hirsh, I.J. 1948. The influence of interaural phase on interaural summation and inhibition. *Journal of the Acoustical Society of America* 20:761–66.

Hotchkiss, D.R. 1989. *The Hearing Impaired Elderly Population: Estimation, Projection, and Assessment* in Monograph Series A, No. 1. Washington, D.C.: Gallaudet Studies and Research Institute.

Humes, L.E. 1983. Spectral and temporal resolution by the hearing-impaired. In *The Vanderbilt Hearing-Aid Report*, eds. G.A. Studebaker and F.H. Bess. Upper Darby: Instrumentation Associates, Inc.

Humes, L.E., and Kirn, E.U. 1990. The reliability of functional gain. *Journal of Speech and Hearing Disorders* 55: 193–97.

Irwin, R.J., and McCauley, S.F. 1987. Relations among temporal acuity, hearing loss, and the perception of speech distorted by noise and reverberation. *Journal of the American Acoustical Society* 81:1557–1565.

Jeffress, L.A. 1972. Binaural signal detection. Vector theory. In *Foundations of Modern Auditory Theory*, Vol. 2, ed. J. Tobias. New York: Academic Press.

Jerger, J., and Hayes, D. 1977. Diagnostic speech audiometry. *Archives of Otolaryngology* 103:216–22.

Jerger, J., Brown, D., and Smith, S. 1984. Effect of Peripheral hearing loss on the masking level difference. *Archives of Otolaryngology* 110:290–96

Jerger, J., Jerger, S., Oliver, J., and Pirozzolo, F. 1989. Speech understanding in the elderly. *Ear and Hearing* 10:79–89.

Kaplan, H., and Pickett, J.M. 1981. Effects of dichotic/diotic versus monotic presentation on speech understanding in noise in elderly hearing-impaired listeners. *Ear and Hearing* 2:202–207.

Kapteyn, T.S. 1977. Satisfaction with fitted hearing aids II. An investigation in the influence of psycho-social factors. *Scandinavian Audiology* 6:171–77.

Katz, J. 1962. The use of staggered spondaic words for assessing the integrity of the central auditory nervous system. *Journal of Auditory Research* 2:327–37.

Kirikae, I. 1969. Auditory function in advanced age with reference to histological changes in the central auditory system. *International Audiology* 8:221–30.

Klein, A.J. 1989. Assessing speech recognition in noise for listeners with a signal processor hearing aid. *Ear and Hearing* 10:50–57.

Klein, A.J., Mills, J.H., and Adkins, W.Y. 1990. Upward spread of masking, hearing loss, and speech recognition in young and elderly listeners. *Journal of the Acoustical Society of America* 87:1266–1271.

Konkle, D.F., Beasley, D.S., and Bess, F.H. 1977. Intelligibility of time-altered speech in relation to chronological aging. *Journal of Speech and Hearing Research* 20:108–115.

Kricos, P.B., Lesner, S.A., Sandridge, S.A., and Yanke, R.B. 1987. Perceived benefits of amplification as a function of central auditory status in the elderly. *Ear and Hearing* 8:337–42.

Kruel, E.J., Nixon, J.C., Kryter, K.D., Bell, D.W., Lang, J.S., and Schubert, E.D. 1968. A proposed clinical test of speech discrimination. *Journal of Speech and Hearing Research* 11:536–52.

Kryter, K.D. 1983. Presbycusis, sociocusis and nosocusis. *Journal of the Acoustical Society of America* 73:1897–1917.

Leijon, A., Eriksson-Mongold, M., and Bech-Karlsen, A. 1984. Preferred hearing aid gain and bass-cut in relation to prescriptive fitting. *Scandinavian Audiology* 13: 157–61.

Levitt, H. 1990. Personal communication.

Levitt, H., Weiss, M., and Rabinowitz, W. 1987. Noise reduction techniques. *ASHA* 20:119.

Milner, B., Taylor, L., and Sperry, R.W. 1968. Lateralized suppression of dichotically presented digits after commissural section in man. *Science* 161:184–85.

Montgomery, A.A., and Edge, R.A. 1988. Evaluation of two speech enhancement techniques to improve intelligibility for hearing-impaired adults. *Journal of Speech and Hearing Research* 31:386–93.

Moscicki, E.K., Elkins, E.F., Baum, H.F., and McNamara, P.M. 1985. Hearing loss in the elderly: An epidemiologic study of the Framingham Heart Study Cohort. *Ear and Hearing* 6:184–90.

Nabelek, A.K., and Mason, D. 1981. Effect of noise and reverberation on binaural and monaural word identification by subjects with various audiograms. *Journal of Speech and Hearing Research* 24:375–83.

Nabelek, A.K., and Robinson, P.K. 1982. Monaural and binaural speech perception in reverberation for listeners of various ages. *Journal of the Acoustical Society of America* 71:1242–1248.

Noffsinger, P.D., and Kurdziel, S.A. 1979. Assessment of central auditory lesions. In *Hearing Assessment*, ed. W.F. Rintelman. Baltimore: University Park Press.

Olsen, W.O., Noffsinger, P.D., and Carhart, R. 1976. Masking level differences encountered in clinical populations. *Audiology* 15:287–301.

Otto, W.C., and McCandless, G.A. 1982. Aging and auditory site of lesion. *Ear and Hearing* 3:110–117.

Patterson, R., Nimmo-Smith, I., Weber, D., and Milroy, R. 1982. The deterioration of hearing with age: frequency selectivity, the critical ratio, the audiogram, and speech threshold. *Journal of the Acoustical Society of America* 72:1788–1803.

Picheny, M.A., Durlach, N.I., and Braida, L.D. 1986. Speaking clearly for the hard of hearing II: Acoustic characteristics of clear and conversational speech. *Journal of Speech and Hearing Research* 29:437–46.

Picheny, M.A., Durlach, N.I., and Braida, L.D. 1989. Speaking clearly for the hard of hearing III: An attempt to determine the contribution of speaking rate to differences in intelligibility between clear and conversational speech. *Journal of Speech and Hearing Research* 32:600–603.

Resnick, S.B., Dubno, J.R., Hoffnung, S., and Levitt, H. 1975. Phoneme errors on a nonsense syllable test. *Journal of the Acoustical Society of America* 58(Suppl.1):114.

Ries, P.W. 1982. Hearing ability of persons by sociodemographic and health characteristics: United States. *Vital and Health Statistics (National Center for Health Statistics)* Series 10, Number 140. Washington, D.C.: Public Health Service/U.S. Government Printing Office.

Rodriquez, G., DiSarno, N., and Hardiman, C. 1990. Central auditory processing in normal-hearing elderly adults. *Audiology* 29:85–92.

Rubenstein, A., and Boothroyd, A. 1987. Effect of two approaches to auditory training on speech recognition by hearing-impaired adults. *Journal of Speech and Hearing Research* 30:153–60.

Ryals, B.M., and Auther, L.L. 1990. Differences in hearing instrument gain as a function of age. *Hearing Instruments* 41:26–28.

Salomon, G., Vesterager, V., and Jagd, M. 1988. Age-related hearing difficulties I. Hearing impairment, disability, and handicap—a controlled study. *Audiology* 27:164–78.

Salthouse, T.A. 1980. Age and memory: Strategies for localizing the loss. In *New Directions in Memory and Aging: Proceedings of the George A. Tallard Memorial Conference,* eds. L.W. Poon, J.L. Fozard, L.S. Cermak, D. Arenberg, and L.W. Thompson. Hillsdale NJ: Lawrence Erlbaum Associates.

Schmitt, J.F. 1983. The effects of time compression and time expansion on passage comprehension by elderly listeners. *Journal of Speech and Hearing Research* 26:373–77.

Schmitt, J.F., and Carroll, M.R. 1985. Older listeners' ability to comprehend speaker-generated rate alteration passages. *Journal of Speech and Hearing Research* 28:309–312.

Schon, J.D. 1970. The effects on speech intelligibility of time compression and expansion on normal hearing, hard of hearing, and aged males. *Journal of Auditory Research* 10:263–68.

Schum, D.J. 1990. Noise reduction strategies for elderly, hearing-impaired listeners. *Journal of the American Academy of Audiology* 1:31–36.

Speaks, C., and Jerger, J. 1965. Method for measurement of speech identification. *Journal of Speech and Hearing Research* 8:185–94.

Speaks, C., Niccum, N., and Van Tasell, D. 1985. Effects of stimulus material on the dichotic listening performance of patients with sensorineural hearing loss. *Journal of Speech and Hearing Research* 28:16–25.

Stach, B. 1990. Age and the binaural advantage. Paper presented at the annual meeting of the American Academy of Audiology, New Orleans, April, 1990.

Sticht, J., and Gray, B. 1969. The intelligibility of time-compressed words as a function of age and hearing loss. *Journal of Speech and Hearing Research* 12:443–48.

Tillman, T., and Carhart, R. 1986. An expanded test for speech discrimination utilizing CNC monosyllabic words. Northwestern University Auditory Test Number 6. Brooks Air Force Base, Texas: USAF School of Aerospace Medicine Technical Report.

Tyler, R., and Kuk, F. 1989. The effects of "noise suppression" hearing aids on consonant recognition in speech-babble and low-frequency noise. *Ear and Hearing* 10:243–49.

Tyler, R., Summerfield, Q., Wood, E., and Fernandes, M. 1982. Psychoacoustic and phonetic temporal processing in normal and hearing-impaired listeners. *Journal of the Acoustical Society of America* 72:740–52.

Upfold, L., and Wilson, D. 1983. Factors associated with hearing aid use. *Australian Journal of Audiology* 5:20–26.

Van Tasell, D., Larsen, S., and Fabry, D. 1988. Effects of an adaptive filter hearing aid on speech recognition in noise by hearing impaired subjects. *Ear and Hearing* 9:15–21.

Walden, B., Demorest, M., and Hepler, E. 1984. Self-report approach to assessing benefit derived from amplification. *Journal of Speech and Hearing Research* 27:49–56.

Warren, L.R., Wagener, J.W., and Herman, G.E. 1978. Binaural analysis in the aging auditory system. *Journal of Gerontology* 33:731–36.

Wingfield, A., Poon, L., Lombardi, L., and Lowe, D. 1985. Speed of processing in normal aging: Effects of speech rate, linguistic structure and processing time. *Journal of Gerontology* 40:579–85.

CHAPTER 22

Hearing Aids and the Elderly
Audiologic and Psychologic Considerations

Barbara E. Weinstein

Advances in biomedical technology enable older adults with sensorineural hearing loss to benefit substantially from personal hearing aids. Contemporary devices are individualized, miniaturized, flexible, and equipped with controls that are easily manipulated by most older adults (Glass 1990). Further, hearing aids facilitate communication efficiency, enhance emotional/social function, promote a more positive self-concept, and improve affect as well as cognitive status in the elderly (Malinoff and Weinstein 1990; Newman and Weinstein 1988; Mulrow et al. 1990; Harless and McConnell 1982). Although the handicapping effects of hearing loss are remediable, the majority of older adults are reluctant to purchase a hearing aid. Only 18% to 20% of hearing-impaired older adults possess a hearing aid (Gallup 1980). As few as 25% of older adults in need of amplification own a hearing aid (Davies and Mueller 1987). One study—a survey of 482 senior citizens in North Dakota—revealed that, although 83% of the subjects acknowledged a hearing problem, only 24% had tried a hearing aid, and only 11% were using amplification at the time of the survey (Shepel 1980).

A host of biopsychosocial variables account for the incongruity between the high prevalence of hearing loss and the underutilization of hearing aids among the elderly. The hearing-impaired elderly maintain that they have a foreshortened future, and that their hearing loss and word recognition problems are minimal. The general attitude of society toward the disabled and older persons further reinforces their pessimism about the virtues of hearing aid use (Kemp 1990a). Thus, audiologists are faced with the challenge of identifying and motivating the elderly to seek assistance in overcoming handicapping hearing impairments. The goal of this chapter is to discuss the behavioral

(e.g., audiologic) and psychologic (e.g., motivation) factors instrumental in the older adult's decision to pursue amplification. A motivational model, drawn from geriatric psychiatry, which may hold promise as a means of recruiting hearing aid users from the ranks of the more than 7.5 million older adults with hearing loss, is included.

Nonaudiologic Correlates of Hearing Aid Rejection

Older adults have a disproportionate burden of chronic conditions including sensory impairments, arthritis, and heart disease, relative to younger adults (Brummel-Smith 1990). They represent the vast majority of persons requiring rehabilitative intervention. Notwithstanding the observation that they derive as much benefit from rehabilitation as their younger counterparts, the elderly represent a small proportion of the caseloads of departments of rehabilitation (Brummel-Smith 1990; Kemp 1990a). Understanding the obstacles to utilizing rehabilitation services, and convincing the elderly of the benefits of early intervention is a challenge to the rehabilitation professions. Why is it that more than half of all hearing-impaired persons fail to seek assistance for their hearing loss (Brooks 1982)? Why is it that the elderly tolerate hearing loss for such a long time (e.g., ten years on the average) prior to seeking audiologic assistance (Brooks 1982)? Finally, why is it that the degree of hearing loss that precipitates audiologic action is greater in older than younger individuals (Brooks 1982; Dodds and Harford 1982)?

In an attempt to highlight obstacles to utilizing speech and hearing services, Shadden and Raiford (1984) conducted a comprehensive survey of clinicians and older adults. Inadequate referrals, lack of awareness of service availability, and advice that hearing-related services are of little benefit were high on the list of reasons for the underutilization of

The author is grateful to Craig Newman, Ph.D. for providing some of the data presented in the manuscript.

speech and hearing services (Shadden and Raiford 1984). A lack of awareness about the benefits to be derived from hearing aids and naïveté regarding modern technology available to remediate hearing loss are additional deterrents to service utilization (Hardick and Gans 1982).

Data from the work of Franks and Beckman (1985) and Fino, Bess, and Lichtenstein (1989) shed light on additional nonaudiologic factors influencing the apparent pessimism about amplification. As indicated in this volume, Chapter 21, finances, the fact that hearing aids amplify noise, and that they call attention to one's handicap rank high on the list of reasons for hearing aid rejection by older adults (Franks and Beckman 1985). Fino, Bess, and Lichtenstein (1989) concurred that the economics of the hearing health care delivery system, cosmetic factors, psychosocial variables, and properties inherent in present-day hearing aids (e.g., noise) influence the decision against hearing aid use. The importance of social, economic, and technologic factors relative to audiometric considerations remains an issue of debate.

Audiologic Correlates of Hearing Aid Use

Isolating the audiologic correlates of hearing aid use in older adults is an especially fruitful area of inquiry. These data may contribute to our understanding of the onset of communication and psychosocial difficulties derived from hearing loss. In addition, this information may have implications for health promotion activities designed to identify probable candidates for hearing aids. The work of Brooks (1982), Dodds and Harford (1982), and Fino, Bess, and Lichtenstein (1989) has contributed to our understanding of the extent to which degree of hearing loss serves as a trigger for persons to seek audiologic assistance.

Brooks (1982) noted that the average degree of hearing loss of first time users of hearing aids was 50 dB HL. Dodds and Harford (1982) contrasted hearing levels of younger and older adults self-referred to a clinic for professional advice about amplification with those of a sample of older adults seeking information about hearing status as part of a community outreach program. Two interesting trends emerged. The mean hearing threshold levels of the younger adults considering hearing aid use were comparable to the mean thresholds of older adults participating in the community outreach program (i.e., those not interested in amplification). Fur-

ther, mean thresholds of the seniors self-referred to the clinic for advice regarding amplification were approximately 15 dB poorer than the thresholds of an age-matched group tested in the field as part of a community service. Based on the preliminary trends apparent from their study, Dodds and Harford (1982) concluded that the elderly do not consider using amplification until the hearing loss is considerably poorer than that of a younger sample.

Fino, Bess, and Lichtenstein (1989) attempted to further clarify some of the audiometric characteristics of elderly hearing aid users. They compared a small sample of older adults electing to seek hearing aid assistance ($n = 25$) to a sample declining intervention ($n = 45$). Hearing aid users and non-users were contrasted across the dimensions of hearing loss and self-assessed hearing handicap. The screening version of the Hearing Handicap Inventory for the Elderly (HHIE-S) was used as an index of perceived handicap. Three interesting trends emerged from their investigation. First, the proportion of hearing aid users with mean pure-tone averages greater than 40 dB HL exceeded the proportion of persons who did not obtain hearing aids (i.e., 40% versus 9%). Second, the percentage of non-users judging themselves to be minimally handicapped by the hearing loss was greater than the proportion of hearing aid users (54% versus 8%). Finally, irrespective of degree of hearing loss, individuals rejecting hearing aids did not perceive themselves to be as handicapped as hearing aid users. That is, within each category of hearing loss (e.g., mild, moderate, etc.), non-users had lower HHIE-S scores than hearing aid users. Fino, Bess, and Lichtenstein (1989) concluded that their findings underscore the importance of viewing functional measures of hearing handicap as a potential indicator of hearing aid candidacy in the elderly.

Fino, Bess, and Lichtenstein (1989) recommended caution in interpreting and generalizing their findings because subjects were recruited exclusively from the practices of primary care physicians in Tennessee. In an attempt to replicate their study using a more diverse sample, I collected data on a sample of 75 non-hearing aid users recruited from selected senior citizen centers and 71 hearing aid users who purchased their hearing aids from one of two hospital clinics in large metropolitan areas. Table I shows the mean hearing levels and standard deviations in the right ear of hearing aid users and nonusers. It is apparent that mean threshold levels in the low- and mid-frequencies (250–2000 Hz) were virtually identical for the two groups, with slightly poorer hearing levels in the

Table I. Mean Thresholds and Standard Deviations in dB HL for Right Ears of Hearing Aid Users (n = 71) and Nonusers (n = 75)

	Frequencies in Hz						
	250	500	1000	2000	3000	4000	6000
Non-users							
Mean	27	30.4	35.7	41.2	50	54.5	59.4
(SD)	(16.5)	(17.8)	(18.6)	(20.2)	(21.7)	(23.5)	(23.4)
Users							
Mean	26.8	30.8	35.5	45.8	57.2	61.5	66.6
(SD)	(14.2)	(15.9)	(16.6)	(13.4)	(13.7)	(14.8)	(16.5)

higher frequencies for the hearing aid users. The latter differences, which are on the order of 5 to 7 decibels, were not significant. Mean pure-tone thresholds at octave frequencies for the left ear were comparable in the two samples, as well.

The performance of the two groups on selected audiometric tests is shown in table II. The mean age of the hearing aid users was 76 years and the non-users 75.6 years. Mean three frequency pure-tone averages in the better and poorer ears were quite similar for the two groups. While word recognition scores appear to be slightly poorer in non-users than in hearing aid users, the differences are too small to be considered clinically significant. Mean HHIE scores of older adults with hearing aids were indicative of significantly greater emotional and social handicaps than that experienced by non-hearing aid users. The finding that persons with hearing aids tend to perceive greater psychosocial

Table II. Means and Standard Deviations on Selected Audiometric Measures in Hearing Aid Users and Non-users

	Subject Group	
Audiometric Measure	Non-Hearing Aid Users	Hearing Aid Users
PTA–Better ear	30.7 dBHL (12.8)	32.6 dBHL (9.6)
PTA—Poorer ear	37.5 dBHL (15.1)	42.2 dBHL (15.1)
Word Recognition Score in % right ear	82.7 (16.9)	89.5 (11.3)
Word Recognition Score in % left ear	81.1 (14.6)	89.5 (14.5)
HHIE Score in %	21.2 (21.5)	35.1 (22.3)

Note: Sample size for each group ranges from 71 to 79 subjects.

handicap is consistent with the data of Fino, Bess, and Lichtenstein (1989).

Given the disparity in mean HHIE scores, and the overlap in mean pure-tone averages and word recognition ability, it is not surprising that the correlations among these variables differed between the two groups of subjects. As is evident in table III, the correlation between HHIE scores and audiometric measures was moderate for the non-hearing aid users and minimal for the hearing aid users. The fact that audiometric measures accounted for more of the variability in response to handicap perceived by non-hearing aid users suggests that other audiologic/nonaudiologic factors are probably operating to influence an older adult's decision to purchase a hearing aid. These data are in keeping with the conclusions of Gilhome-Herbst (1983), who speculated that degree of hearing loss, namely impairment, is one of the least significant determinants of perceived hearing handicap. It may well be that the extent to which the hearing loss "actually matters and is bothersome" to the individual is a powerful influence on handicap judgments among hearing aid users (Gilhome-Herbst 1983, p. 186).

Finally, Gates et al. (1990) recently broadened the database emanating from the hearing testing of the Framingham cohort. One thousand six hundred sixty-two subjects obtained a biennial auditory examination that included completion of an auditory questionnaire, word recognition testing, immittance testing, and pure tone testing. Only 10% of subjects judged likely to benefit from hearing aids were using them at the time of the evaluation. Gates et al. (1990) compared the hearing aid users and former users on selected audiometric variables in an attempt to identify audiometric factors influencing the decision to use a hearing aid. The current hearing aid users and former users were contrasted on mean AMA handicap scores (i.e., audiometric based definition of hearing handicap), mean word recognition scores at conversational level, and mean pure-tone averages. None of the differences in mean scores obtained on the hearing tests between users and former users achieved statistical significance. Once again, their

Table III. Correlations Between Audiometric Measures and HHIE Scores in Hearing Aid Users and Non-Hearing Aid Users

	Non-Hearing Aid Users	Hearing Aid Users
PTA × HHIE	.56*	.22
WRS × HHIE	−.42*	−.12

data point to the overlap in performance on audiometric tests routinely used to decide upon hearing aid candidacy.

In sum, a number of investigators have attempted to delineate the audiometric similarities and differences among older adults who use hearing aids and those who do not. It appears that, audiometrically, the similarities among the groups with respect to mean pure-tone thresholds and mean word recognition scores, are more noteworthy than the differences. In contrast, as suggested by Kapteyn (1977), and reinforced by the aforementioned studies, psychosocial variables, including expression of the extent of hearing handicap, appear to be a strong indicator of hearing aid candidacy in older adults.

Audiologic Correlates of Hearing Aid Benefit

To further explore the influence of audiometric variables on hearing aid use, Newman et al. (1991) administered the screening version of the Hearing Handicap Inventory for the Elderly (HHIE-S) to 91 new hearing aid users prehearing aid fitting and three weeks posthearing aid fitting. Overall, a significant reduction in self-perceived hearing handicap was noted for the entire sample, following a brief interval of hearing aid use. The change in HHIE-S scores before and after hearing aid fitting as a function of hearing level category are shown in table IV. Three trends are apparent. First, a significant reduction in mean HHIE-S scores was noted for those with normal to mild hearing levels and for those with moderate to severe hearing loss. Next, the absolute amount of change in mean HHIE-S

scores was comparable for both groups of hearing aid users, as well. Finally, despite differences in hearing level, prefitting, postfitting, and difference scores on the HHIE-S were comparable. The latter finding suggests that hearing level did not influence the perceived handicap in this sample of new hearing aid users. Similar trends were noted when subjects were classified according to monosyllabic word recognition scores. The 91 new hearing aid users were divided according to mean suprathreshold word recognition scores obtained using the W-22 word lists. As is clear from table V, mean word recognition scores did not appear to influence the perception of hearing handicap. Prefitting HHIE-S scores, postfitting HHIE-S scores, and difference scores on the HHIE-S were comparable. The fact that hearing level category and word recognition ability did not appear to influence the perception of hearing handicap, and the reduction in perceived handicap following a brief interval of hearing aid use, lends additional support to the hypothesis that nonaudiologic variables, most notably the perceived psychosocial handicap, influences hearing aid candidacy and benefit.

Motivational Dynamics and Hearing Aid Candidacy

In their discussion of decision making in rehabilitative audiology, McCarthy, Montgomery, and Mueller (1990) acknowledged that "when fitting hearing aids, the goal of maximizing speech reception is usually thought of in the context of obtaining de-

Table IV. Means and Standard Deviations on HHIE-S Pre- and Post Hearing Aid Fitting as a Function of Hearing Level Category in a Sample of Older Adults ($n = 91$)

	HHIE-S Scores	
	Prefitting	Postfitting[1]
Normal to Mild ($n = 54$)		
Mean*	16.6	3.0
(SD)	(8.3)	(3.8)
Moderate to Severe ($n = 37$)		
Mean*	18.8	3.6
(SD)	(8.3)	(5.1)

[1]Three weeks postfitting

*$p < .001$

(From Newman et al. 1991.)

Table V. Means and Standard Deviations Associated with Pre- and Post Hearing Aid Fitting HHIE-S Scores as a Function of Word Recognition Category in a Sample of Older Adults ($n = 91$)

	HHIE-S Scores	
Word Recognition Score	Prefitting	Postfitting[1]
90–100% ($n = 42$)		
Mean*	16.0	3.2
(SD)	(7.8)	(4.3)
80–88% ($n = 29$)		
Mean*	17.9	2.4
(SD)	(9.0)	(3.0)
$<$/= 78% ($n = 20$)		
Mean*	18.0	4.5
(SD)	(9.7)	(5.6)

[1]Three weeks postfitting

*$p < .001$

(From Newman et al. 1991.)

sired gain at selected frequencies throughout the speech spectrum" (p. 23). What is overlooked frequently by audiologists is the more rudimentary form of maximizing speech reception ability, namely encouraging hearing aid use (McCarthy, Montgomery, and Mueller 1990). As older persons tend to make choices that are in keeping with the status quo, and require more time to make decisions, they often are not motivated toward hearing aid use (Brummel-Smith 1990). Brooks (1982) speculated that lack of motivation is a likely cause of unwillingness on the part of the elderly to seek audiologic assistance. Motivation affects rehabilitation outcome, adaptation to disability, and represents the "single most important problem facing the rehabilitation worker" (Kemp 1990b, p. 295). Until recently, motivation has been an elusive and enigmatic psychological variable. A theory of motivation that accounts in part for why behavior persists, why behavior is initiated, and why behavior attenuates was described by Kemp (1990b) in his text on geriatric rehabilitation.

Kemp (1990b) suggested that motivation, which means "to move," is multifactorial, resulting from the interplay among four variables—wants, beliefs, rewards, and costs. The formulation of motivation applies to a wide range of behaviors (Kemp 1990b). The discussion below describes the application of motivation to hearing aid use in the elderly. The motive system can be expressed as an equation wherein:

$$\text{Motivation} = \frac{\text{Wants} \times \text{Beliefs} \times \text{Rewards}}{\text{Costs}}$$

The term *wants* refers to one's needs and goals relative to the disability and the intervention. Specifically, one's wants are integrally related to initiating behavior and toward achieving a positive outcome. Audiologists are encouraged to obtain very specific information about what exactly patients expect to gain from a hearing aid. The more explicit the goal, the greater the likelihood individuals will achieve it (Kemp 1990b; Mento, Steele, and Karrem 1987). One strategy that has proved successful in eliciting information about goals is questioning the individual about the perceived problems that derive from a hearing loss. An understanding of the communicative difficulties and the handicap in the psychosocial domains of function, can assist audiologists in coming to grips with what an older adult may want from a hearing aid. For example, an individual complaining of difficulty understanding the television or radio may simply need a hearing aid or assistive listening device that facilitates television under-

standing. Similarly, an individual frustrated by the inability to understand speech in less than optimal listening situations may require a hearing aid with noise reduction circuitry. Finally, older adults may be frustrated by the fact that hearing loss interferes with overall function and hence compromises independence. Restoration of functional abilities seems to be at the crux of what older adults want from rehabilitation, and it is incumbent on audiologists to impress upon hearing-impaired persons how assistance can help achieve this goal (Brummel-Smith 1990).

Beliefs reflect an individual's subjective view of his or her expectations and perceptions (Kemp 1990b). It is important to note that an individual's views often run counter to a professional's opinions. Beliefs represent the cognitive component of motivation and in large part influence that which a person will act upon (Kemp 1990b). The classic example in audiology would be a 75-year-old retired individual with a pure-tone average of 55 dB HL, who denies being handicapped by his or her hearing loss, and refuses to purchase a hearing aid, despite provocations from family members.

Individuals' beliefs about their capabilities, regarding the possibility of improvement from a given intervention (e.g., hearing aid) and about the future, are powerful determinants of motivation (Kemp 1990b). In order to influence this component of motivation, the subjective viewpoint of individuals may be more important than the clinician's appraisal (Kemp 1990b). Communication specific assessment tools may be helpful in uncovering situation specific difficulties that can serve as a focus of discussion regarding the potential for improvement with a hearing aid or assistive listening device. Similarly, completion of a handicap scale can assist audiologists in exploring individuals' reactions or adaptations to the hearing loss. It is often helpful to link the benefits derived from amplification systems to the specific emotional and situational reactions expressed by the hearing impaired. Such an approach may be clarifying to the point of influencing subsequent behavior (Kemp 1990b).

Frequent feedback about the rewards associated with hearing aid use are necessary to influence the decision to obtain a hearing aid and to continue wearing it once purchased. Word recognition testing in quiet can be instrumental in providing immediate reinforcement about the potential benefit from hearing aids. Real ear measures wherein the patient can visualize the capability and flexibility of the hearing aid can demonstrate improved performance and promote feelings of success, as well.

Newman et al. (1991) and Malinoff and Weinstein (1989) documented that self-perceived emotional and social handicaps were reduced dramatically after only three weeks of hearing aid use. Mulrow et al. (1990) demonstrated that the improvement in HHIE scores following six weeks of hearing aid use tends to be sustained after a four month interval. Any objective evidence of reduction in psychosocial handicap associated with hearing aid use, as demonstrated by self-report scales, should be shared with the client. Frequent and immediate feedback tends to promote a sense of self-confidence and often helps to maintain the desired behavior (e.g., continued hearing aid use). A family member who completes a self-assessment scale, and confirms the view that the hearing aid is in fact beneficial, provides an additional sense of success. It is important to note that older persons are easily discouraged and require frequent feedback to ensure that they recognize and appreciate the progress being made.

Finally, the social, physical, and psychological costs associated with handicapping hearing loss may in fact influence the decision to obtain a hearing aid. Accordingly, audiologists should share information about personal adaptations to and consequences of unremediated hearing loss with the hearing impaired and their families. It should be made clear that a defeatist attitude, not assuming responsibility for the disability, and lack of assertiveness about overcoming hearing loss will increase the costs exacted by hearing loss (Kemp 1990b). The psychologic costs associated with unremediated hearing loss are often compelling, as in many cases an older adult is unaware of the burden hearing loss poses. Glass (1990) described hearing loss as a "glass wall" that forms a barrier between individuals. The invisible handicap of hearing loss is associated with decreased self-esteem, loss of independence, depressed affect, and reduced enjoyment of routine leisure activities (Glass 1990).

The social consequences of hearing loss are often "unrecognized adaptations" on the part of hearing-impaired adults (Glass 1990). They may include unconscious or conscious avoidance of previously enjoyed activities, offering inappropriate reactions during conversation, or a reduction in the frequency with which one participates in recreational and leisure activities. The fact that hearing loss may pose a threat to personal safety, especially among nonambulatory and confused older adults, is often reason enough to pursue a hearing aid or assistive listening device.

Finally, a major obstacle to hearing aid use remains the excessive cost associated with purchasing a hearing aid and related services. Mulrow et al. (1990) suggest that the cost of a hearing test, hearing aid selection, hearing aid, and dispensing fee may amount to $1,000. They advocate cost analyses, wherein the economic impact of a hearing aid is considered in the context of financial outlay coupled with psychosocial benefit to the individual and his or her family. Mulrow et al. (1990) computed the cost of a hearing aid in terms of hearing quality adjusted life years (HQALYS). That formula considers actual financial outlay for hearing health care services, along with some measure of benefit from amplification. Using percent improvement in the HHIE score as an outcome/benefit measure, Mulrow et al. (1990) projected the actual cost effectiveness estimate for an individual receiving a hearing aid to be $200. Therefore, when the cost-benefit is considered, hearing aids represent a relatively inexpensive form of intervention (Mulrow et al. 1990). If the patient is acquainted with the cost of a hearing aid, relative to its long-term utility and benefit, this may be a powerful influence on the decision to proceed with amplification.

Kemp (1990b) acknowledged that motivation is understandable and can be improved. Accordingly, he recommended that the rehabilitation worker examine and analyze each of the components of motivation in the context of aging, of the disability (i.e., hearing loss), and of the rehabilitative intervention (hearing aid). When assessing and attempting to manipulate one's motivation toward hearing aid use, the following considerations are important (Kemp 1990b):

1. One's subjective viewpoint on each of the components of motivation will influence behavior and rehabilitative outcome.
2. The viewpoints of significant others regarding the extent of disability and the philosophy about audiologic intervention is a powerful influence on the hearing aid candidate. Indeed "motivational problems seldom arise unless there is more than one person involved" (Kemp 1990b, p. 304).
3. Each individual has a critical variable (e.g., physical cost, social cost) preventing better motivation. Accordingly, each component of the model should be thoroughly explored to insure that the key deterrent to the desired behavior emerges.
4. It is crucial to uncover the rewards necessary to sustain hearing aid use. Once these are under-

stood, feedback regarding the rewards should be frequent and time-linked to the desired behavior.

In sum, hearing aids are the primary rehabilitation tool for the population of elderly persons with handicapping hearing impairments (Bess, Lichtenstein, and Logan 1990). They are a beneficial form of therapy, which can improve the quality of life of elderly persons with handicapping hearing loss (Mulrow et al. 1990). Yet, even if a patient acknowledges a hearing loss, there is a 50% chance he or she will be referred for audiologic intervention (Bess, Lichenstein, and Logan 1990). Audiologists are encouraged to experiment with motivational dynamics as a means of increasing the relatively small pool of individuals benefitting from hearing aids.

References

Bess, F., Lichtenstein, M., and Logan, S. 1990. Audiologic assessment of the hearing-impaired elderly. In *Hearing Assessment*, ed. W.B. Rintelmann. Austin: Pro-Ed.

Brooks, D.N. 1982. Pre- and post-hearing aid provision management. In *The Vanderbilt Hearing Aid Report: State of the Art-Research Needs*, eds. G. Studebaker and F.H. Bess. PA: Monographs in Contemporary Audiology.

Brummel-Smith, K. 1990. Introduction in *Geriatric Rehabilitation*, eds. B. Kemp, K. Brummel-Smith, and J. Ramsdell. Boston: College-Hill Press.

Davies, J.W., and Mueller, H.G. 1987. Hearing aid selection. In *Communication Disorders in Aging*, eds. H.G. Mueller and V.C. Geoffrey. Washington, DC: Gallaudet University Press.

Dodds, E., and Harford, E. 1982. A community hearing screening program for senior citizens. *Ear and Hearing* 3:160–66.

Fino, M.S., Bess, F.H., and Lichtenstein, M. 1989. Attitudes and characteristics differentiating elderly hearing aid users and nonusers. Paper presented at the Annual American Speech-Language-Hearing Association, St. Louis.

Franks, J.R., and Beckman, N.J. 1985. Rejection of hearing aids: Attitudes of a geriatric sample. *Ear and Hearing* 6:161–66.

The Gallup Organization, Inc. 1980. A survey concerning hearing problems and hearing aids in the United States. Princeton, NJ: Author.

Gates, G., Cooper, J., Kannel, B., and Miller, N. 1990. Hearing in the elderly: The Framingham Cohort, 1983–1985. Part I. Basic audiometric tests. *Ear and Hearing* 11:247–57.

Gilhome-Herbst, K. 1983. Psycho-social consequences of disorders of hearing in the elderly. In *Hearing and Balance in the Elderly*, ed. R. Hinchcliffe. New York: Churchill Livingstone.

Glass, L. 1990. Hearing impairment in elderly. *Geriatric Rehabilitation*, ed. B. Kemp, K. Brummel-Smith, and J. Ramsdell. Boston: College-Hill Press.

Hardick, E.J., and Gans, R.E. 1982. An approach to rehabilitation with amplification. *Ear and Hearing* 3:178–82.

Harless, E., and McConnell, F. 1982. Effects of hearing aid use on self concept in older persons. *Journal of Speech and Hearing Disorders* 47:305–309.

Kapteyn, T.S. 1977. Satisfaction with fitted hearing aids II. An investigation in the influence of psycho-social factors. *Scandinavian Audiology* 6:171–77.

Kemp, B. 1990a. The psychosocial context of geriatric rehabilitation. In *Geriatric Rehabilitation*, eds. B. Kemp, K. Brummel-Smith, and J. Ramsdell. Boston: College-Hill Press.

Kemp, B. 1990b. Motivational dynamics in geriatric rehabilitation: Toward a therapeutic model. In *Geriatric Rehabilitation*, ed. B. Kemp, K. Brummel-Smith, and J. Ramsdell. Boston: College-Hill Press.

Malinoff, R., and Weinstein, B.E. 1990. Measurement of hearing aid benefit in the elderly. *Ear and Hearing* 10:354–56.

McCathy, P.A., Montgomery, A., and Mueller, H.G. 1990. Decision making in rehabilitative audiology. *Journal of the American Academy of Audiology* 1:23–30.

Mento, A., Steele, R.P., and Karrem, R.J. 1987. A meta-analytic study of the effects of goal setting on task performance: 1988–1984. *Organ. Behav. Hum. Decision Process* 39:52.

Mulrow, C., Aguilar, C., Endicott, J., Tuley, M., Valez, R., Charlip, W., Rhodes, M., and Hill, J. 1990. Quality of life changes and hearing impairment: Results of a randomized trial. *Annals of Internal Medicine* 113:189–94.

Newman, C., and Weinstein, B. 1988. The Hearing Handicap Inventory for the Elderly as a measure of hearing aid benefit. *Ear and Hearing* 9:81–85.

Newman, C., Jacobson, G., Hug, G., Weinstein, B., and Malinoff, R. 1991. A practical method for quantifying hearing aid benefit in older adults. *Journal of the American Academy of Audiology*.

Shadden, B.B., and Raiford, C.A. 1984. Factors influencing service utilization by older adults. *Journal of Communication Disorders* 17:209–224.

Shepel, F. 1980. Geriatric hearing health care for the future. *Hearing Instruments* 31:7–8.

CHAPTER 23

Hearing Aid Selection for High-Frequency Hearing Loss

H. Gustav Mueller, Margaret P. Bryant, Wayne D. Brown, and Ann Calkins Budinger

Hearing aid selection for individuals with high-frequency sensorineural hearing loss has been discussed in the audiology literature since at least the 1940s, when several early investigators reported on earmold venting experiments for this patient population (e.g., Schier 1941; Grossman 1943; Grossman and Molloy 1944). The interest in earmold acoustics and high-frequency amplification increased in the late 1960s as a result of a series of publications by Harford and colleagues describing the benefits of the CROS hearing aid and the CROS-type (open) earmold (e.g., Harford and Barry 1965; Harford and Dodds 1966). Following these publications, clinicians began to use the CROS-type earmold routinely with conventional behind-the-ear hearing aids, and this type of fitting was dubbed an IROS— *i*psilateral *r*outing *o*f *s*ignal. Although the IROS term is a rather poor descriptor of an open mold fitting or hearing aid style, as nearly all hearing aid fittings are an ipsilateral routing, it remains the most popular description of this type of fitting; therefore, this term is used throughout this chapter.

While the technology for fitting individuals with high-frequency hearing loss has changed significantly since the 1960s, so has our definition of what constitutes a high-frequency hearing loss. Jetty and Rintelman (1970) reported the use of modified earmolds for three different types of hearing loss groups; one of these groups was described as having a "precipitous high-frequency hearing loss." The Jetty and Rintelman high-frequency loss group had mean thresholds of 35 dB at 1000 Hz and 60 dB at 2000 Hz. Today, when audiologists state that they are fitting hearing aids to someone with a high-frequency loss, it is often true that the patient's hearing loss at 1000 and 2000 Hz is no worse than *10 dB*.

While it can be argued that almost any hearing loss sloping downward from 500 Hz is "high frequency," the high-frequency hearing loss configuration that seems to attract the most interest today is one with normal hearing through 2000 Hz. Discussions among colleagues concerning this group usually are mildly controversial—some audiologists consider these patients excellent candidates for hearing aids and fit them binaurally, whereas other audiologists consider them poor candidates and do not fit them at all. The focus of this chapter, therefore, is on the group of individuals with high-frequency hearing loss beginning at 3000 Hz.

If one believes that someone with hearing loss beginning at 3000 Hz is indeed a candidate for hearing aids, several considerations must be made during the fitting and rehabilitative process. First, the advantages and disadvantages of various hearing aid styles must be weighed. Second, a theoretical fitting strategy must be formulated and implemented. Third, the theoretical hearing aid selection model needs to be tested and possibly modified. And finally, consideration must be given to establishing some type of postfitting verification of the fitting process. Each of these factors is discussed in the following four sections.

Selection of Hearing Aid Style

In the day-to-day fitting of hearing aids, the greatest emphasis usually is placed on the selection and verification of the hearing aid's electroacoustic features. For many patients, however, the selection of the hearing aid style deserves equal attention, as this single factor may determine whether or not the hearing aid is used. In some work settings, the audiologist chooses the hearing aid style with little input from the patient—the logic being that "the audiologist knows what's best." In other work settings, the patient often is allowed to choose the hearing aid style. The thought here is that the patient will be more apt to use and be satisfied with hearing aids that are his or her style choice. Because most patients are concerned about receiving a "modern" hearing aid, when both the audiologist and the patient believe that a small custom in-the-ear (ITE) instrument is the best, style selection is a smooth process. Compromise often is necessary, however, when the audiologist prefers to fit a behind-the-ear (BTE) model.

The need for compromise can be even greater when the patient has a high-frequency hearing loss. When patients know that they have a "mild" handicap, they are more apt to believe that only a small hearing aid is necessary. Paradoxically, audiologists are more likely to encourage the use of a BTE hearing aid, as they know that this high-frequency hearing loss configuration calls for prescriptive gain that is very difficult to achieve with small ITE or in-the-canal (ITC) instruments.

When decisions are made, therefore, regarding the hearing aid style for these high-frequency loss patients, the trade-offs center on two important questions: (1) Will hearing aid style affect the ability to achieve prescriptive target gain? and (2) Will hearing aid style affect long-term hearing aid use and patient satisfaction?

Achieving Target Insertion Gain

The majority of audiologists fit hearing aids using some type of prescriptive fitting technique. This may be accomplished directly, by specifying 2-cm³ coupler gain following mathematical calculations, or indirectly, by sending an audiogram to a custom ITE manufacturer. Regardless of which ordering or prescriptive method is used, the desired result for the high-frequency loss patient is little or no gain at 2000 Hz and below, with gain equal to ⅓ to ½ the hearing loss for 3000 Hz and above. How does hearing aid style affect one's ability to achieve this real ear response?

We examined the real ear insertion response (REIR) for four different hearing aid styles on ten individuals. The hearing aid styles that were used were a BTE (high-frequency earmold), ITE-Helix, ITE-IROS, and ITC-IROS. These styles represent the common options available to and used by hearing aid dispensers for this type of hearing loss.

The mean REIR results of the four instruments are shown in figure 1, with gain matched at 3000 Hz so that relative differences in the frequency response configurations can be observed easily. Clearly, hearing aid style is a dominant factor when achieving target gain is the goal of the hearing aid selection procedure. If we consider the audiogram of a typical patient with thresholds no worse than 10 dB through 2000 Hz, 40 dB at 3000 Hz, and 60 dB at 4000 Hz, then the mean REIR of the BTE is a near perfect fit for a prescriptive formula such as the National Acoustic Laboratories (NAL) method (Byrne and Dillon 1986). Observe that the ITE and ITC models all would provide excessive gain in the 1500–2000 Hz region, and also substantially fail to achieve target gain in the higher frequencies. The ITE-Helix, for example, provides mean real ear insertion gain (REIG) 20 dB below that of the BTE for 4000 Hz.

The results shown in figure 1 might suggest to

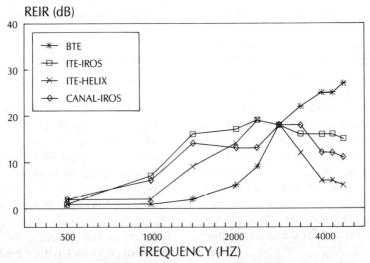

Figure 1.   Mean real ear insertion response (REIR) measures for ten individuals fitted with four different hearing aid styles: behind-the-ear (BTE), in-the-ear (ITE)-IROS, ITE-Helix, and in-the-canal (ITC)-IROS. Mean REIRs matched at 3000 Hz.

some, at least those who are advocates of prescriptive fitting techniques, that patients with hearing loss beginning at 3000 Hz always should be fitted with BTE instruments. If target insertion gain were the only issue, this notion would be hard to refute. But, what is the role of patient style preference?

Consideration of Patient Preference

As stated earlier, some audiologists believe that patients should be allowed to choose their hearing aid style. When given this choice, a patient will almost always select the smaller custom ITE instrument. In a 1988 article, Surr and Hawkins reported that even when the advantages and disadvantages of BTEs and ITEs are explained to the patients, 73% of new users select the ITE style. In a separate study of 153 first time hearing aid users, Mueller and Budinger (1990) reported that 90% of their patients selected the ITE style over a BTE instrument. If providing the patient with the style of his or her choice enhances long term use of and benefit from hearing aids, then a compromise between desired gain and patient preference may be necessary. On the other hand, if the patient can be convinced that "the BTE is really the best for you," then fitting these high-frequency loss patients with BTEs would have no long-term negative consequences.

We recently addressed the issue of ITE/BTE preference by comparing the opinions of hearing aid users one year after the hearing aid fitting. All subjects participating in this study were males, new users of hearing aids, and were receiving their hearing aids free of charge as an entitlement for military service. Consecutive patients reporting to our clinic for a hearing aid fitting were arbitrarily divided into two groups. One group was fitted with ITE hearing aids and the other group was fitted with BTE instruments. All subjects were fitted binaurally. Patients considered to be poor candidates for binaural use were not included as subjects.

At the time of the hearing aid fitting, the subjects were not given any information regarding the advantages or disadvantages of one style over another. Their opinions were not solicited regarding the hearing aid style that they preferred. When subjects asked why they were being fitted with a given style, they were told simply, "It's the style that's best for you and you will have the best speech understanding with this type of hearing aid." The subjects in the BTE group were fitted with the minicase size, and the ITE fittings were the full-concha style.

The frequency response for both styles of hearing aids was selected based on the National Acoustic Laboratories' (NAL) prescriptive fitting approach. At the time of the fitting, REIR measures were conducted, and appropriate alterations were made until the frequency response fell within our clinic tolerances of the NAL target. No significant differences were observed in the direction or degree of deviation from NAL target gain between the two different groups.

One year after the last subject was issued his hearing aids, a short questionnaire was mailed to all the subjects asking them to rate their use of, benefit and satisfaction from the hearing aids. Additionally, they were asked to answer a series of questions about the "other style" of hearing aid, (i.e., the style that they were *not* issued). Data analyses were based on the resulting responses from 52 individuals from the BTE group (88% return rate) and 43 replies from the ITE group (84% return rate). Although the subjects in the two different groups were not matched for hearing loss or age, there were no significant differences between groups for these two variables.

The data from the questionnaires were divided into specific areas pertaining to hearing aid use, perceived benefit in a variety of listening situations, and overall satisfaction from the hearing fitting. Hearing aid use was categorized according to percent of use on an average day. Because all patients from both groups were fitted binaurally, the patients reported the percent of daily use of at least one hearing aid (total use) and the percent of time that they used two hearing aids.

Figure 2 shows the percent of total and binaural hearing aid use for both groups. Observe that both the ITE and BTE users report using at least one hearing aid 70% of their average day. If, however, binaural use is examined (see figure 2), the ITE users report nearly 20% greater use of two hearing aids (2–3 hours per day) than the BTE group. In agreement with this hearing aid use data, 84% of the ITE users stated that they understood speech better with binaural hearing aids, whereas only 66% of the BTE users gave this report.

While the increased use of binaural hearing aids for the ITE group might suggest that these individuals would report greater benefit, there was no difference in reported hearing aid benefit between the two groups. Satisfaction ratings, however, did indicate that the BTE users were less satisfied. As shown in figure 3, 49% of the BTE users reported that they were only "somewhat satisfied."

Perhaps the most revealing differences between the two groups were observed when their re-

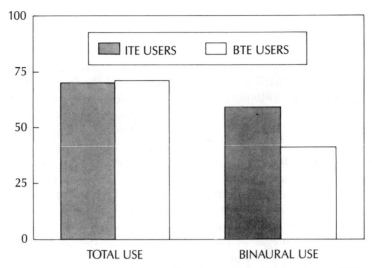

Figure 2. Percent of hearing aid use/average day that in-the-ear (ITE) and behind-the-ear (BTE) users reported for at least one hearing aid (total use) or for two hearing aids (binaural use).

sponses concerning the "other style of hearing aid" were compared. These responses are shown in table I (the patients were given the option of stating "unsure," and therefore, the "agree" and "disagree" responses do not total 100%). Note the general dissatisfaction of the BTE users. Nearly 100% of them believe that the other style is less obvious, 88% believe that the other style is more modern, and 80% state that they would use their hearing aids more if they had the other style. On the other hand, over 90% of the ITE users *disagreed* with these three statements.

These findings cannot be ignored when hear-

ing aid style is selected. Achieving target gain may be inconsequential if the patient believes that he or she received a second-rate product and uses this as a reason for not using the hearing aid. As shown in figure 1, however, the trade-offs that are made when REIG is sacrificed for style can be significant. For the readers who are proponents of prescriptive selection methods, but who really would like to fit ITE and ITC hearing aids to these patients, the following thought might be considered. If high-frequency loss patients actually use less gain than predicted from prescriptive methods, then the frequency response trade-off would not be as great as

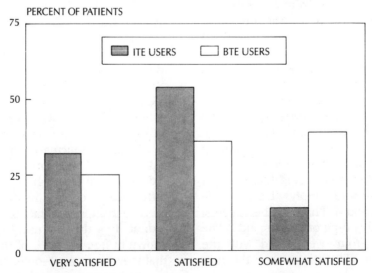

Figure 3. Distribution of satisfaction ratings for in-the-ear (ITE) and behind-the-ear (BTE) hearing aid users.

Table I.   Hearing Aid Users' Ratings of the "Other Style"*

	Agree		Disagree	
	BTE Users	ITE Users	BTE Users	ITE Users
1. The other style of hearing aid would be less obvious to others.	94	2	2	91
2. The other style of hearing aid would cause less interference with my glasses.	94	0	2	93
3. The other style of hearing aid is more modern.	88	0	0	93
4. I would use my hearing aid(s) more if I had the other style of hearing aid.	80	0	10	91
5. The other style of hearing aid would be more comfortable to wear.	70	5	0	54
6. I would be more apt to use two hearing aids if I had the other style of hearing aids.	68	0	4	88
7. The other style of hearing aid would be easier to insert and remove.	58	14	4	68
8. The other style of hearing aid would be more stable.	46	0	0	41
9. The other style of hearing aid is more durable.	41	2	4	23
10. I could understand speech better with the other style of hearing aid.	26	2	0	51
11. The other style of hearing aid has better electronics.	24	7	0	32
12. The other style of hearing aid would have fewer repair problems.	24	0	2	22

*Percent BTE ($n = 52$) and ITE ($n = 43$) users responding in each category for the twelve statements. The "other style" refers to the instrument the patient was *not* fitted with.

suggested by figure 1, as it may be possible to approximate desired gain with an ITE instrument. This is addressed in a later section of the chapter.

Establishing Pass/Fail Criteria

Few audiologists would argue with the notion that the selection of a frequency response that maximizes the patient's ability to understand speech is the goal of nearly all hearing aid fittings. It follows logically, therefore, that speech testing should be part of the custom ITE verification process. It usually is not, however, because it commonly is believed that the variability of clinical speech measures is too great to allow for the detection of small but important changes in the hearing aid's frequency response characteristics. This reported shortcoming of speech audiometry has encouraged audiologists to rely more heavily on prescriptive hearing aid fitting methods. The belief, of course, is that if the prescriptive targets are met, then speech understanding has been maximized, and to attempt to determine empirically if this is true is not necessary.

Computerized probe microphone measures fit nicely into the prescriptive method/custom ITE

verification protocol. This is especially true when fitting high-frequency loss patients, because the masking effect of the hearing aid prevents reliable functional gain measures at frequencies where the patient has normal hearing (see Haskell 1987, for review). Probe microphone measures provide an efficient and reliable method of determining real-ear hearing aid output. The real ear aided response (REAR), or more commonly the real ear insertion response (REIR), can be compared to the prescriptive targets and the goodness of the hearing aid then can be judged. Even after the audiologist has made all possible in-house modifications, however, it is unusual for the REAR or the REIR to meet target for all frequencies of interest. For the high-frequency loss patient, frequently there is too much gain at 1500–2000 Hz and not enough gain at 3000–4000 Hz. The clinician, therefore, must establish what is an acceptable dB deviation from target and what is not (i.e., a pass/fail criterion for the verification process). Presumably the ITE hearing aids that pass are fitted to the patient, and the ones that fail are returned to the manufacturer for alteration of the frequency response, if indeed there is a circuitry that would result in an improved REIR. Obviously, a criterion that is too lax could result in an unacceptable number of patients being fitted with hearing aids that, at least theoretically, are not maximizing speech understanding. On the other hand, a pass/fail standard that is too rigid could result in an unacceptable number of hearing aids being returned to the manufacturer.

Regarding the issue of returning custom ITE hearing aids for the purpose of changing the frequency response, the entire pass/fail verification procedure is based on the assumption that the audiologist is aware of the limitations of ITE circuitry. As mentioned earlier, it is counterproductive to request a change, such as additional gain at 4000 Hz, if the instrument in question already contains the best circuitry available from a given manufacturer to accomplish this goal.

When fitting the patient with a high-frequency loss, there appear to be two different approaches that could be used to establish reasonable dB cutoff values for the REIR/target gain differences. The most ideal, but least practical, approach would be to fail the hearing aid if the deviation from target was great enough to cause a significant decrease in the patient's speech understanding ability. For example, if NAL target gain for a given patient at 2000 Hz was 5 dB, and the real ear insertion gain (REIG) was 15 dB, and if it was known that 10 dB above target would cause a significant decrease in speech understanding, then the hearing aid would fail and be returned to the manufacturer. Whereas in theory this method seems sound, implementation is difficult as the precise dB deviations that begin to cause a reduction in speech understanding are not known. The use of a simplified Articulation Index (AI) procedure, such as that suggested by Mueller and Killion (1990), possibly could help solve this problem. But again, one would have to determine what is the maximum AI possible for a given patient, and then determine what percent below this value would warrant a hearing aid return.

A second approach for establishing an insertion gain pass/fail protocol is to compare the REIG/target gain differences for a given patient to similar measures obtained from a large pool of hearing aid fittings. The hearing aid is judged as good or bad therefore, based on how similar the deviations from target are to previous findings. For example, as in the previous case, if REIG at 2000 Hz was 10 dB above target, but in 70% of similar fittings for high frequency loss patients the deviation from target was greater than 10 dB, then for obvious practical reasons, the hearing aid likely would pass the verification process for that frequency. Until the data or clinical test procedures are available to allow for the implementation of the first mentioned pass/fail procedure, we believe the alternative approach will

provide a reasonable method of maximizing speech understanding for the patient, yet will prevent an unreasonable return rate for custom hearing aids.

To evaluate the relationship between the REIR and desired gain values for individuals with high-frequency hearing loss, we reviewed the REIR findings from 38 custom ITE-IROS hearing aid fittings. All subjects had hearing loss beginning at 3000 Hz, and the mean audiogram is shown in figure 4. The hearing aids were ordered from a major custom hearing aid manufacturer using the National Acoustic Laboratories' (NAL) prescriptive method and correction factors for 2-cm³ coupler (Byrne and Dillon 1986). Two modifications to the Byrne and Dillon NAL procedure were employed when the hearing aids were ordered. First, only 10 dB reserve gain was requested, rather than the 15 dB called for by Byrne and Dillon (1986). And second, using the real ear unaided response (REUR) correction procedure described by Mueller (1989), the requested 2-cm³ coupler gain was altered when the patient's REUR deviated from average (i.e., more 2-cm³ gain was requested at 3000 and 4000 Hz if the patient's REUR was larger than average for these frequencies). This latter modification, in effect, usually did not alter the hearing aid's frequency response, as maximum high-frequency emphasis circuitry was selected by the manufacturer even without the REUR correction. The 38 subjects reviewed here normally were fitted with a 2-cm³ coupler response that peaked at 3000 Hz with a 12 dB/octave slope (Knowles microphone EK 3029).

When evaluating the accuracy of a prescriptive fit, the primary concern is the slope of the REIR rather than the actual REIG at a given frequency (e.g., a REIR that falls 5 dB below target at all frequencies usually is considered a perfect fit). To calculate the appropriateness of the REIR, therefore, it is necessary to match REIG to target at a given frequency so that the slope error can be measured for the other frequencies of interest. For individuals with normal hearing through 2000 Hz, it is most logical to match REIG to target at 3000 Hz, and that is the approach utilized for the present review.

Figure 5 shows the mean NAL target compared to the mean REIR for the 38 subjects. Comparison values are not shown for 500 and 1000 Hz, as these REIG values are very dependent on the skills of the dispenser for conducting in-house ITE modifications. Almost always, the hearing aid can be modified so that little gain is present at 1000 Hz and below, and therefore it is unlikely that a hearing aid would be judged unacceptable based on the REIG findings at these lower frequencies. The mean re-

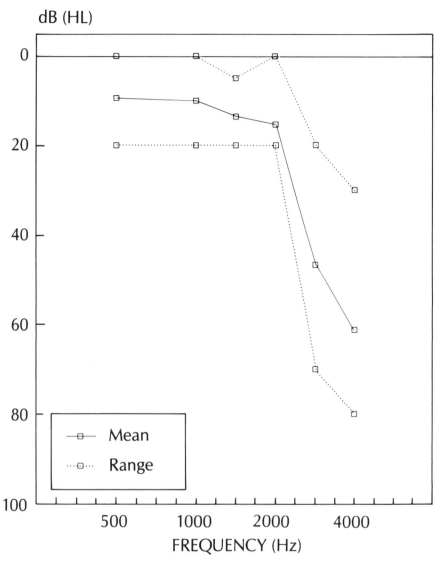

Figure 4. Mean audiometric thresholds and ranges for 38 individuals fitted with ITE-IROS hearing aids.

sults for the higher frequencies show that 3 to 6 dB excess gain was present for 1500 and 2000 Hz, and that mean REIG at 4000 Hz fell 7 dB below target.

For day-to-day clinic practice, individual REIG variations from target are more important than mean data, because this is what determines if the hearing aids meet the predetermined standard. Again, by matching REIG to NAL target gain at 3000 Hz, we calculated individual deviations from target for 1500, 2000, and 4000 Hz. These results are shown in figures 6, 7, and 8. For each frequency, the REIG deviation from target is plotted relative to the amount of NAL target gain. As predicted from the mean REIGs of figure 5, individual deviations usually exceeded target at 1500 and 2000 Hz and were below target at 4000 Hz. Figure 8 also shows the ex-

pected trend that REIG deviation from target at 4000 Hz increases as a function of desired gain. Note that when desired gain was only 15 to 20 dB, the REIG for several subjects was at or near target. When desired gain was 25 dB, REIG values usually fell below target by 10 dB or more.

Some dispensers select an arbitrary dB value as a cutoff for their REIG pass/fail criteria. Figure 9 summarizes the data points of figures 6, 7, and 8, showing percent of REIG deviations from target that were greater than 5 dB. Total deviations are shown, as well as the percent of deviations above and below target. Figure 9 clearly illustrates that 5 dB would be a pass/fail tolerance value that is too small, because 50% of the hearing aids would be rejected based on the REIG findings of 2000 Hz

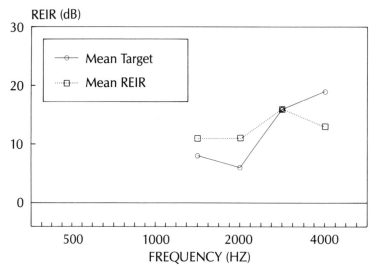

Figure 5. Comparisons of mean NAL prescriptive target and real ear insertion response (REIR) for 38 custom ITE fittings.

alone. While the >5 dB errors at 2000 Hz could be reduced by simply turning down the gain of the hearing aids, this would serve only to increase the >5 dB deviations at 4000 Hz.

As mentioned earlier in this section, one possible way to establish pass/fail criteria is to view the dB deviations that commonly are obtained when a "best case" fitting scenario is used (e.g., careful ordering procedure, conscientious manufacturer using the most appropriate circuitry available). Using this method, it is then possible to calculate percentile REIG deviations for the frequencies of interest. These data for our 38 high frequency fittings are shown in table II. Table II can assist with the practical management of accepting or rejecting the

REIR for a custom hearing aid. For example, if a given clinic decides not to reject more than 5% of their ITE-IROS hearing aids because of too much gain at 2000 Hz, then it will be necessary to use a value as large as 14 dB as the pass/fail criterion. Similarly, table II shows that if an audiologist cannot tolerate deviations from target that are greater than 10 dB at 4000 Hz, probably 20% of the ITE-IROS fittings will be rejected. Importantly, recall that the values shown in table II are for the NAL prescriptive method. If a different prescriptive approach were used, these values would be altered. If the prescription of gain/output (POGO) method (McCandless and Lyregaard 1983) were employed, for example, the 4000 Hz value would be even larger,

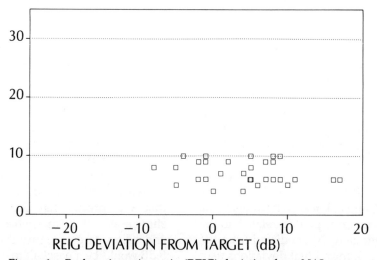

Figure 6. Real ear insertion gain (REIG) deviation from NAL target at 1500 Hz for 38 ITE-IROS fittings. Calculations obtained by matching REIG to NAL target at 3000 Hz.

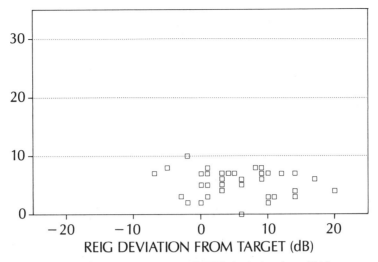

Figure 7. Real ear insertion gain (REIG) deviation from NAL target at 2000 Hz for 38 ITE-IROS fittings. Calculations obtained by matching REIG to NAL target at 3000 Hz.

because the POGO procedure always calls for more gain than the NAL at this frequency.

It must be emphasized that the values shown in table II do not represent our theoretical acceptable tolerances, but only the values that we probably must accept given 1990 custom ITE technology. This is not to suggest that we should be satisfied with falling below our target by 9 dB at 4000 Hz for 30% of our fittings. In this regard, it is encouraging to report that the numbers shown in table II are smaller than our 1989 calculations, and we fully anticipate that these numbers again will be smaller in 1991.

Determining Use Gain

A third consideration when fitting individuals with high-frequency hearing loss is making a reasonable prediction of actual use gain. Assuming that the patient's use gain is within the range of the hearing aid's capabilities, one might believe that a prefitting estimate of use gain is not very critical, because the patient simply will adjust the volume control wheel until a desired setting is obtained. Knowledge of probable use gain, however, can have a significant effect on the decision-making strategies at the time

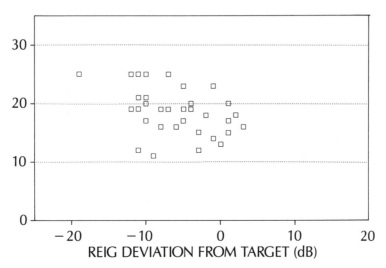

Figure 8. Real ear insertion gain (REIG) deviation from NAL target at 4000 Hz for 38 ITE-IROS fittings. Calculations obtained by matching REIG to NAL target at 3000 Hz.

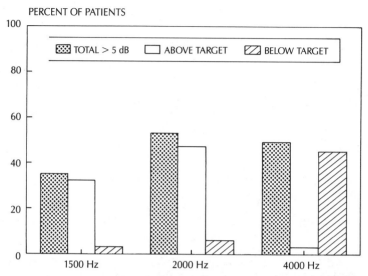

PERCENT OF PATIENTS

TOTAL > 5 dB   ABOVE TARGET   BELOW TARGET

Figure 9.   Percent of 38 patients whose real ear insertion gain (REIG) deviated from NAL target by more than 5 dB. Percent of deviations above and below target also are shown. Calculations obtained by matching REIG to NAL target at 3000 Hz.

of the hearing aid fitting. In fact, this information can dictate whether a hearing aid is accepted or rejected.

If a patient's use gain is below target gain, which seems to be the case for most high-frequency fittings, hearing aids often will be judged more acceptable during the clinical evaluation. For example, if target gain is 20 dB at 3000 Hz and a custom ITE hearing aid begins to produce feedback just as gain approaches this level, some dispensers will return this hearing aid to the manufacturer because of "feedback problems." If, however, this patient's use gain is only 10 dB at 3000 Hz, then there is no feedback problem, and the patient has the desired 10 dB of reserve gain.

As mentioned in the preceding section, use gain also can influence the pass/fail criteria for a prescriptive fitting method. Although use gain does not influence the slope of the REIR, which is

the most important attribute of the prescriptive fit, it does alter the dB error values when target is not achieved, which, at least superficially, makes the fitting more acceptable. For example, as shown in the mean results of figure 5, a common deviation from target in fitting high frequency losses is to obtain too much gain at 1500 and 2000 Hz. If target gain for a given individual is 20 dB at 3000 Hz and 5 dB at 2000 Hz, and the REIG of the hearing aid is equal for 2000 and 3000 Hz, then target at 2000 Hz will be exceeded by 15 dB when desired gain is achieved at 3000 Hz. Some audiologists consider it inappropriate to give a patent 15 dB gain over target, especially for a frequency where the patient has normal hearing. If the patient actually uses less gain at 3000 Hz, such as 10 dB, then the excess gain for the midfrequencies becomes proportionately smaller and is less of a concern.

It has been suggested that some prescriptive methods such as the NAL might call for more gain than necessary for selected hearing loss populations. Lejon et al. (1990), for example, recently reported that the NAL overestimated preferred gain by 5 to 10 dB for a group of elderly subjects fitted monaurally.

Our clinical experience with patients with high-frequency hearing loss has agreed with the work of Lejon et al. (1990), and therefore we recently sought to determine average use gain levels for a group of patients with high-frequency hearing loss. A second purpose of this study was to evaluate two different types of hearing aid circuitry. In the

Table II.   Percentile Deviations from NAL Target*

	Percentile			
	70th	80th	90th	95th
1500 Hz	7 dB	8 dB	10 dB	11 dB
2000 Hz	9 dB	10 dB	12 dB	14 dB
4000 Hz	9 dB	10 dB	11 dB	12 dB

*Amount of deviation from the National Acoustic Laboratories' (NAL) prescriptive target gain that falls within the 70th, 80th, 90th, and 95th percentiles of measured Real Ear Insertion Gain (REIG) for patients with normal hearing through 2000 Hz. REIG was matched to target gain at 3000 Hz.

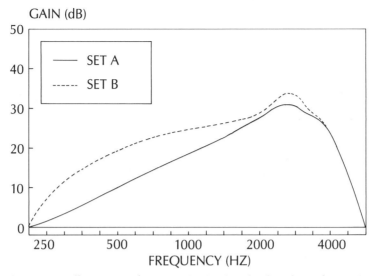

Figure 10.   Illustration of variance in circuitry (re: 2-cm³ coupler gain) used in two different sets of ITE-IROS hearing aids fitted to twelve subjects with high-frequency hearing loss.

past, as described in the preceding section, we have fitted individuals having high-frequency loss with hearing aids utilizing a microphone with a 12 dB/octave slope (Knowles EK 3029). A major manufacturer reported to us that when they were allowed to choose the circuitry, they selected a microphone with a 6 dB/octave slope (Knowles EK 3028) for this type of hearing loss. In the present study, therefore, two sets of custom ITE-IROS hearing aids were built for each subject; one set containing the 12 db/octave slope (Set A), and the other containing the 6 dB/octave slope (Set B). The 2-cm³ coupler responses for the two different hearing aids are shown in figure 10.

Both sets of ITE hearing aids were ordered for twelve subjects, all new hearing aid users with hearing loss beginning at 3000 Hz bilaterally. On the day of fitting, subjects were instructed on the use of the instruments, and then each subject adjusted the hearing aids for desired gain. While all subjects were fitted binaurally, volume control adjustments were made for monaural use. For the use gain adjustment, the subjects listened to continuous discourse of a female talker presented from a loudspeaker at 55 dB SPL one meter from the subject in a mildly reverberant room. Each of the four hearing aids was adjusted separately, and REIR measures were made following each adjustment. Following the initial fitting, the subjects were asked to use the two sets of hearing aids for a six-week period, alternating sets from day-to-day and during different listening situations.

Following the six-week trial of the hearing aids,

each subject returned to the clinic, and monaural use gain REIRs again were measured for each of the four instruments. REIRs also were measured for binaural use gain at this time, and the subject's subjective comparisons of the two different hearing aid sets were obtained.

Figure 11 shows the mean use gain REIRs obtained at the time of the initial fitting for the two different hearing aid sets for the right (top panel) and left (bottom panel) ears of the twelve subjects. This figure clearly shows that although the frequency response of the Set A hearing aids differs substantially from Set B in the 2-cm³ coupler, this difference in gain in the low frequencies is not present in the real ear (recall that these all were IROS fittings). Real ear aided response (REAR) values also were recorded, and as expected, the mean differences between sets also were minimal for this measure.

Although little difference in mean REIRs between the A and B hearing aid sets was observed, we continued to conduct separate measures for the different hearing aids throughout the experiment. Neither the subjects nor the investigators knew which sets were A or B until after the final real ear and subjective responses were obtained.

The relatively low gain shown in the REIRs (see figure 11), suggests that the NAL 3000 Hz prescription, the value used in the preceding section for matching REIG to target, probably is more gain than normally used by individuals with this hearing loss configuration. The mean hearing loss at 3000 Hz for these subjects was 48 dB, and hence, mean use gain for this initial fitting measurement

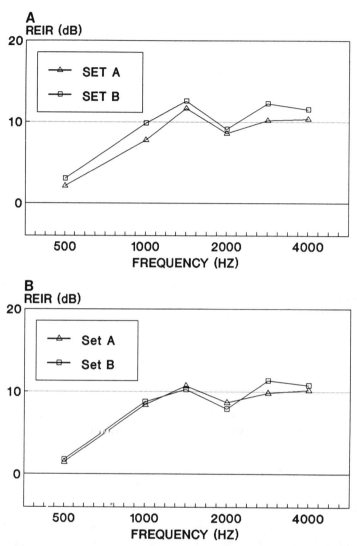

Figure 11.   Mean real ear insertion response (REIR) findings for use gain for the right ear (top panel) and left ear (bottom panel). REIRs shown for hearing aids with different 2-cm³ coupler gain for the low frequencies (see figure 10).

was only about 20% of the hearing loss. It justifiably could be argued that if these subjects had been fitted with the BTE shown in figure 1, they might have chosen to use more gain at 3000 Hz, as the presumably undesired gain in the lower frequencies would not have been present. We do not know, however, if indeed the subjects selected this lower volume control wheel setting because of the gain in the 1500 to 2000 Hz range, or simply because the overall gain across frequencies satisfied their amplification needs. Regardless, patients with this type of hearing loss typically are fitted with ITE instruments, and therefore these use gain values must be considered.

After the six-week trial period, REIR measures were repeated. As before, the subjects adjusted the

hearing aid gain to a comfortable listening level. Shown in figure 12 are the results for both Set A and Set B for the six week postfitting findings compared to the initial REIG measures. Because insertion gain was relatively equal for 1500, 2000, 3000, and 4000 Hz, the values depicted in figure 12 represent an average of these four frequencies. Observe that for both the right and left ears, average use gain decreased by 1 to 3 dB from the initial gain settings. We offer no explanation for the somewhat lower settings for the left ear, as mean audiograms for the right and left ears were essentially identical.

As mentioned, these subjects were all fitted binaurally, and all but one subject reported using both hearing aids whenever hearing aids were

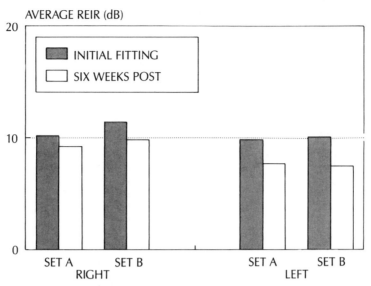

Figure 12. Comparison of mean real ear insertion response (REIR) use gain (average of 1500, 2000, 3000, and 4000 Hz) for the initial hearing aid fitting and six weeks postfitting. REIRs shown for hearing aids with different 2-cm³ coupler gain for the low frequencies (see figure 10).

used. It is important, therefore, also to consider the hearing aid gain settings for binaural use, as all previous measures were conducted for a monaural fitting. The same user adjustment procedure was repeated again, with one exception. For this final measure, the subjects selected their desired listening levels for both hearing aids while fitted binaurally. The results of this measure are shown in figure

13. Note that average use gain values are reduced 1 to 3 dB from the monaural levels. Results for the two different hearing aid sets continued to be very similar.

Even though no difference in REIRs was noted between sets of hearing aids for either individual ears or group data, the subjects were asked to comment on the two sets. The subjects rated their preference

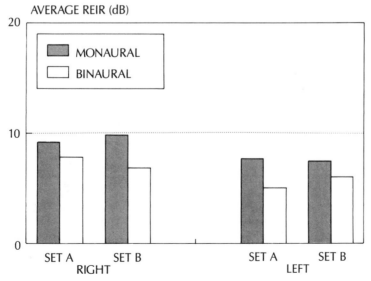

Figure 13. Comparison of mean real ear insertion response (REIR) use gain (average of 1500, 2000, 3000, and 4000 Hz) for monaural and binaural hearing aid use measured six weeks postfitting. REIRs shown for hearing aids with different 2-cm³ coupler gain for the low frequencies (see figure 10).

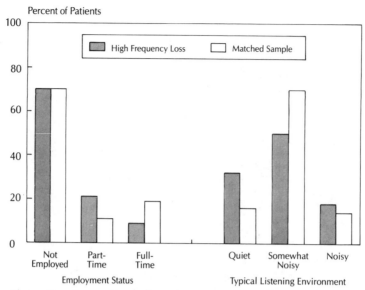

Figure 14. Comparison of employment status and typical listening environment for a group of patients with high-frequency hearing loss and a matched group of patients with significant hearing loss across all frequencies.

for both speech quality and intelligibility for a variety of listening conditions. As might be expected, 10 of the 12 subjects had a clear preference, with the ten votes split evenly between Set A and Set B.

In summary, the results shown in figure 13 suggest that these patients with high-frequency hearing loss use much less gain than is often believed. Average values shown for the binaural fitting REIGs are as low as *5 dB* for the left ear. It is important to point out that 10 of the 12 new hearing aid users were enthusiastic regarding hearing aid use, and stated that the use of hearing aids had significantly improved their communication ability. This finding leads us to our final area of consideration: verification of the hearing aid fitting.

Verification of Hearing Aid Fitting

As with all types of hearing aid fittings, some type of verification process other than probe microphone measures must be implemented with patients having high-frequency loss to assure that they indeed are successful hearing aid users. As we review the preceding section of this chapter, and relate these findings to a typical dispensing practice, consider that we first might sacrifice the best BTE REIR because the patient wants a small ITE instrument. Next, we see that practical factors force us to use a

window of tolerance of 10 dB or more for our NAL targets. And finally, we discover that these patients having high-frequency loss may not be using more than 5 to 8 dB of gain. Are these really successful hearing aid fittings?

We recently compared the use of, benefit of, and satisfaction with hearing aids for a group of patients with high-frequency loss to a group of patients with mild-to-moderate hearing loss across all frequencies. As before, the patients with high-frequency loss all had normal hearing bilaterally through 2000 Hz and were fitted binaurally with ITE-IROS hearing aids. These individuals were fitted with the same style of ITE hearing aids as discussed earlier in this chapter, and therefore deviations from target similar to those shown in figures 6, 7, and 8 were present. The comparison group had gradually downward-sloping audiometric configurations, with hearing loss at 500 Hz of 25–40 dB (mean PTA of 44 dB). This group also was fitted binaurally with ITE hearing aids having either small or medium vents.

Fifty subjects from each hearing loss group were selected randomly from our clinical database of patients who had been fitted with their first hearing aids 6 to 8 months prior to the time of the survey. Only individuals retired from the military were used as subjects. This resulted in a close match in age and employment status between the two hearing loss groups (mean age of 67 years for the high-

TOTAL HEARING AID USE

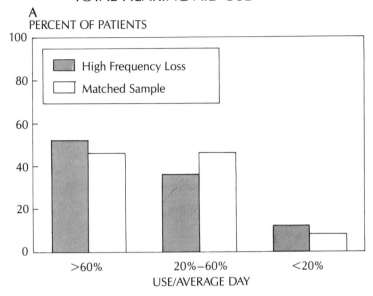

BINAURAL HEARING AID USE

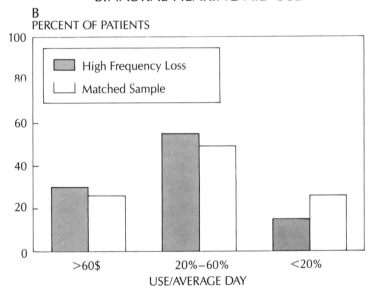

Figure 15. Comparison of hearing aid use/average day for a group of patients with high-frequency loss and a matched group of patients with significant hearing loss across all frequencies. Distribution shown for the use of at least one hearing aid (total use: A) and the use of two hearing aids (binaural use: B).

frequency loss group, 68 years for the matched sample). A ten-question questionnaire was mailed to the 50 subjects in each group. The first 35 replies from each group were used for the analysis that follows.

Because all the subjects were retired military servicemen, we expected close agreement between their employment status and typical listening envi-

ronment, two factors besides age that easily could affect use, benefit, and satisfaction ratings. Figure 14 confirms that the two groups were very similar in their employment status (e.g., 70% not employed) and average listening environment. It should be noted that motivation to obtain amplification was not a major factor for either group. The subjects all received their hearing aids free of charge as an en-

HEARING AID BENEFIT

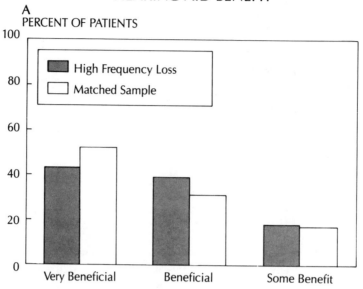

HEARING AID SATISFACTION

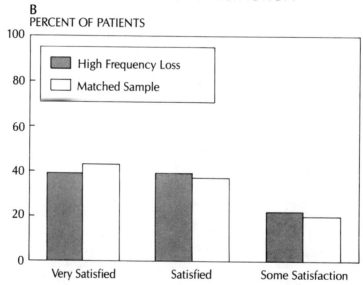

Figure 16. Comparison of successful hearing aid use for a group of patients with high-frequency loss and a matched group of patients with significant hearing loss across all frequencies. Distribution shown for benefit (A) and satisfaction (B) ratings.

titlement for military service. The majority of the patients reported for their hearing aid evaluation because an audiologist told them that they needed hearing aids. The direction from the audiologist was the same whether the hearing loss began at 500 or 3000 Hz.

The data shown in figure 14 suggest that we had perhaps achieved our goal of comparing two groups of subjects whose only major difference was their degree of hearing loss in the low and midfrequencies. If true, then the results of the subsequent

use, benefit, and satisfaction ratings take on added meaning.

The subjects reported percent of hearing aid use per average day for the use of at least one hearing aid (total use) and the use of binaural hearing aids. Mean use values for both conditions revealed no significant differences between groups, and distributions for total use (top panel) and binaural use (bottom panel) are shown in figure 15. Note that 45 to 50% of the subjects report using at least one hearing aid for more than 60% of their average day, and

25 to 30% report daily use of binaural amplification for this amount of time. Most important, however, is that a nearly identical hearing aid use distribution was obtained for each group.

The questionnaire contained six questions relating to benefit or satisfaction, which were rated on a scale of 1 to 5 (5.0 = most positive rating). The responses to the questions were then averaged to obtain a mean rating for each subject for both benefit and satisfaction (e.g., 4.7–5.0 = very satisfied, 3.7–4.3 = satisfied, 3.3 and below = some satisfaction). The distribution of these findings for benefit (top panel) and satisfaction (bottom panel) are shown in figure 16. No averaged score fell below 2.7 for any subject, and therefore "little" and "no" benefit/satisfaction ratings do not appear on the charts.

Consistent with the results relating to hearing aid use, the most notable finding of the benefit/satisfaction ratings was that the two different hearing loss groups reported almost identical success with hearing aids. Because these subjects received their hearing aids free of charge, it is possible, of course, that they might have inflated the ratings shown in both figures 15 and 16. But, even if this is true, there would be little reason to believe that one hearing loss group would inflate their ratings more than the other, and therefore the relative similarity of the ratings maintains its significance.

Verification of the hearing aid selection process often is difficult to quantify. Obviously, we would like to see all ratings in the very beneficial and very satisfied category. For the purposes of this chapter, however, it is most important to focus on the conclusion that the high-frequency loss patients reported the same hearing aid use, benefit, and satisfaction as those individuals with a 25 to 40 dB hearing loss in the low and midfrequencies. This finding was in spite of (or maybe *because of*) the fact that these individuals were fitted with a REIR slope that differed significantly from what would be called for by most prescriptive fitting approaches.

Summary

Our amplification strategies have changed significantly in recent years regarding the patient with high-frequency hearing loss. Today, most would agree that the individual with hearing loss beginning at 2000 Hz is a good candidate for hearing aids, and few audiologists would fit hearing aids to patients with hearing loss beginning at 4000 Hz. Mixed opinions, however, usually are voiced concerning the patient with hearing loss beginning at 3000 Hz, and therefore this chapter has focused on this hearing loss population.

We have discussed the insertion gain/prescriptive target trade-offs that sometimes must be made as the dispenser attempts to accommodate the patient's choice of hearing aid style. Clearly, if we choose to fit these individuals with ITE instruments, the data suggest that we can expect to observe relatively large deviations from prescriptive target gain. Prescriptive target, however, must be viewed carefully, as indicated by the use gain results reported here.

The final section of this chapter presents data that to some, might be somewhat surprising. When we compared a group of older individuals with hearing loss beginning at 3000 Hz to a matched group of hearing aid users with hearing loss beginning at 500 Hz, there was no difference in reported hearing aid use, benefit, or satisfaction. These results suggest that these patients with high-frequency loss are not "marginal candidates," as they often are told, but rather are just as likely to be successful hearing aid users as their counterparts with significantly more hearing loss. This good news needs to be relayed to the patients, and also to the professionals who advise them.

References

Byrne, D., and Dillon, H. 1986. The National Acoustic Laboratories' (NAL) new procedure for selecting the gain and frequency response of a hearing aid. *Ear and Hearing* 7(4):257–65.

Grossman, F.M. 1943. Acoustic sound filtration and hearing aids. *Archives of Otolaryngology* 38:101–112.

Grossman, F.M., and Molloy, C.T. 1944. Acoustic sound filtration and hearing aids. *Journal of the Acoustical Society of America* 16:52–59.

Harford, E., and Barry, J. 1965. A rehabilitative approach to the problem of unilateral hearing impairment: The contralateral routing of signals (CROS). *Journal of Speech and Hearing Disorders* 30:121–138.

Harford, E., and Dodds, E. 1966. The clinical application of CROS. *Archives of Otolaryngology* 83:455–64.

Haskell, G. 1987. Functional gain. *Ear and Hearing* 8(5): 95S–99S.

Jetty, A.J., and Rintelmann, W.F. 1970. Acoustic coupler effects on speech audiometric scores using a CROS hearing aid. *Journal of Speech and Hearing Research* 13(1): 101–113.

Leijon, A., Lindkvist, A., Ringdahl, A., and Israelsson, B. 1990. Preferred hearing aid gain in everyday use after prescriptive fitting. *Ear and Hearing* 11(4):299–305.

McCandless, G., and Lyregaard, P. 1983. Prescription of gain/output (POGO) for hearing aids. *Hearing Instruments* 34(1):16–21.

Mueller, H.G. 1989. Individualizing the ordering of custom hearing instruments. *Hearing Instruments* 40(2): 18–22.

Mueller, H.G., and Budinger, A.C., 1990. Selection of hearing aid style. *Reports in Hearing Instrumentation and Technology* 2(1):5–10.

Mueller, H.G., and Killion, M.C. 1990. An easy method for calculating the articulation index. *Hearing Journal* 43(9):14–17.

Schier, M.B. 1941. The earpiece-in testing for and fitting hearing aids. *Laryngoscope* 51:52–60.

Surr, R., and Hawkins, D.B. 1988. New hearing aid users' perception of the "hearing aid effect." *Ear and Hearing* 9(3):113–18.

CHAPTER 24

Hearing Aid Bandwidth for Sloping, High-Frequency Losses

Jean A. Sullivan, Cathy A. Allsman, and Lars B. Nielsen

Hearing scientists, engineers, and hearing aid manufacturers focused much of their research and development efforts of the past two decades on increasing hearing aid bandwidth. The products of these efforts are new hearing aid transducers, new acoustic coupling materials and techniques, and new sound measuring instruments. As hearing aid bandwidth has increased, the need to examine the relationship between bandwidth and listener performance has become apparent. An issue of particular interest is the identification of candidates for these new aids. Not surprisingly, listeners with hearing loss limited to 1000 Hz and higher frequencies have been primary candidates. The hearing aids of the 1950s and 1960s were not appropriate for these patients because they amplified primarily at the frequencies of normal hearing sensitivity. Today, hearing aids can deliver significant acoustic gain at the higher frequencies where the majority of hearing-impaired listeners have the greatest hearing loss: 2000 to 5000 Hz. The important question now is whether this type of amplification is useful to the population of impaired listeners with high-frequency losses.

This chapter briefly discusses studies in the past two decades that explored the effects of signal bandwidth and high-frequency gain on speech recognition and on sound quality for listeners with hearing loss above 1000 Hz. In addition, this chapter describes experiments in our laboratory with a subgroup of these listeners who are distinguished by the severity of their hearing loss at 2000 Hz and higher frequencies. We conclude with suggestions for future research and a discussion of the implications for clinical practices of hearing aid fitting.

This work was supported by the Margaret W. and Herbert Hoover, Jr. Foundation. The authors acknowledge the contributions of the following House Ear Institute employees: Diane Knudsen, J. Phil Mobley, Sigfrid D. Soli, and Janet Stoeckert.

Bandwidth Effects

Effects on Speech Recognition and Judgments of Speech Intelligibility

One of the first questions a potential hearing aid user asks is whether the proposed aid will improve speech understanding. Methods that were common to all of the experiments carried out over the past two decades that are included in this chapter (Barfod, Christensen, and Pedersen 1971; Lippmann, Braida, and Durlach 1981; Murray and Byrne 1986; Rankovic 1989; Skinner 1980; Sullivan et al. 1990) may be important to clinical practice but may require modification for clinical situations because of practical considerations. All researchers used subjects with normal hearing at 250 and 500 Hz and hearing loss beginning at either 1000 Hz or 2000 Hz. All data were collected in laboratories, and all of the studies used laboratory equipment rather than commercial hearing aid components to manipulate bandwidth. Signals were delivered to the sound-field or headphones rather than through hearing aid transducers. All but one study evaluated a linear amplification system.

A consistent finding of these studies was that speech recognition scores improved as audible bandwidth increased, particularly when tests were administered in noise. Four studies showed that listeners with high-frequency hearing loss obtain better speech recognition scores with high-frequency gain than with uniform gain, regardless of the amount of uniform gain (Barfod, Christensen, and Pedersen 1971; Lippmann, Braida, and Durlach 1981; Skinner 1980; Sullivan et al. 1990). This result is presumably because only the high-frequency emphasis aid amplifies high-frequency speech energy to audible levels. For example, Lippmann and his colleagues (1981) indicated that speech energy above

287

2000 Hz was inaudible to their subjects with high-frequency loss with the uniform frequency response and that most speech energy was audible to at least 4000 Hz with high-frequency emphasis. In other words, the upper cutoff frequency of the audible signal increased from 2000 to 4000 Hz. Percentage correct scores for sentences improved 29 points with the wider bandwidth.

Our work with steeply sloping hearing loss was motivated by a colleague with this type of hearing loss who had not found a hearing aid that improved his speech understanding. His hearing thresholds are normal at 250 and 500 Hz and severe at 2000 Hz and higher frequencies. Few subjects in past studies had such severe hearing loss at 2000 Hz. Indeed, few hearing aid users have this type of hearing loss: only about 3% of the patients referred for hearing aid evaluations at our clinical affiliate, The House Ear Clinic, fit this description.

We have found that the hearing aids of many listeners with severe high-frequency loss do not provide enough gain to achieve audibility, despite research demonstrating the advantages of amplifying high-frequency speech energy to audible levels. We measured the insertion gain of the personal aids of five people with high-frequency loss. All personal aids provided less gain at use gain settings than would be specified by the National Acoustics Laboratories (NAL) prescription method. Figure 1 illustrates the effect of insertion gain on the relationship between thresholds and amplified speech levels for one subject whose hearing aid gave the best match to the NAL prescription. Note that high-frequency components of speech are below threshold for this subject. A similar pattern was observed for the other four subjects.

There are two possible reasons these aids had insufficient high-frequency gain. First, technical difficulties such as hearing aid bandwidth limitations and feedback may have prevented the desired high-frequency gain. Second, aids fitted with no technical problems or with solutions to technical problems to achieve adequate high-frequency amplification still did not benefit the patient. Because we felt that it is important to know whether the prescribed amplification would be useful, we explored the second alternative.

Figure 2 shows means and standard deviations for hearing levels on the test ears of 17 men who participated in our first study. All subjects had acquired hearing loss with a history of military or occupational noise exposure. Thirteen subjects wore hearing aids: eleven binaurally and two monaurally.

The first experiment examined the effects

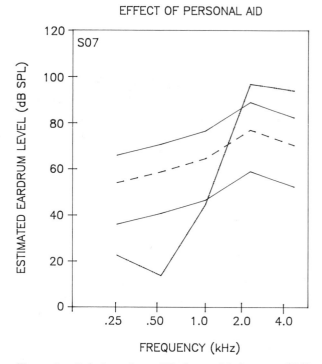

Figure 1. Relation of amplified one-third octave RMS sound pressure levels of speech to hearing thresholds. The dot-dashed line shows the estimated eardrum sound pressure levels associated with threshold. The dashed line shows the estimated eardrum sound pressure levels of the average spectrum of a male voice at a normal vocal effort (Pearsons, Bennett, and Fidell 1976) after amplification by the subject's personal hearing aid. The solid lines denote normal distributions of level within the one-third octave bands.

of bandwidth on speech recognition and ratings of speech intelligibility. A digital master hearing aid created the test frequency responses and headphones were used as the transducer (see Nielsen 1989, for a detailed description of the master aid). Four frequency responses were tested: a flat response and three shaped responses. The flat response had a bandwidth of 6000 Hz and uniform gain as a function of frequency. The shaped responses were the low cutoff response (LCO), the mid-cutoff response (MCO), and the high cutoff response (HCO); bandwidths were 710 Hz, 1798 kHz, and 6000 Hz, respectively. For the shaped responses, we prescribed the coupler gains to amplify one-third octave bands of our test speech signals to sound pressure levels associated with comfortable loudness. Figure 3 shows the relationship between thresholds, amplified speech levels, and loudness discomfort levels for one subject. The appendix to this chapter describes the procedures for measuring and specifying the illustrated signals.

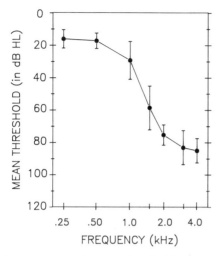

Figure 2. Mean headphone thresholds and standard deviations of the 17 subjects of experiment 1.

Each frequency response was evaluated at three overall coupler gain settings: the prescribed gain (PG) setting, the prescribed gain minus 10 dB (PG −10) setting, and the prescribed gain plus 10 dB (PG +10) setting. The speech recognition test was the City University of New York Nonsense Syl-

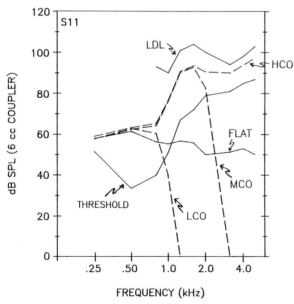

Figure 3. Relation of the 1% cumulative levels of continuous discourse to hearing thresholds and loudness discomfort levels of one subject. Solid lines show hearing thresholds and loudness discomfort levels. The dashed lines and dot-dashed line indicate the 1% cumulative levels of speech in one-third octave bands for the subject's frequency responses at his prescribed gain settings (see Appendix). The upper cutoff frequencies for the FLAT, LCO, MCO, and HCO conditions were 6000, 710, 1798, and 6000 Hz, respectively.

lable Test (NST) (Resnick et al. 1975). A 25-second recording of continuous discourse spoken by the same talker of the NST was used to obtain speech ratings. The calibration signals of the speech materials were presented to the digital master hearing aid at a voltage that produced 65 dB SPL in the coupler when the aid was set to its reference calibration configuration (i.e., 0 dB gain). For each subject, the coupler sound pressure level varied as a function of the combined effects of the prescribed frequency response and the gain setting condition.

Figure 4 presents the mean NST scores for the test conditions. Results indicated that as the bandwidth increased from 710 Hz to 6000 Hz, performance improved. As expected, performance differed significantly with changes in gain setting: as gain increased from the PG −10 setting to the PG +10 setting, performance improved. (We were not able to collect data for 16 of the 17 subjects at the PG +10 setting for the HCO condition due to loudness intolerance.) Statistical analyses indicated a significant bandwidth effect ($p<.001$) and a significant overall gain effect ($p<.001$).

Figure 4 also shows mean intelligibility ratings. Ratings ranged from five (every word understood) to one (no words understood). With the exception of the HCO response, the rank order of hearing aid performance from best to worst was the same for the rating task and the NST: MCO, FLAT, and HCO. Note that the intelligibility ratings were near maximum, although speech recognition scores were only fair. Differences among the bandwidth conditions were significant only at the PG −10 setting ($p<.01$).

A second experiment was conducted to examine the effects of the experimental frequency responses on the NST administered with competing noise. Ten subjects participated: 9 of the 17 in experiment 1 and a tenth subject who met the hearing loss criteria.

We evaluated the two-test frequency responses that gave superior performance in experiment 1: MCO and HCO. Each was tested at the signal level corresponding to maximum performance in experiment 1 and at a comfortable listening level. Speech signals were mixed with cafeteria noise at signal-to-noise ratios of +7 dB and +12 dB.

Figure 4 also shows the mean NST scores and intelligibility ratings in this experiment. For comparison of the results in quiet and in noise, the quiet test results of experiment 1 are shown for the nine subjects who participated in both experiments. Although the two responses yielded similar mean NST scores in quiet, mean scores differed for tests

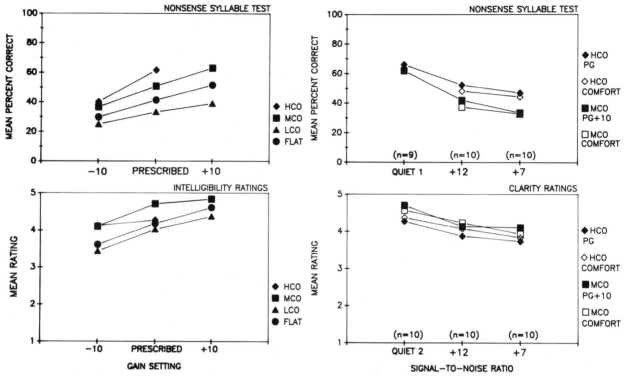

Figure 4.   Mean NST scores and mean intelligibility ratings by frequency response condition. The left side of the figure shows the results of tests conducted in quiet for the 17 subjects of experiment 1. The right side of the figure shows the results of tests conducted in noise for the 10 subjects of experiment 2

in noise. Recognition was significantly higher for the HCO response than for the MCO response ($p<.001$). As expected, noise had a significant effect on recognition performance: scores were significantly poorer in the more adverse listening condition, +7 dB S/N. Gain setting did not have a significant effect on performance. The pattern of results for the intelligibility ratings was essentially the same as the NST results; ratings were higher for the HCO response than for the MCO response. However, we found no significant effects of bandwidth, overall gain, or noise.

The results of the two experiments demonstrate that subjects with severe loss at 2000 Hz, like listeners with less severe loss at this frequency, experience improved speech recognition with the addition of spectral information above 2000 Hz. If improved speech recognition is the primary goal of the hearing aid fitting, it is important to amplify high-frequency signals to audible levels for these listeners.

Given evidence that large changes in upper cutoff frequency (2000 to 6000 Hz) improve speech recognition, the next issue is the effect of smaller changes within the high-frequency region. Is the widest possible bandwidth always desirable for subjects whose hearing loss is restricted to frequencies above 1000 Hz? This is an important question because additional clinical time is often needed to ensure that the hearing aid provides adequate high-frequency gain. The high frequencies are susceptible to probe measurement error (Dirks and Kincaid 1987; Hawkins 1987) and are affected greatly by acoustic coupling methods (Lybarger 1985). Both factors increase the probability that the desired high-frequency gain will not be achieved.

To our knowledge, Murray and Byrne (1986) conducted the only published study to examine the effect of several cutoff frequencies above 1000 Hz. The experimental conditions were four frequency responses shaped according to the procedure of the NAL (Byrne and Dillon 1986) and with upper cutoff frequencies of 1500, 2500, 3500, and 4500 Hz. Subjects judged the intelligibility and pleasantness of the conditions in pairwise comparisons. In addition, they adjusted the ratio between the test speech and test noise for each frequency response condition until 50% of the speech was judged intelligible. Improvements in performance on both measures with increased bandwidth were observed for normal-hearing listeners, while few significant effects were found for the hearing-impaired subjects for bandwidths greater than 2500 Hz. Unfortunately, the authors did not report whether the high frequency signals were audible for all subjects in the widest bandwidth condition. Comfortable listening levels chosen by subjects may have been too low to

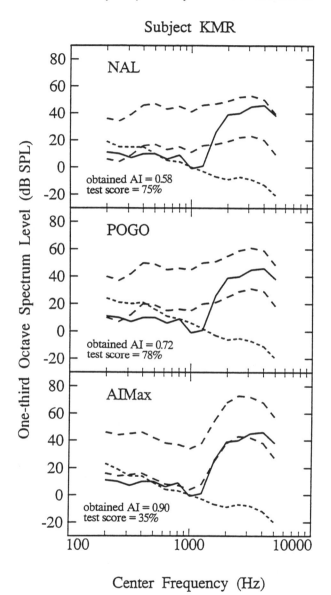

Figure 5. Amplified speech spectra of the three hearing aids conditions for one subject of the Rankovic (1989) study. The solid line indicates thresholds represented in dB SPL spectrum level, the dashed lines indicate the estimated level distribution of the amplified test stimuli, and the short dashed lines indicate the equipment noise floor. Articulation indices are shown in relation to actual test scores for the three hearing aid conditions: POGO, NAL, and AIMax. From "An Application of the Articulation Index to Hearing Aid Fitting" by C.M. Rankovic, in press, *Journal of Speech and Hearing Research, 34.* Copyright 1991 by the American Speech-Language-Hearing Association. Reprinted with permission.

ensure audibility of the signal in the high frequencies. In this case, subjects would not have been able to detect differences in the experimental conditions. Additional information about the sensation levels of signals in different frequency regions for the test conditions would enhance the interpretation of these research findings.

The shape of the widened frequency response and the magnitude of high-frequency gain also appear to be related to recognition performance. Skinner (1980) found that increasing high-frequency gain to more than 20 dB above the low-frequency gain caused a decrement in performance for some listeners. She speculated that spectral balance is necessary to maintain optimum recognition performance.

Rankovic (1989) reported that maximizing the audibility of speech within the widest bandwidth does not improve speech recognition for all listeners. She evaluated speech recognition for frequency responses prescribed by the NAL procedure, the prescription of gain/output (POGO) procedure (McCandless and Lyregaard 1983), and for a frequency response that attempted to maximize the Articulation Index. The important difference among the conditions was the proportion of audible high-frequency speech energy. For the majority of the subjects, speech recognition increased as the proportion of high-frequency energy increased. However, the subjects with sloping high-frequency hearing loss obtained a decrement in performance with the condition that gave the greatest high-frequency gain.

Figure 5 shows the amplified spectra of the three experimental hearing aid conditions for one subject with steeply sloping hearing loss. Note that the subject obtained a substantially lower score with the hearing aid with the highest speech sensation levels in the high frequencies.

The experimental results discussed in this section indicate that speech recognition performance of listeners with high-frequency hearing loss improves as the audible bandwidth increases above 2000 Hz. In contrast, increasing the audible bandwidth does not always appear to improve subjective judgments of speech intelligibility.

Effects on Sound Quality

At the first Vanderbilt Hearing Aid conference, Killion (1982) argued that researchers should shift emphasis from the effects of hearing aids on speech discrimination to the effects on sound quality. He pointed out the importance of knowing whether the goal of maximizing speech understanding was compatible with the goal of achieving good sound quality. Of the six cited studies on speech recognition with high-frequency amplification, two did not measure impressions of sound quality, one study reported subjects' descriptions of the sound quality of the experimental aids, and only three studies obtained a direct measure of sound quality. The results indicate that extending the bandwidth of a hearing aid causes either no change or a decrement in the sound quality for listeners with hearing loss restricted to the high frequencies.

This result is disturbing for two reasons. First, it appears to be a unique characteristic of sloping hearing losses, and perhaps of hearing loss in general, because normal-hearing listeners (Murray and Byrne 1986; Killion 1982) realize improvements in sound quality as bandwidth increases. Second, there seems to be a trade-off between speech intelligibility and sound quality for listeners with sloping loss: the response that gives the best speech understanding may not give the best sound quality.

Studies in our laboratories clearly show the negative association between speech recognition and sound quality. In addition to rating speech intelligibility, the subjects rated the sound quality of the hearing-aid-processed continuous discourse presented in quiet and in noise. Figure 6 shows the mean quality ratings of experiments 1 and 2. Quality ratings ranged from five (excellent) to one (poor sound quality). Ratings of speech in quiet increased as cutoff frequency increased from 710 to 2000 Hz, but decreased as it increased from 2000 Hz to 6000 Hz. The HCO response was rated poorest of all responses. Differences among the responses for the quality ratings were significant at the PG −10 and the PG settings ($p<.001$). The pattern of results was the same for ratings of the hearing aids tested in noise: HCO was rated poorer then MCO. However, this difference was not statistically significant.

Given the apparent conflict between the optimum bandwidth for speech understanding and the optimum bandwidth for sound quality, it is important to examine the reasons for poor quality ratings. Electroacoustic characteristics of the hearing aids, other than frequency response, may have contributed to perceptions of sound quality in the cited studies. Nonlinear distortion and internal noise are often present in hearing aids with high gain levels. Yet, none of the studies reported these characteristics for their experimental hearing aids. More comprehensive electroacoustic measurements and extensive ratings of the perceptual dimensions of sound quality might help identify the acoustic pa-

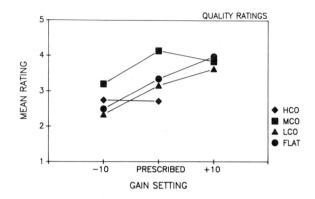

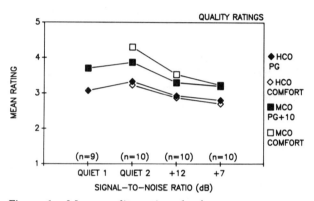

Figure 6. Mean quality ratings by frequency response condition. The upper box shows the results of tests conducted in quiet for the 17 subjects of experiment 1 and the lower box show the results of tests conducted in noise for the 10 subjects of experiment 2.

rameters that contribute to overall judgments. Poor ratings of sound quality may also be the result of listening to high-frequency signals at excessive sound pressure levels. In this case, technical improvements would not improve sound quality.

Summary

Future Research Needs

A hearing aid with the widest possible bandwidth may not always be superior to a hearing aid with a narrower bandwidth for listeners with hearing loss limited to frequencies above 1000 Hz. Before these listeners are rejected as candidates for wideband hearing aids, we need to know if we can reduce the discrepancy between speech recognition performance and judgments of sound quality. In particular, can sound quality be improved by signal processing techniques or by more appropriate fitting algorithms? For example, signal distortion could be reduced with compression in the high frequencies, thereby resulting in improved sound quality. In addition, it is important to know whether laboratory tests of speech recognition and sound quality predict benefit in actual use conditions, both when the patient first tries the aid and after the patient has worn the aid for several months.

Clinical Implications

Research data so far are insufficient to formulate firm rules for prescribing the bandwidth or other hearing aid characteristics for listeners with hearing loss above 1000 Hz. Findings of previous research can be used to develop a fitting approach.

Research findings reveal that, for maximum speech recognition, a wideband, high-frequency hearing aid should be considered for patients with high-frequency hearing loss, even for patients with severe hearing loss at 2000 Hz. However, the amount of gain in the high frequencies should be carefully selected. For reasons still not known, performance will be affected by the shape of the gain contour.

It is premature to recommend the exact upper cutoff frequency above 2000 Hz. The data of Murray and Byrne (1986) indicate flexibility in choosing a cutoff frequency; some listeners might not benefit from the widest possible frequency response.

Regardless of the hearing aid bandwidth, speech recognition will not always be restored to normal performance levels. Furthermore, the listener may not perceive overall improvements in speech understanding, as shown in the Sullivan et al. (1990) study. This result is not surprising given the redundancy of the continuous speech used to rate intelligibility. Yet the clinician, when counseling patients, should specify possible improvements. For example, our subjects recognized a greater number of fricatives and affricates with amplification above 2000 Hz than with amplification only below 2000 Hz. Once these improvements are noted, the patient can determine their importance.

Negative impressions of the sound quality from a hearing aid should be expected for some listeners with a high-frequency-emphasis hearing aid. Nevertheless, this problem should not discourage the clinician from considering such high-frequency amplification. The research results to date do not identify the cause of poor quality ratings. If internal hearing aid noise or nonlinear distortions are the cause of poor quality, they are likely to vary with the gain requirements of individual

patients and specific characteristics of individual hearing aids. Therefore, not all listeners will experience poor sound quality. In cases in which sound quality cannot be improved, a hearing aid with user control of two frequency responses might be indicated. The listener could use the wideband response in noisy environments for optimum speech recognition and a narrower response in quiet environments for good sound quality.

Given the uncertainty of achieving a frequency response that will provide both the desired speech recognition performance and acceptable sound quality, flexibility is important when working with a patient with hearing loss restricted to the high frequencies. Because more time might be required to meet the needs of these patients, they might be classified as difficult-to-fit for several years to come. We hope, however, that the number of clinical studies with this population will increase. The new programmable hearing aids could be a useful tool for such studies. Because their characteristics can be adjusted in seconds, the clinician can easily test the patient with several bandwidths at both the initial evaluation and over time. Clinical studies will contribute to a better understanding of the relationship between speech recognition and sound quality with high-frequency-emphasis hearing aids.

Appendix

All signals in the Sullivan et al. 1990 study were specified with reference to the 6-cm³ coupler. Thresholds, most comfortable listening levels, and uncomfortable listening levels were obtained for one-sixth octave narrowbands of noise. The digital master hearing aid (DMHA) was set to produce a flat response in the coupler, and the noise stimuli were input to the DMHA at a constant voltage. The signal level was varied for a particular measurement (e.g., threshold) by adjusting the programmable attenuator of the DMHA. Figure 3 shows for one subject, the corresponding coupler sound pressure levels of the noise bands at threshold and loudness discomfort.

The speech values shown in figure 3 correspond to the 1% cumulative levels of speech for the talker of the test materials. For these measurements, the frequency response of the DMHA was set for the four test conditions: FLAT, LCO, MCO, and HCO. The calibration signal of the continuous discourse sample was input at a constant voltage and the overall gain of the aid was adjusted so that the signal in the coupler was equal to 65 dB plus the prescribed system gain for the subject at that frequency. A General Radio 1955 Integrating Real-Time Analyzer was used to measure the one-third octave band sound pressure levels. The analyzer has an RMS detector with a 125 ms averaging time. The distribution of levels in each band was analyzed statistically to identify the 1% cumulative level (i.e., the level exceeded by 1% of the samples). We plotted each of eight band levels analyzed at their center frequencies: 800, 1000, 1250, 1600, 2000, 3150, 4000, and 5000 Hz.

References

Barfod, J., Christensen, ATh., and Pedersen, O.J. 1971. Design of hearing aid frequency response for maximum speech intelligibility of patients with high-tone loss. *Scandinavian Audiology* Supplement 1:54–60.

Byrne, D., and Dillon, H. 1986. The National Acoustics Laboratories' (NAL) new procedure for selecting the gain and frequency response of a hearing aid. *Ear and Hearing* 7:257–265.

Dirks, D.D., and Kincaid, G.E. 1987. Basic acoustic considerations of ear canal probe measurements. *Ear and Hearing* 8:605–75.

Hawkins, D. 1987. Clinical ear canal probe tube measurements. *Ear and Hearing* 8:745–815.

Killion, M.C. 1982. Transducers, earmolds and sound quality considerations. In *The Vanderbilt Hearing-Aid Report: State of the Art-Research Needs*, eds. G.A. Studebaker and F.H. Bess. Upper Darby: Monographs in Contemporary Audiology.

Lippmann, R.P., Braida, L.D., and Durlach, N.I. 1981. Study of multichannel amplitude compression and linear amplification for persons with sensorineural hearing loss. *Journal of the Acoustical Society of America* 69:524–34.

Lybarger, S.F. 1985. Earmolds. In *Handbook of Clinical Audiology*, ed. J. Katz. Baltimore: Williams and Wilkins.

McCandless, G.A., and Lyregaard, P.E. 1983. Prescription of gain/output (POGO) for hearing aids. *Hearing Instruments* 34:16–21.

Murray, N., and Byrne, D. 1986. Performance of hearing-impaired and normal hearing listeners with various high frequency cut-offs in hearing aids. *Australian Journal of Audiology* 8:21–28.

Nielsen, L.B. 1989. A computer controlled digital master hearing aid. *Proceedings of the International Symposium of Circuits and Systems*. Piscataway, NJ: IEEE 1291–1294.

Pearsons, K.S., Bennett, R.L., and Fidell, S. 1976. Speech levels in various environments. Prepared for Office of Resources and Development, Environmental Protection Agency. *Bolt Beranek and Newman Inc. Report No. 3281*.

Rankovic, C.M. 1989. An application of the articulation index to hearing aid fitting. Ph.D. diss., University of Minnesota, Minneapolis.

Resnick, S.B., Dubno, J.R., Hoffnung, S., and Levitt H. 1975. Phoneme errors on a nonsense syllable test. *Journal of the Acoustical Society of America* 58(Suppl. 1):114.

Skinner, M.W. 1980. Speech intelligibility in noise-induced hearing loss: Effects of high-frequency compensation. *Journal of the Acoustical Society of America* 67:306 17.

Sullivan, J.A., Allsman, C.S., Nielsen, L.B., and Mobley, J.P. 1990. Amplification for listeners with steeply sloping, high-frequency hearing loss. Paper read at Annual Convention of the American Speech-Language-Hearing Association, November 1990, St. Louis.

CHAPTER 25

Modified Hearing Aid Selection Procedures for Severe/Profound Hearing Losses

Denis Byrne, Aaron Parkinson, and Philip Newall

There are many hearing aid selection procedures, some of which are supported by a considerable body of research. Most such research has considered mainly the amplification needs of mildly and moderately hearing-impaired persons. However, there are reasons to believe that the principles that apply to the moderately hearing-impaired population may need to be varied for at least *some* of those who are severely and profoundly hearing impaired. One reason concerns the frequency range of available hearing. In most procedures there is an assumption, explicit or otherwise, that it is desirable to provide an audible signal over a wide frequency range and that, within limits, speech intelligibility should improve with increases in the frequency range and the amount of audible signal. Another principle, embodied in many procedures, is to restrict the amount of low-frequency amplification to avoid any risk of upward spread of masking and to avoid increasing the loudness of the signal excessively. This may induce the client to turn down the hearing aid volume control to a point where the mid- and high-frequencies are inadequately amplified. Both of these principles, namely, maximizing the frequency range of audible signal and limiting the low-frequency amplification, need to be reexamined when we are considering the severely and profoundly hearing impaired because the logic behind these principles ceases to apply, or is less applicable, for clients with little or no useful hearing at the higher frequencies. A further consideration is that severely hearing-impaired persons may need a combination of auditory and visual cues to function satisfactorily. It has been argued that when this is so, the high-frequency auditory information largely is redundant with visual information (Lindblad, Haggard, and Foster 1983), and it becomes more important to use amplification to provide adequate low-frequency information. In other words, the optimum frequency response may depend on whether the client can function satisfactorily by au-

dition alone or on whether he or she is heavily dependent on lipreading.

Gain Requirements

The overall gain required by severely hearing-impaired persons is examined before considering the more complex issue of frequency response requirements. It is well established that clients with moderate hearing losses use gain equal to half, or somewhat less than half, of hearing threshold level (HTL). However, if this principle were applied to the severely hearing-impaired population, it can be shown that they would receive very little of a speech signal at audible levels.

Figure 1 shows the sensation levels (SL) of the peaks of speech, presented at the most comfortable listening level, and amplified by the gain preferred by a group of mildly to moderately hearing-impaired adults. According to the Articulation Theory, the speech peaks would need to be 30 dB above threshold to maximize the potential for understanding speech. This, in fact, only occurs for mild hearing losses, and if we extrapolate the regression line to severe losses, say over 70 dB, we would conclude that not very much of the speech signal would be audible. However, it is *not* generally true that severely hearing-impaired persons are unable to hear amplified speech. We must suspect, therefore, that the gain rule implied in this figure must cease to apply when we reach severe degrees of hearing loss.

Now some recent National Acoustic Laboratories' (NAL) data, together with data from other studies, are examined to suggest what rules may be needed when prescribing gain and frequency response for those with severe and profound hearing impairment. We recently have published a study of the gain and frequency response requirements of 46 severely and profoundly hearing-impaired adults

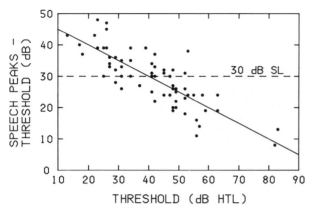

Figure 1. Sensation levels of the speech peaks (rms level + 12 dB) as a function of three-frequency-average HTL for speech at the preferred listening level of sensorineurally hearing-impaired listeners. (Reprinted with permission from Byrne and Cotton 1987.)

(Byrne, Parkinson, and Newall 1990a). We have also completed a similar but smaller study of 14 children, aged from 6 to 14 years. For each client, we estimated the optimal frequency response slope, from the low frequencies to 2000 Hz, using intelligibility judgments and speech recognition testing and, for the adults, home trials with different hearing aid tone settings. We also measured the real-ear gain that the clients preferred to use.

Figure 2 shows the used gain for the tone setting estimated to be best. The three-frequency-average used gain is plotted against the gain prescribed by the NAL procedure. The diagonal line would indicate agreement between used and pre-

scribed gain. Clearly, most subjects, whether adults or children, used more than the prescribed gain. On the average, they used about 10 dB more than the NAL gain. For example, for a 90 dB HTL, the NAL-prescribed gain was 40 dB, whereas used gain averaged 50 dB. These data raise two questions. First, at what hearing level do we need to change the gain rule; and, second, what is the appropriate rule for severe hearing losses? These questions may be examined by considering these data in conjunction with data from another NAL study and from two studies from other laboratories (figure 3).

In figure 3 the squares represent the present studies, and the solid circles represent a previous NAL study. These show the average used gain plotted against the average prescribed gain for subjects grouped according to six ranges of hearing level. The diagonal line shows agreement of used with prescribed gain or, in other words, it shows gain increasing at 46% of the rate that hearing level increases. The solid circles all fall very close to the diagonal line, indicating that, for these moderately hearing-impaired subjects, used gain agreed almost perfectly with prescribed gain, on the average. The open squares are the adult data for the present studies and the solid squares are the child data. These show that the severely hearing-impaired subjects used substantially more gain than the prescribed gain. If we disregard the solid circle that is based on two subjects only, our data show that the half-gain rule applies to hearing losses up to at least 60 dB, but that it ceases to apply when we reach 80 dB.

The other points on this figure, namely the crosses and the open circles, represent data from two studies that show how the most comfortable

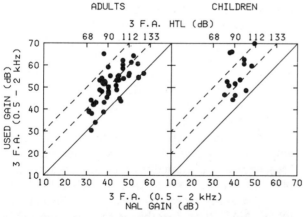

Figure 2. Three-frequency-average used (real-ear) gain as a function of NAL prescribed gain and HTL for adults and children. (Left panel reprinted with permission from D. Byrne, A. Parkinson, and P. Newall. Hearing aid gain and frequency response requirements for the severely/profoundly hearing-impaired. *Ear and Hearing* 11/1:40–49. Copyright by Williams & Wilkins, 1990.)

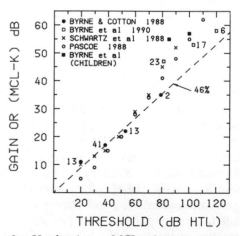

Figure 3. Used gain, or MCL minus a constant, as a function of HTL, from three NAL and two other studies. Broken line indicates gain prescribed by NAL procedure.

loudness level (MCL) increases as a function of hearing level (Schwartz, Lyregaard, and Lundth 1988; Pascoe 1988). The MCL values have been converted to gain values by subtracting a constant. Once again we see that the points are close to the diagonal line for hearing levels up to 60 dB, but are above the line for greater hearing loss levels. Considering the data from all these studies, it is clear that a half-gain rule, or a somewhat less than half-gain rule, applies to hearing levels up to 60 dB but, that for greater hearing losses, the rule needs to change.

Figure 4 may help to clarify what would be an appropriate gain prescription rule for severe hearing losses. The NAL data points are the same, but the 46% gain rule line has been stopped at 60 dB HTL. Above this are regression lines derived from the Pascoe (1988) and Schwartz et al. (1988) data. These lines are slightly less steep than the actual regression lines of the MCL versus HTL data. The reason for this adjustment is that, when addressing more severely impaired people, talkers tend to raise their voices. Consequently, the increase in gain that is required is slightly less than the increase in MCL would suggest. The adjustments were based on some NAL data (Byrne and Cotton 1987) that indicated speech input levels to increase at 7.5% of the rate that hearing levels increased. The slope values of the adjusted regression lines are 0.625 and 0.675. The NAL data are broadly consistent with these values, particularly as the point for the most severely impaired group probably underestimates preferred gain, as there were several subjects in this group who were using the maximum gain available.

Considering all the data, the appropriate gain rule for hearing levels over 60 dB would be to increase gain at about two-thirds of the rate that hearing level increases. This is in keeping with some suggestions in the literature (Libby 1986).

Frequency Response Requirements

The question of frequency response may now be considered. In the NAL studies we estimated the best frequency responses for our subjects by various experimental procedures (Byrne, Parkinson, and Newall 1990a). We then compared the estimated best responses with the responses we would prescribe by the NAL procedure.

Figure 5 shows the best response plotted against the NAL response for responses expressed as the average slope from .25 kHz to 2 kHz. The diagonal indicates agreement between the best slope and the NAL slope. The broken lines are drawn 6 dB/octave either side of the diagonal because, for various reasons, we believe this is a realistic tolerance to allow for imprecision in estimating the best responses. In other words, we can only be confident that the best response differed from the NAL response when that difference was at least 6 dB/octave. On this basis, the best response agreed with the NAL response for the majority of subjects. However, there was a proportion of subjects for whom the best response was less steeply sloping than the NAL response; that is, some subjects required relatively more low frequencies than the NAL response prescribed.

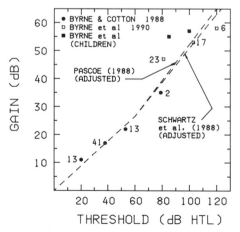

Figure 4. NAL data as in figure 3 and data from other studies represented by regression lines (see text for explanations). Figure illustrates how 46% gain rule applies to HTLs up to 60 dB but needs to change to about 66% for greater HTLs.

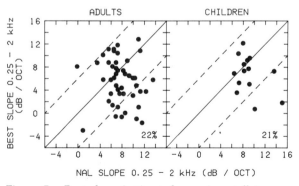

Figure 5. Best slope (estimated experimentally) versus NAL prescribed slope for slopes from .25 kHz for 2 kHz, for adults and children. (Left panel reprinted with permission from D. Byrne, A. Parkinson, and P. Newall. Hearing aid gain and frequency response requirements for the severely/profoundly hearing-impaired. *Ear and Hearing* 11/1:40–49. Copyright by Williams & Wilkins, 1990.)

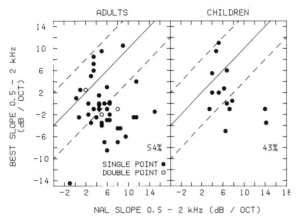

Figure 6. Best slope versus NAL slope for slopes from .5 kHz to 2 kHz, for adults and children. (Left panel reprinted with permission from D. Byrne, A. Parkinson, and P. Newall. Hearing aid gain and frequency response requirements for the severely/profoundly hearing-impaired. *Ear and Hearing* 11/1:40–49. Copyright by Williams & Wilkins, 1990.)

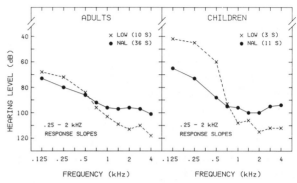

Figure 7. Average audiograms of those subjects who were suited by the NAL response and those who required more low frequencies. (Left panel reprinted, slightly modified, from D. Byrne, A. Parkinson, and P. Newall. Hearing aid gain and frequency response requirements for the severely/profoundly hearing-impaired. *Ear and Hearing* 11/1:40–49. Copyright by Williams & Wilkins, 1990.)

Figure 6 is the same as figure 5, except that the frequency responses have been expressed as slopes from .50 kHz to 2 kHz. Here we see that about half of the subjects required more low frequencies than would be prescribed by the NAL procedure. This is about twice as many as there were when we considered the slopes from .25 kHz to 2 kHz. The main reason for the difference is that the frequency response curves are irregular. Consequently, the calculated values for slope are highly dependent upon which frequencies are used in the calculation. We think it would be realistic to say that between a third and a half of our subjects required more low frequencies than the NAL response. Obviously, the precise proportion is not critical and it depends entirely on the composition of the subject group.

A more important question is: What kind of clients will require more low frequencies than would be prescribed by the NAL procedure or, as will be explained later, by *any* of the commonly used procedures? To get a first impression of what the answer might be, we calculated the average audiograms for those clients who did and those clients who did not require more low frequencies than the NAL procedure. These are shown in figure 7.

The crosses show the audiograms of the clients who required more low frequencies than the NAL response. We see that they tended to have more sloping audiograms and, more importantly, poorer hearing at the high frequencies. If we consider the adult subjects, the group with the more steeply sloping audiograms required, on the average, a flat frequency response, whereas the subjects who had the flatter audiograms required a frequency response slope of 6 to 7 dB/octave. Of course, this is opposite to the usual prescription principle that the steeper audiograms require the steeper frequency response slopes.

We found that the required frequency response slope was moderately predictable from hearing level at either 1 kHz or 2 kHz (Byrne, Parkinson, and Newall 1990a). Considering both the adults and the children, the correlations ranged from −.34 to −.63. The negative correlations mean that the greater the hearing loss, the less the slope that was required.

Next we asked the question: At what point do we need to vary the rule for selecting frequency response? Figure 8 shows the difference between the NAL slope and the best slope as a function of hearing level at 2 kHz. The horizontal line indicates that the NAL and best slopes agreed. The points above the line indicate that the best slope was less steep than the NAL slope. We see that, for hearing levels above 95 dB, the best slope was nearly always less steep than the NAL slope. In other words, these subjects consistently needed more low frequencies than the NAL prescription. On the other hand, for hearing levels less than 95 dB, there was no consistent trend for the best slope to be either less or more steep than the NAL slope. We suggest that a reasonable rule of thumb would be that, when the 2 kHz hearing level exceeds 95 dB, then the client will need more low frequencies than would be prescribed by the NAL procedure.

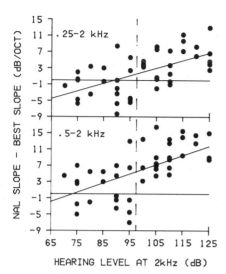

Figure 8. The difference between the NAL slope and the Best slope as a function of HTL at 2 kHz for the adults. (Reprinted with permission from D. Byrne, A. Parkinson, and P. Newall. Hearing aid gain and frequency response requirements for the severely/profoundly hearing-impaired. *Ear and Hearing* 11/1:40–49. Copyright by Williams & Wilkins, 1990.)

Prescriptive Procedures for the Severely Hearing-Impaired

So far we have related our data to the NAL prescriptive procedure, but have hinted that our conclusions also apply to other procedures. The basis for this assertion is a comparison of prescriptions from the NAL procedure with prescriptions derived from MCL measurements. We measured MCLs for all of our adult cases, although there were some for whom we could not make the comparison because we could not reach MCL at 2 kHz. This study showed close agreement between the NAL and MCL responses and showed that when the NAL procedure prescribed too little low-frequency amplification, then the MCL procedure also did so (Byrne, Parkinson, and Newall 1990b). Thus, the NAL procedure was doing what it was supposed to, namely amplifying all frequency bands to MCL, but that rationale ceased to apply to some of the severely hearing-impaired persons. This finding is not at all unexpected but it deserves to be emphasized. It means that *all* procedures based on an MCL, or similar, rationale need to be modified when applied to the severely and profoundly hearing impaired. Furthermore, virtually all of the commonly used procedures do have an MCL rationale either

expressed explicitly or included in their derivation (Byrne, Parkinson, and Newall 1990b).

To conclude, we shall consider the practical matter of how we might modify prescriptive procedures to accommodate the requirements of the severely hearing impaired. Provisionally, we have altered the NAL procedure in two ways (see figure 9), according to the principles suggested earlier (Hodgson and Dillon 1989).

First, the overall gain is varied using a new table for calculating the "X" factor in the prescription formula. For three frequency average hearing levels of 60 dB or less, X continues to be 5% of the combined hearing levels. However, for average hearing levels exceeding 60 dB, X has been modified so that gain will increase at 66% of the rate that hearing loss increases for that part of the hearing loss that exceeds 60 dB. In other words, the usual 46% gain rule applies up to 60 dB hearing level but, thereafter, it becomes a 66% rule.

A set of correction figures is also used so that, when the 2 kHz hearing level equals or exceeds 95 dB, the average frequency response slope below 2 kHz is decreased. The amount of decrease is proportional to the extent by which hearing level exceeds 95 dB. For example, if the 2 kHz hearing level were 105 dB, then the slope would be reduced by 4 dB/octave whereas, if the hearing level were 115 dB, the reduction in slope would be about 7 dB/octave.

We have not attempted any calculations for other prescriptive procedures. However, for the reasons mentioned, virtually all of them would need to be modified along similar lines to be generally applicable to the severely and profoundly hearing-impaired population.

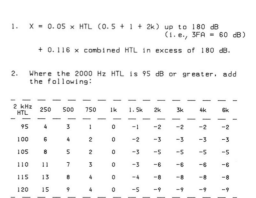

1. X = 0.05 × HTL (0.5 + 1 + 2k) up to 180 dB
   (i.e., 3FA = 60 dB)

   + 0.116 × combined HTL in excess of 180 dB.

2. Where the 2000 Hz HTL is 95 dB or greater, add the following:

2 kHz HTL	250	500	750	1k	1.5k	2k	3k	4k	6k
95	4	3	1	0	-1	-2	-2	-2	-2
100	6	4	2	0	-2	-3	-3	-3	-3
105	8	5	2	0	-3	-5	-5	-5	-5
110	11	7	3	0	-3	-6	-6	-6	-6
115	13	8	4	0	-4	-8	-8	-8	-8
120	15	9	4	0	-5	-9	-9	-9	-9

Figure 9. Modifications to NAL hearing aid selection procedure (Byrne and Dillon 1986) for application to severe/profound hearing losses.

References

Byrne, D., and Cotton, S. 1987. Preferred listening levels of sensorineurally hearing-impaired listeners. *Australian Journal of Audiology* 9:7–14.

Byrne, D., and Cotton, S. 1988. Evaluation of the National Acoustic Laboratories' new hearing aid selection procedure. *Journal of Speech and Hearing Research* 31:178–86.

Byrne, D., and Dillon, H. 1986. The National Acoustic Laboratories' (NAL) new procedure for selecting the gain and frequency response of a hearing aid. *Ear and Hearing* 7:257–65.

Byrne, D., Parkinson, A., and Newall, P. 1990a. Hearing aid gain and frequency response requirements for the severely/profoundly hearing-impaired. *Ear and Hearing* 11:40–49.

Byrne, D., Parkinson, A., and Newall, P. 1990b. Comparisons of NAL and MCL based hearing aid frequency response prescriptions for severely/profoundly hearing-impaired clients. *Australian Journal of Audiology* 12:1–9.

Hodgson, F., and Dillon, H. 1989. Modified hearing aid gain and frequency response requirements for severe/profound losses. *NAL Audiology Circular* 1989/23.

Libby, E.R. 1986. The 1/3–2/3 insertion gain hearing aid selection guide. *Hearing Instruments* 37:27–28.

Lindblad, A-C., Haggard, M.P., and Foster, J.R. 1983. Audio versus audio-visual—implications for hearing aid frequency responses. *Report TA 108*. Stockholm: Karolinska Institute.

Pascoe, D.P. 1988. Clinical measurements of the auditory dynamic range and their relation to formulae for hearing aid gain. In *Hearing Aid Fitting: Theoretical and Practical Views* ed. J.H. Jensen. Copenhagen: Stougaard Jensen.

Schwartz, D., Lyregaard, P.E., and Lundth, P. 1988. Hearing aid selection for severe/profound hearing loss. *Hearing Journal* 41 (2):13–17.

CHAPTER 26

Clinical Management of Assistive Technology Users
Issues to Consider

Cynthia L. Compton

Over the past decade, the audiology profession has witnessed dramatic changes in the provision of services to the hearing-impaired consumer. Technological advances in the personal hearing aid, coupled with improved fitting techniques, have provided us with solutions to communication problems that in the past could not have been resolved. Hearing aid selection considerations now include a variety of electroacoustic parameters, such as frequency response, gain, and saturation sound pressure level (SSPL90), and a myriad of special features such as type of microphone (directional or omnidirectional), type of compression circuit, noise suppression circuits, type of earmold plumbing, and programmability. Still, even this arsenal of hearing aid technology cannot always be counted on to solve every client's receptive communication difficulties (Beck and Nance 1989).

A significant number of clients require alternative technologies to the hearing aid to assist them in understanding speech in noise, in reverberant conditions, from a distance, over the telephone, or when listening to a dictation machine, portable tape player, or other electronic device. We have known about these technologies—assistive devices—for several years now, and, until recently, have not paid much attention to them. Today, however, there is considerably more emphasis being placed on assistive *listening* devices (ALDs). One need only open an audiology trade journal, newspaper, or tabloid and one will see advertisements touting miraculous feats of sound enhancement made possible by devices that pick up everything from a whisper to a deer snort. In the May 1990 issue of *The Hearing Journal* it was reported that an increased emphasis on ALDs is contributing to behind-the-ear (BTE) hearing aids maintaining a respectable 20% share of the market (Mahon 1990).

Three forces seem to be at work in promoting the popularity of assistive technology. Consumer self-help groups have been instrumental in popularizing the need for this technology. Concerned, rehabilitation-oriented audiologists also have stressed the need for assistive devices. As a result of these forces, governmental support for assistive devices is having a positive impact on the use of this technology. With legislation and increased state funding available, more and more public areas are being made accessible through the use of telecommunications and large area assistive technology. Perhaps the most significant piece of legislation is the Americans With Disabilities Act (ADA) of 1990, which requires communication accommodation for hearing-impaired persons requiring access to public transportation, services, accommodations, employment, and telephone services. With assistive technology becoming more and more popular, it becomes imperative that clinicians be competent in the needs assessment process.

The purpose of this chapter is to provide clinicians with a framework for identifying the potential assistive device user and his or her specific equipment needs, but two important points must be made. First, *improving speech recognition should not be our only goal in the rehabilitative process.* Second, *the hearing aid fitting should not necessarily be the "terminal activity of audiological case management"* (Binnie and Hession 1990, p. 37).

Hearing-impaired people have communication needs in three basic areas: (1) interpersonal communication and enjoyment of media, (2) telecommunications, and (3) communication of the occurrence of alerting signals (figure 1). The personal hearing aid cannot always completely meet the needs in each of these areas. It is common for a hearing aid user to experience difficulty understanding speech in noise, from a distance, and on the telephone. A person with even a mild to moder-

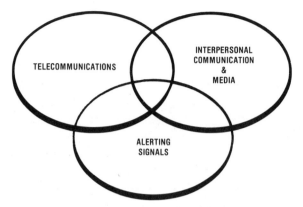

Figure 1. Communication needs of hearing-impaired people.

ate hearing impairment might be functionally deaf to a smoke alarm located down the hall and behind a closed door when sleeping with the hearing aid(s) removed. The same person might miss the doorbell when using an infrared system plugged into the television earphone jack.

Numerous auditory and nonauditory, hardwired and wireless technologies (Compton 1990) are available to meet these needs. As a profession, we must be able not only to fit hearing aids appropriately, but also to evaluate their place within the larger framework of maximizing the communication skills of the hearing-impaired person in all aspects of his or her daily life. Accordingly, we must be able to demonstrate and recommend appropriate auditory and nonauditory assistive technology as well as provide the ongoing training and counseling necessary to assure success in its use.

Assistive Technology: A Review

Before describing needs assessment procedures, a review of the available technology might be helpful. As mentioned previously, assistive devices for hearing-impaired people are designed to meet communication needs in three areas: (1) interpersonal communication and enjoyment of media, (2) telecommunications, and (3) communication of the occurrence of alerting signals. A quick review of the technology available for each area follows. For a more detailed review, see Compton (1989, 1991).

Assistive Listening Devices (ALDs)

The term *ALDs* is used here to describe a group of products that are designed to improve the signal-to-noise ratio (S/N ratio) for the listener by as much as

15 to 19 dB in moderate noise and reverberation (Hawkins 1985). ALDs can be used alone or in conjunction with a hearing aid and can be helpful in a variety of listening situations, including listening alone (radio, television, stereo, dictaphone), listening in a one-to-one conversation (in person or on the phone), or listening in groups of varying sizes. Customized ALDs can also be fashioned for specific applications.

Hardwired Systems   Hardwired systems physically tether the listener to the sound source. The sound source—a person talking, the television, a radio—may be picked up via a remote hand-held, lapel, or velcro-attached microphone. For electronic sound sources, an electrical plug/jack connection can also be used. The signal then is delivered to the listener's ears via a headset or earbuds or to a personal hearing aid via direct audio input (DAI) or inductive coupling (neckloop or silhouette inductor). Separation from the sound source is limited by the length of the cord.

Hearing aid dependent DAI systems. DAI systems, available from most behind-the-ear (BTE) hearing aid companies, plug directly into BTE hearing aids via an audio shoe. In some cases, the technology can be adapted to ITE and body aids. Lightweight and inexpensive, these systems can be used to gain access to media such as television, radio, and stereo via a direct plug-in connection or remote microphone. Microphones of various types (omnidirectional, directional, and directional boom) may be used. These systems can be used with the hearing aid's environmental microphone (EM) activated or deactivated. Depending upon the manufacturer's philosophy, control of the EM is accomplished via the hearing aid's switch, audio shoe, or DAI cords. At this time, it cannot be assumed that any DAI system can be used with any brand of hearing aid due to impedance variations. Although there are exceptions and custom modifications are possible, in general, brand "A" hearing aid must be used with its own audio shoe, cord, and microphone.

Hearing aid dependent inductive systems. Plug-in neckloops and silhouette inductors are available that connect directly to televisions, radios, dictaphones, and other electronic devices via a plug/jack connection (and extension cord, if desired) and are powered by the voltage from the device.

Acoustic-to-magnetic (A/M adapters). A/M adapters pick up an acoustic telephone signal and change it to electromagnetic energy for pick-up by a hearing aid's telecoil. One of these devices also can be ordered with a monaural cord terminating in a silhouette inductor to allow diotic telephone listening as well as use of the device as a remote microphone system.

Personal amplification systems (PAS). PAS are battery-powered hardwired systems that can stand alone or can be used with a hearing aid. Depending on the individual user's personal preference, the level of hearing loss present, and whether the listener will use the PAS in conjunction with a hearing aid, the auditory signal can be provided by connecting an earphone headset, earbuds, a DAI cord, a neckloop, or a silhouette inductor to the amplifier. PAS can serve as part-time or full-time amplification systems for those people who for various reasons do not use a hearing aid. For those who do, PAS offers the only way a hearing aid equipped with a telecoil but without a DAI connection can be coupled to a remote microphone system. Several brands of PAS are available; two are available with built-in telecoils that allow them to be used as induction loop receivers also. PAS can be ordered with corded microphones or extension cords for use with neckloops or headphones to allow for remote microphone placement. Some brands on the market do not have this feature and thus are limited in their ability to easily increase the environmental signal-to-noise ratio—the *raison d'etre* of an ALD.

Wireless Systems   Wireless systems consist of a battery- or AC-powered transmitter that sends some type of radio signal to a battery-powered receiver, avoiding the need for a cord between the sound source and the listener. Although more expensive than hardwired systems, wireless systems are superior when mobility and versatility are concerns. Applications include large areas such as concert and lecture halls, classrooms, and houses of worship. Wireless systems also function well at home, in the office, and in other situations involving small group, one-to-one, or listening alone situations (e.g., TV) where the user would rather not be tethered to the sound source.

Induction. Induction (or audio) loop systems are relatively inexpensive, require little maintenance, and work well in the home and in meeting rooms where the listeners have telecoil equipped hearing aids. Unlike other wireless systems, a separate receiver (and maintenance program) is not needed, provided the listener is wearing a telecoil-equipped hearing aid. Use of the hearing aid telecoil as a wireless receiver also is cosmetically appealing to many people. For those without telecoil circuits, portable telecoil receivers can be used (but must be maintained). Induction systems are vul-

nerable to interference (60 cycle hum) from various sources such as fluorescent light, transformers, and electrical power wiring within a building. In addition, electromagnetic energy from a loop system can travel through solid surfaces, causing spillover into adjacent rooms. Another problem is that the strength of the magnetic signal decreases sharply with distance. Finally, sensitivity of hearing aid telecoil reception often is dependent on the spatial positioning of the coil within the hearing aid chassis. Reduction in output has been noted simply by changing the plane of the telecoil in relation to the induction source (Matkin and Olsen 1970).[1]

Infrared. Infrared technology is popular in large area, as well as home television, applications. As with FM transmission, there are no seating restrictions, provided the room has a sufficient number of infrared transmitters and provided that they are oriented properly. In addition, because infrared light will not penetrate solid barriers, it can be used simultaneously in adjacent rooms without interference and is ideal for use in the legitimate theatre, courtrooms, larger conference rooms, cinema houses, and other areas where security of the signal is a concern. Currently, most (but not all) large area infrared systems designed for use by the hearing impaired are monophonic and transmit on a carrier frequency of 95 kHz. Small transmitters are available in monaural and stereo configurations for television listening at home as well as at business meetings and other small group or one-to-one situations. Because most systems use a 95 kHz carrier frequency (IEC standard), an infrared user can take his or her receiver from home and use it at the theatre in order to avoid waiting in line for the theatre's receivers. The limitations of infrared technology are as follows: (1) infrared systems cannot be used outside because they are subject to interference from sunlight; (2) infrared light also travels in a straight line, meaning that the strongest and clearest signal is obtained when received from direct line of transmission; (3) in most applications, the infrared signal is also reflected by walls, ceiling, furnishings, clothing, and so forth, and the reception of the signal is not completely directional. However, in large area applications where the coverage area of the

---

[1]Field testing of a new 3-dimensional induction system currently is being carried out. Consisting of a prefabricated configuration of three audio loops (varying in amplitude and phase) embedded in a flexible foam mat, the "3-D pad" is placed under a carpet. The inventor, Norman Lederman of Oval Window Audio, reports that testing thus far demonstrates excellent uniformity throughout a 24' × 24' room, ± 3 dB, irrespective of hearing aid telecoil positioning. Attenuation of spillover from room to room is in excess of 30 dB. This is a 20dB improvement over conventional audio loops and is hoped to be increased.

emitters may be pushed to its maximum, the infrared signal may prove to be more directional, requiring the user to face in the direction of the emitters in order to receive a clear signal.

Infrared transmitters cannot be efficiently operated by battery power due to their comparatively high power needs. Even personal transmitters must be powered by electricity from a wall outlet, limiting their use as portable ALDs. Finally, the performance of an infrared transmitter is determined by the correlation between the number of transmitting diodes and the physical and lighting conditions in a given room. Attempting to use a personal transmitter in larger rooms without the addition of remote emitters may provide a limited signal and potentially inferior performance.

Frequency modulation (FM). FM systems are perhaps the most versatile of all listening systems. Easy to install, they can be used indoors or outdoors, in large areas or in small groups, in one-to-one listening situations, or while listening to media. Systems can be purchased that allow the listener to enjoy a lecture while recording it at the same time. FM receivers also can be ordered with environmental microphone jacks to allow the receiver to be used as a PAS when preferred. Some contain personal amplification devices (auditory trainers) and some do not (personal FM). FM technology is being employed in the education of hearing-impaired children as well as children and adults with central auditory processing disorders.

FM systems broadcast between 72 and 76 MegaHertz on 32 narrowband (NB) or eight wideband (WB) channels. Limitations of FM systems include the fact that the 72 MegaHertz band is no longer reserved solely for use by hearing-impaired people. As a result, interference from other radio transmissions (pagers, taxis, etc.) may occur. In fact, this problem has become so pronounced that FM manufacturers are investigating the possibility of using another FM band for transmission (Anderson 1990; Mendosa 1990).

Another problem involves the fact that so many different frequencies can be used to transmit the signal. Narrowband (NB) and wideband (WB) systems operate on different channels from each other, use different frequency spacing, and possess different transmission characteristics. Because of these differences, they are essentially incompatible with each other. For example, the signal produced by an NB transmitter may not be detected by a WB receiver or may not produce the same output signal as when used with the complimentary NB receiver.

Conversely, depending on the channel used, a small portion of the signal produced by a WB transmitter might happen to align with an NB receiver. However, depending on the selectivity of the NB receiver, reception could be distorted. Because of this, it is not necessarily true that a user of FM transmission at home can necessarily use his or her personal FM receiver in an FM-equipped theatre.

Telecommunications Devices and Systems

Auditory Telephone Devices

Replacement handsets. These devices can be used with modular handset telephones only and must be matched electronically to the telephone to avoid distortion and to provide adequate gain. Replacement handset amplifiers can be used with or without a hearing aid, depending upon the user's preference and particular hearing impairment. When used with a hearing aid telecoil, the handset must, of course, be hearing aid compatible. A person with even profound hearing impairment often can use a voice telephone successfully if fitted with a hearing aid with an adequate telecoil and a hearing aid compatible replacement handset.

In-line Amplifiers. As with replacement handsets, in-line amplifiers must be used with modular phones. On some electronic (as opposed to carbon bell ringers) telephone systems, line-powered in-line amplifiers will reduce the loudness of the user's voice to the person on the other end of the line due to power drain. In this case, a transformer- or battery-powered in-line amplifier can be employed to alleviate the problem.

Portable amplifiers. There are two types of battery-powered portable amplifiers—those that couple magnetically to the telephone and those that couple acoustically. Magnetically coupled amplifiers can be used only on hearing aid compatible phones. Legislation has mandated that all new corded telephones manufactured or imported for use in the United States must be hearing aid compatible after July 16, 1989. The same holds true for cordless telephones as of August 16, 1991.[2] However, this legislation exempts telephones used with public mobile services, private radio services, and secure telephones—telephones used for the transmission of classified or sensitive information. In addition, this legislation does not require home owners to replace their noncompatible telephones with compatible models. Consequently, to ensure a consumer tele-

---

[2]Hearing Aid Compatibility Act of 1988–Public Law 100-394.

phone access, it is prudent to recommend a portable amplifier that couples acoustically. As of this writing, there is only one device on the market that couples to the phone acoustically and can be used without a hearing aid (up to a moderate loss) or with a hearing aid's telecoil.[3]

Portable induction systems. As of this writing, two acoustic-to-magnetic adapters are available that couple acoustically to any telephone. One is used with a hearing aid telecoil only. The other, AT&T's Portable Amplifier,™ can be used with the naked ear or coupled acoustically or inductively to a hearing aid.

Interpersonal ALDs with telephone interface. Several hardwired and wireless interpersonal ALDs have modular telephone interfaces, enabling the user to listen to the telephone monotically or diotically and can be used with earphones or hearing aids (DAI or inductively).[4] DAI and earphone coupling to these devices is also useful when a hearing aid's telecoil is rendered useless due to electromagnetic interference from fluorescent lights and/or computers. These devices can be particularly useful for hearing-impaired people who rely on heavy telephone use for occupational reasons and can make the difference between retaining or losing such employment.

Acoustic Telepads/Couplers The feedback that occurs when coupling a hearing aid acoustically to the telephone can often be eliminated through the use of an inexpensive foam telepad or plastic coupler that slips over the telephone receiver speaker. A shortened styrofoam cup minus its bottom can also be used for this same purpose!

Telephones Designed for the Hearing Impaired Two companies (Walker and Williams Sound) market hearing aid compatible telephones that provide increased amplification over that of traditional telephone amplifiers via an adjustable gain-control built into the body of the telephone. These specialty telephones also provide enhanced high frequency responses, much like a hearing aid. One of the companies (Williams Sound) markets two models with adjustable frequency responses and signal processing circuitry.[5] The more powerful model also allows

the connection of a hearing aid via DAI or induction. Both brands of telephones also contain built-in low frequency ringers.

NonAuditory Telephone Devices The primary means of telephone communication by people who cannot understand speech, even amplified speech on the telephone, is the Telecommunication Device for the Deaf (TDD). The term *TDD,* although ostensibly a generic term for any device used by deaf people for telephone communication, actually applies only to a narrow category of devices. Descendants of teletypewriters, today's TDDs are small terminals approximately 9″ by 12″ in size and weighing between two and five pounds. TDDs translate typed input into an acoustic code (called Baudot) that is carried across the telephone line to another location, where a compatible TDD decodes the message and displays the text to the other caller. Although TDDs are used mostly by deaf people, they are also used by hard-of-hearing and speech-impaired people.

Dual party relay systems also are available that allow the user of a voice telephone to communicate with a TDD user via a TDD-using operator. The Americans with Disabilities Act of 1990 mandates all telephone companies provide intra- and interstate relay services within three years of enactment of the bill.

Other visually based telephone technologies include computers equipped with modems and telecommunications software, touch-tone technology, message relay systems, and facsimile (FAX) transmission. Research is being done toward the eventual introduction of video telephones, which would permit the use of sign language and speech-reading over phone lines (Harkins in press).

Television Devices
ALDs. Any of the hardwired and wireless devices mentioned previously can be used for television viewing. Microphone pick-up is desired when other family members want to listen to the broadcast. Plug-in pick-up is desired for private listening. Some televisions have two jacks, one deactivates the external TV speaker and one that allows the speaker to continue functioning. Hardwired systems are the least expensive; wireless systems are excellent if the client prefers not to be tethered to the television.

Closed captioned decoder. Closed captioned decoders provide television access to deaf as well as hard-of-hearing individuals. For many hard-of-hearing individuals, closed captioning can fill in the gaps of comprehension that amplification and

---

[3]AT&T Portable Amplifier™.

[4]Audex SounDirector, Williams Sound PockeTalker, and Comtek FM receiver, option two.

[5]Because of the power requirements of its amplifier, this telephone operates in half-duplex, causing the user's voice to fade slightly if interrupted by the person on the other end of the line.

speechreading cannot.[6] And, even people who use amplification for awareness only can often enjoy the music tracks of movies, music videos, and other shows by using an ALD along with the decoder. Legislation requires that by July 1, 1993, all new televisions with screens larger than 13 inches must contain decoder circuitry.[7] This would alleviate the need for a separate decoder box and would make captioning accessible to millions of Americans.

Alerting Devices

Electronic Alerting devices, often thought of as used by only severely to profoundly hearing-impaired people, are gaining in popularity with hard-of-hearing people who want to remain independent. The first alerting devices focused on common signals to be monitored such as telephone rings, doorbells, smoke alarms, wake-up alarms, and baby cries. While these are still the most common requests, even mildly hearing-impaired people may need assistance in monitoring the increasing number of soft auditory signals used today. These include microwave timers, telephone ring "chirps," computer prompts, intercom prompts, apartment intercom buzzers, and so forth. Because of the great variety of sounds used in our environment, the audiologist is often involved in the recommendation of an appropriate signalling system. In many instances, a hearing aid enables a person to hear most sounds. But, if a person is not wearing his or her hearing aid (e.g., while sleeping), is in another room, is amid background noise, or is hooked up to the television with ALD, then, at these times, visual or vibrotactile alerting systems can serve as a backup system to the hearing aid.

Alerting devices monitor sounds using a microphone, a direct electrical connection, or inductive pick-up. Signal transmission occurs using hardwired or wireless technology. Types of alerting stimuli include visual (bright light, strobe light), auditory (louder or lower pitched signal), or tactile. Tactile stimuli include vibration (e.g., bed shakers, pocket pagers) or an air stream (fan). Figure 2 illustrates the various options available for monitoring, transmitting and receiving information about environmental events. Wireless systems are available that can monitor various signals in an entire home

or office. Portable vibratory pagers are also available. Some of these pagers transmit over short distances (100 feet), whereas others can reach out thousands of miles, using sophisticated telecommunications systems comprising telephone lines, satellite down-links, and local pager antennas. Some paging systems also are available that alert the wearer via sound or vibration and display an alpha-numeric message.

Wake-up systems include small, portable, battery-powered clocks that shake a person awake as well as AC-powered clocks that can be connected to a lamp, a strobe, a bed shaker, or a fan. A very inexpensive system consisting of a lamp, a lamp timer, and a flasher button placed in the lamp socket can be recommended.

The monitoring of computer prompts can be accomplished through the use of a hearing aid or special visual display programmed to appear on the computer monitor.

Research at the Graduate Center of the City University of New York (CUNY) is being done toward the eventual development of a visual alerting system that, using a signal processor, warns hearing-impaired drivers of important sounds such as sirens from emergency vehicles and close by car horns, but ignores all other normal traffic noise. This type of technology eventually may be used in all microphone pick-up alerting systems, virtually eliminating the occurrence of false positive warning signals (Weiss 1990).

Visual alerting technology that meets National Fire Protection (NFPA) criteria is available to warn hearing-impaired people in the event of a fire or other emergency. This life saving protection is accomplished using relatively inexpensive high intensity strobe lights, often combined with compatible smoke detectors. Many states and the U.S. Department of Housing and Urban Development Consolidated Supply Program require a minimum effective intensity of 100 candela. This specification is based upon findings and criteria provided by the NFPA[8] and the Illuminating Engineering Society (IES)[9] (Sievers 1990). Unfortunately, this technology is not always utilized in public accommodations, apartments, and other occupancies, many of which are mandated to do so by law. Many alerting devices for fire on the market do not meet NFPA standards, yet they are purchased and are giving a false sense of security to consumers.

---

[6]Clients who plan to use captioning as well as speechreading and audition to receive television programming should be warned that captioned and spoken words do not occur simultaneously. Initially, this may create confusion and frustration for the television viewer.

[7]Television Decoder Circuitry Act.

---

[8]NFPA 72G, Sections 3-2.4.1 and 3-2.4.1.3.

[9]IES Handbook Section 3-24.

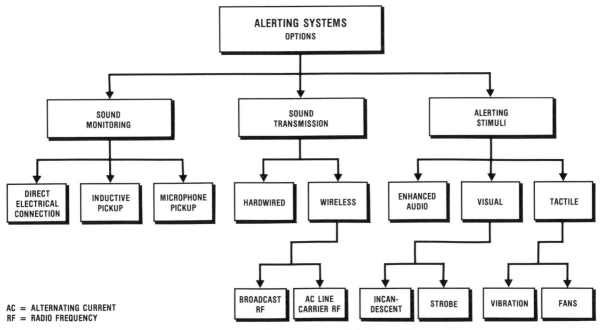

Figure 2.   Methods for the monitoring, transmission, and reception of warning signals.

Mammalian   The Hearing Ear Dog is a viable alternative to electronic alerting technology. Warm and fuzzy, a hearing ear dog is powered by food, water, and love, and can provide important companionship as well as communication access and safety to its owner. Hearing ear dogs are trained professionally to alert their owners to various pertinent sounds. Almost all states have hearing ear dog legislation. Although the vast majority of states may give legal status equivalent to seeing eye dogs, many require some form of certification and have some limitations.

The Needs Assessment/Selection Process

The identification of candidacy for assistive technology and the subsequent recommendation for use of specific technology may occur at several points along a continuum of audiologic care (figure 3). The needs assessment/selection process for assistive technology begins with a thorough audiologic and communication needs assessment. This sets the stage for the selection of appropriate personal amplification that can be used in conjunction with assistive technology. The actual selection of assistive technology may occur during the counseling session preceding the hearing aid/assistive device evaluation or during or following the hearing aid trial. Follow-up is essential to successful use of assistive

technology and aural rehabilitation may be required as well.

Let us examine each of these points as they involve issues and decisions that have direct impact on our goal—improving a client's ability to communicate in everyday life.

Audiologic/Communication Needs Assessment

Undoubtedly, the most important part of the needs assessment process is the time one spends with a client taking a case history. Thorough assessment of a client's communicative difficulties with respect to his or her specific lifestyle needs is essential because this will determine not only whether a hearing aid and/or assistive device is necessary, but what specific type of technology should be recommended.

Evaluation of Client's Communicative Needs With Respect to Lifestyle   A client's lifestyle may dictate the level of communication needs in various situations: on the job, at home, in a group home, at school, while traveling, or while engaging in a recreational activity. Communication concerns for each of these situations are addressed below:

Job.   When querying a client about communication on his or her job, one must appraise the following areas:

1. Telephone communication (in office, while traveling);

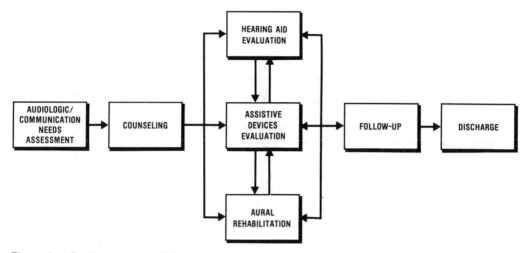

Figure 3.   Continuum of audiologic care.

2. Office conversation (one-to-one, meetings within office);
3. Lectures/seminars within or outside of office;
4. Casual conversation with colleagues or clients, (office, car, restaurants, etc.);
5. Speech recognition from a dictaphone or telephone answering machine; and
6. Reception of important warning signals in the office and while traveling (e.g., fire alarm, telephone ring, pager, doorbell/door knock, computer prompts).

Needs analysis for each situation can lead the way toward the selection of an appropriate hearing aid and/or assistive device. For example, the need to hear on a dictaphone may point out the need for a hearing aid equipped with a DAI connection or telecoil to allow the hearing aid to be used with a DAI or neckloop interface to the dictaphone. Difficulty hearing incoming messages on an answering machine (even with a hearing aid) may point out the need for an answering machine retro-fitted with a hearing aid compatible telephone receiver (and telecoil-equipped hearing aid). Electrical interference from computer monitors and fluorescent lighting might preclude the use of a hearing aid telecoil with telephones and interpersonal ALDs, thereby making it necessary to recommend that a DAI hearing aid be used with the telephone and interpersonal ALDs. An employee who must attend seminars as well as group meetings might be more appropriately fitted with a wireless listening device than a hardwired one since the former allows for mobility whereas the latter limits movement and distance from the sound source.

Visual emergency alarms may also be needed. If so, a sufficient number of alerting signals must be installed in all areas of the building where the hearing-impaired employee might go, including restrooms and storage areas.

Home.   Home communication needs may be similar to those on the job and include:

1. Telephone communication;
2. TV reception;
3. Radio, stereo reception;
4. One to one conversation;
5. Group conversation (with family, relatives, friend, associates, etc.); and
6. Reception of warning signals (e.g., telephone ring, doorbell/doorknock, fire alarm, wake-up alarm, appliance signals, monitoring of children's or mate's activities from another room, security signals, etc.).

Group home (nursing home, half-way house, etc.).   Communication needs in this situation may be similar to those in the home with the addition of:

1. Receptive conversation in common dining areas, game rooms, media rooms, chapel, conferring with medical personnel and other care givers, etc.; and
2. Reception of warning signals also apply unless under 24-hour supervision (wherein group home personnel would be responsible for client's safety, security, and for admission of visitors to client's room or apartment).

In addition to hearing aids and ALDs, acoustical treatment of common areas can do much to reduce the negative effects of noise and reverberation on communication.

School/College.   Communication needs here may include:

1. Speech recognition in classrooms, lecture halls;
2. Speech-language therapy;
3. Auditory training;
4. Meetings with teachers and other personnel;
5. One-to-one or group conversation in dormitory, apartment, etc.;
6. Telecommunications in dormitory, apartment, on and off campus; and
7. Reception of warning signals as mentioned previously, including local (client's room, apartment) and general (hallway, common areas) fire alarm systems in dormitory and/or apartment.

Recreation and travel. Recreational and travel activities include:

1. Telephone conversation (pay phone, hotel, car);
2. One-to-one, small or large group conversations in hotels, lecture halls, restaurants;
3. Speech recognition while on indoor and outdoor tours (bus, train, plane, boat, on foot, bicycles, horses, skis, etc.); and
4. Instruction (any type of hobby or activity where the hearing-impaired person must be able to hear instructor/guide).

As more and more theatres, movie houses, houses of worship, and other large areas install wireless listening systems, accessibility to these locations increases. However, it becomes even more important that hearing aid users be fitted with hearing aids that can be used in conjunction with these large area systems. Regardless of how well a hearing aid is fitted, if it does not contain a telecoil, it cannot be used with a large area listening system. This is not to say that all clients will need telecoils in their hearing aids. However, when fitting personal amplification, one must make sure that, if needed or desired, the client can benefit from large area listening systems in his or her community—either via a telecoil circuitry or by removing the hearing aid and using a headset.

Many hearing-impaired people can benefit from ALDs when engaging in recreational activities. The listening device of choice can be determined by the type of activity. For example, skiing, horseback riding, hiking, and golfing occur outdoors and are mobile activities; therefore, a personal FM system would be a convenient and an effective choice for the transmission of an instructor's voice to a hearing-impaired student (or vice versa). On the other hand, quilting, usually an indoor and stationary activity, could be handled with an infrared system. One-to-one instruction in a foreign language might be handled with a less expensive hardwired system because the activity could occur

across a table and the student's hands would not be in danger of becoming tangled in the cord connecting the teacher's microphone to the students personal amplifier (as might occur with quilting).

Counseling

Following a thorough communication and audiologic assessment, the clinician should have a good foundation on which to base specific decisions concerning the need for personal amplification, assistive devices and aural rehabilitation. Unfortunately, currently there are no empirical data (related to degree of hearing loss, speech recognition scores, etc.) on which to base decisions concerning personal hearing aids and assistive technology. However, based on our experience at the Gallaudet Audiology Clinic, here are some clinical observations that might be helpful in decision-making:

1. In many cases, clients with pure-tone averages of 40 dB HL may require telecoil circuitry. Telephone listening is probably the biggest concern of clients, next to one-to-one communication and TV listening. To decide whether to install a telecoil, observe how well the client performs on the telephone, both without and with an amplifier. If the client experiences difficulty, install a telecoil.
2. There is not always a positive correlation between degree of hearing impairment and the need for assistive listening devices. While this is generally true, life-style often determines the need for an ALD. For example, clients with very mild hearing impairment who work may need the assistance of a remote microphone in staff meetings or in other difficult listening situations. On the other hand, a retired person with a very mild hearing impairment and a quiet life-style may not even require a personal hearing aid.
3. In general, there is a negative correlation between the need for ALDs and speech recognition ability. But, life-style plays an important role here too. An active life-style seems to call for ALDs more often, even for people with better speech recognition scores. Clients with mild high-frequency hearing impairment with good aided speech recognition scores (in S/N ratios of 0 dB) can sometimes benefit from the use of a hearing aid coupled to a remote microphone system in staff meetings. Furthermore, clients who use hearing aids for speech awareness only sometimes find ALDs beneficial, as in the case of deaf clients who use DAI and neckloop

interfaces with portable tape players to enjoy music.

4. In general, there is a positive correlation between degree of hearing impairment and the need for alerting devices. However, even people with mild hearing impairment may need enhanced auditory or visual signalling systems when their hearing aids are not being worn or when they are using an ALD to listen to media (TV, stereo, etc.).

Hearing Aid/Assistive Device Evaluation

If a hearing aid is to be recommended, the clinician must determine whether it will need to be used with other assistive devices. This decision will be based on the communication needs assessment as well as the eventual performance of the hearing aid. While final decisions do not necessarily need to be made at this point, it is a good place to decide what type of hearing aid to fit. The client should be shown models of BTE, ITE (in-the-ear), and ITC (in-the-canal) hearing aids and the pros and cons of each type should be explained. If assistive listening devices appear to be needed, then this should be discussed at this time. It also is important to address the fact that telecoil circuitry and DAI can be incorporated readily into some types of hearing aids but not others. We have found that clients often are willing to sacrifice cosmetics for better hearing, once they understand the advantages and disadvantages of the various hearing aid technologies.

Selection of Appropriate Hearing Aid(s)   Although it is not always possible to achieve, obviously hearing aids should be selected with the goal of solving as many of the client's communication difficulties as possible. One of the most common difficulties experienced by hearing aid users is listening amidst background noise. This problem may be solved using special circuitry. If this is not feasible, then the hearing aid should be equipped with features to allow it to be coupled to ALDs. Telecoil circuitry also may be needed specifically for telephone communication.

Use of hearing aid(s) with the telephone. A client's ability to recognize speech through a telephone should be a major concern of the clinician during the hearing aid selection process. For many people, the telecoil is the single most important hearing aid option, allowing access to not only the telephone but also to interpersonal and large area ALDs. Some considerations for each type of hearing aid include:

I. BTE hearing aids offer stronger telecoil circuits and more sophisticated switching systems (T, M/T, DAI, DAI/M) than do other hearing aids. Therefore, they are easier to use with ALDs and the telephone, and provide many more listening options than do ITE hearing aids. They also allow DAI coupling to the telephone, which may be necessary with clients who have moderate-to-severe hearing impairment and who cannot use inductive coupling on the telephone due to electromagnetic interference from fluorescent lighting, video terminals, etc.

II. ITE hearing aids may be more cosmetically acceptable and may be the only hearing aid of choice in certain cases due to pinna malformation, activity level (sports), etc.

If an ITE hearing aid is chosen, the clinician must decide whether to install a telecoil circuit. Depending upon the degree of the hearing impairment, the ITE may be coupled to the telephone in one of two ways, inductively or acoustically.

A. Inductive coupling

Inductive coupling is recommended for clients with moderate-to-severe hearing impairment. This is because feedback occurs with acoustic coupling and because the installation of a telecoil circuit allows for ALD interface in large areas such as theaters. When installing a telecoil, one must consider proper strength and orientation.

Telecoil performance can be improved by several methods: by adding a preamplifier circuit, by adding additional coils of wire to the telecoil, by wiring two telecoils together, by increasing the size of the telecoil's ferriferous core, and by orienting the telecoil perpendicular to the magnetic field it is trying to receive (Brunved 1989; Preves 1989; Nybakki 1989).

If the hearing aid is to be used with an ALD, the telecoil should be mounted vertically to allow for best reception from a room or neckloop or silhouette inductors.[10] If the hearing aid's telecoil is to be used to pick up electromagnetic leakage from the telephone directly, then the telecoil should be mounted horizontally. If the client desires to use the telecoil next to the

---

[10]Interpersonal ALDs also can be interfaced to the telephone calling for vertical, not horizontal orientation of the hearing aid's telecoil.

telephone receiver, but will also be using ALDs in interpersonal communication situation, then the telecoil can be mounted vertically and the client taught to compensate on the telephone by angling the telephone receiver for the best reception.

One must also consider whether switch modifications are necessary (e.g., does the client need a combination M/T switch?). The client also must be instructed on proper use of the telecoil.

B. Acoustic coupling

Acoustic coupling may be necessary due to ear size or client preference for an in-the-canal (ITC) hearing aid. To eliminate feedback when the hearing aid microphone is held next to the telephone handset, a foam telepad, plastic acoustic coupler, or handset amplifier (amplifier turned up, hearing aid microphone turned down) can be tried. It also may be possible for the client simply to remove the hearing aid and use a telephone amplifier.

If acoustic coupling (with or without a hearing aid) does not result in satisfactory telephone performance, then a hearing aid with an appropriate telecoil must be considered.

C. Direct audio input (DAI)

It is also possible to install a DAI circuit on some brands of ITE hearing aids, allowing them to be coupled to ALDs, which can then be interfaced to the telephone. This might be warranted in the case of a cosmetics-conscious ITE user who cannot couple his or her hearing aid to the telephone—either inductively (due to magnetic interference) or acoustically (due to feedback, etc.) and who cannot use the naked ear with the telephone.

Figure 4 illustrates the various ways the ear can be coupled to the telephone. Note that the use of a hearing aid telecoil increases one's telephone listening options.

Use of hearing aids with ALDs. If it appears that a client's interpersonal communication difficulties will not or are not being solved through the use of a personal hearing aid alone, then one must consider interfacing the hearing aid with an ALD. In fact, some clients' needs may be best met through the use of an ALD only, as in the case of an elderly, hospital-bound person. Figure 5 illustrates the communication options provided by using an ALD with

and without a hearing aid. Some issues to consider are as follows:

I. BTE hearing aids provide the most flexibility with ALDS. Switching systems offer various modes for control of hearing aid environmental microphone (M, T, M/T, DAI, DAI/M). Due to larger chassis, stronger telecoils are available for use with large area audio loops and neck loops.

II. If an ITE hearing aid is chosen, it should be equipped with a proper telecoil. If not, the client should also be counseled concerning his or her future ability to hear and understand speech in interpersonal/media listening situations. The following questions must be considered:

A. If the client continues to have difficulty listening in noise and from a distance, how will he or she use the hearing aid with an ALD?

B. Will it be possible for the person to remove the hearing aid and use a hardwired ALD or wireless ALD receiver with earphones, earbuds, or custom earmold receivers?[11]

C. Or, should the client turn down the hearing aid and place the ALD earphones on top of the hearing aid microphone? (If the hearing aid microphone is turned down, an earphone headset can be placed on top—not the preferred approach, but it sometimes works as a temporary solution.)

III. Does the client need a way of controlling the hearing aid's external microphone? BTE hearing aids allow for more flexible manipulation of the hearing aid's external microphone. A combination M/T or M/DAI mode might be desired for people who want to maintain contact with the outside world while using ALDs. T- and DAI-only modes are desired for especially noisy situations or for people whose speech recognition ability deteriorates significantly in presence of any background competition.

ITE hearing aids can be ordered with M–T toggle switches or combination M/T switches. As mentioned previously, telecoil performance in ITE hearing aids can be im-

[11]Note: All hardwired ALDs and wireless FM and infrared receivers can be ordered with earphones, earbuds, or custom fitted external receivers. Audio loop receivers come in three configurations: connected to earphones or incorporated into a BTE or an ITE hearing aid chassis.

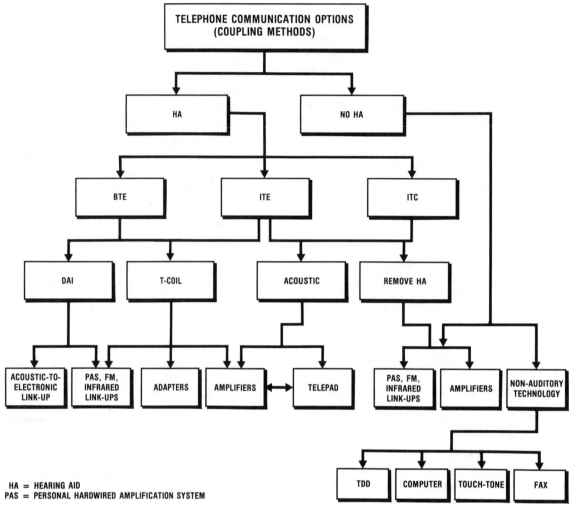

Figure 4. Telephone communication options: Coupling methods.

proved. Adjustments must be done on a case-by-case basis by consulting with each manufacturer's engineering department.

Finally, as mentioned in the section on using hearing aids with the telephone, DAI also is available from some manufacturers.

Selection of Appropriate Assistive Devices   Often, the hearing aid is fitted and the client is given an opportunity to use it in the real world prior to a final decision being made concerning the need for assistive devices. During the hearing aid trial, the needs assessment process can be repeated. If the client continues to have difficulty in certain listening situations, then assistive devices may be indicated. In addition to the life-style considerations already discussed, several other issues need to be weighed when selecting appropriate assistive tech-

nology. Each issue is listed below and is accompanied by several examples:

I. *Portability:*

Some systems are easier to carry around than others. For example, a DAI remote microphone system is lighter in weight and easier to set up than is an FM system (although an FM system is more versatile). A battery-powered portable telephone amplifier is easier to put in one's pocket or purse than is a replacement handset amplifier (which can be used only with a modular telephone).

II. *Versatility:*

Some systems are more versatile than others. While they may cost more, they avoid the need for a different system for each

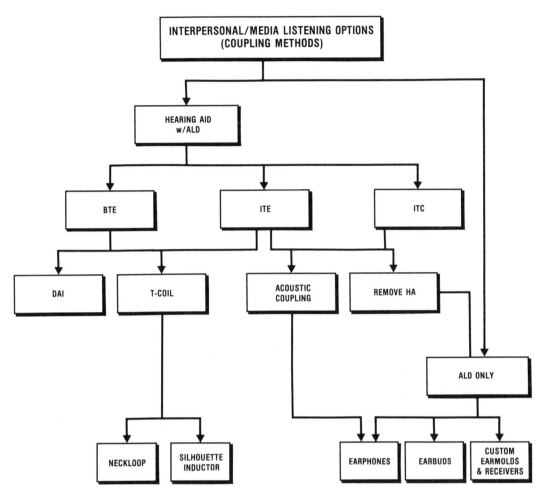

ALD = ASSISTIVE LISTENING DEVICE

Figure 5. Interpersonal/media listening options: Coupling methods.

application—and the training that goes with it. For example, FM is more versatile than other interpersonal listening systems. It works well indoors or outdoors, can be used for TV or telephone listening or for listening to a lecture or meeting. If, however, a client has only TV listening needs, then an inexpensive hardwired system might be the system of choice. All interpersonal listening systems can be equipped with various types of microphones, making them applicable to a variety of listening situations.

III. *Personal mobility:*

Distance and mobility needs will often determine the choice between hardwired and wireless systems (figure 6).

For example, short distance and immobile activities (e.g., TV listening, one-to-one

conversation, small group conversation) can be met with both hardwired or wireless systems. Short distance, mobile, indoor and outdoor activities (e.g., sports, hobbies) can best be met with FM technology although some short distance, mobile activities, such as "working a room" at a party can be met via a hardwired remote microphone system (e.g., DAI directional boom microphone).

Long distance, immobile, indoor, or outdoor (e.g., lectures) needs can best be met with FM technology (although infrared would be appropriate for some indoor activities). If a person appears to need a listening system and has a combination of mobile and immobile needs, then go with a wireless system that can cover all bases. If the client has a limited budget and has mostly indoor, im-

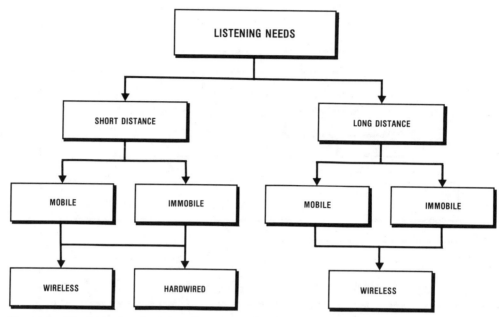

Figure 6.   Hardwired and wireless listening technology: Selection process.

mobile needs, then go with hardwired technology, provided that large area listening needs can be met with wireless systems available in the client's community.

IV. *Cosmetics:*

Clients may require reassurance and possibly assertiveness training to use certain ALDs.

In general, it is best to first demonstrate the equipment before discussing cosmetics. Often the client is so impressed with the assistance provided by the technology that the issue of cosmetics becomes less important.

"More is sometimes less." Sometimes equipment such as an FM system can be less obvious than a small, hardwired DAI remote microphone due to the ability to hide the FM receiver and neckloop under clothing. Audio loop systems are particularly cosmetically acceptable since they allow the listener to use his or her hearing aid telecoil as the ALD receiver. Some people may associate hardwired amplifiers and wireless receivers with portable radios or tape players and may therefore not be adverse to using assistive listening technology.

V. *Compatibility of personal ALD receivers with current and future hearing aid(s)/ALD(s) in the home and community:*

Telecoil-equipped hearing aids or telecoil receivers are compatible with all loop systems. There are usually no compatibility

problems with infrared systems because currently, 95 KHz is used as a de facto standard. (This may change with the introduction of stereo infrared systems.) Compatibility of personal FM receivers is a more difficult issue due to the existence of numerous broadcast bands. It is recommended that the client leave his or her personal FM system at home and use the one provided at the large area facility to avoid interference problems due to his or her system having close to, but not identical, transmission characteristics.

VI. *Previous experience with amplification/ALDs/ hearing health care professionals:*

Previous experiences can have a positive, negative, or neutral effect.

VII. *Possible need for non-auditory telecommunications devices:*

TDDs, computers, FAX machines, and decoders may be needed to augment or even replace auditory devices. Consider standard and optional features in terms of the person's home/work needs. Also consider portability, compatibility with other telecommunications devices, cost, etc.

VIII. *Need for alerting devices:*

Some clients may benefit from alerting devices that can augment or replace hearing aids. These devices employ different methods for monitoring, transmitting, and signalling the occurrence of sounds and other phenomena (figure 2).

Alerting devices might be needed in the home or office while the client is using an ALD to couple to a desired sound source (e.g., dictation machine or TV). They also can be indicated when a personal hearing aid is used in noise, reverberation, from a distance, in another room, or is not being used at all (e.g., while sleeping).

While vibrotactile devices can maintain privacy, some people may, at first, consider them an intrusion into their physical space.

Alerting devices should not be recommended unless they have appropriate UL approval (e.g., #1638 for fire safety devices) and meet safety and housing code standards.

When selecting a device for a client's home, office, or other setting, a floor plan is helpful. Coverage and mobility needs must be addressed (e.g., if sender and receiver must be mobile, then a phone-activated alpha-numeric pager might be best; if both sender and receiver are confined to a particular building, then an AC- or battery-powered inter-office paging system might work, depending upon the transmission range required and the number of metal support beams in the building).

Alerting devices offer various options in terms of the way they monitor, transmit, and signal. The advantages and disadvantages of hardwired and wireless systems should be considered and explained.

IX. *Cost:*

Hardwired listening systems are less expensive but lack the ability to pick up a signal over a larger distance. Realistically speaking, ALDs are simply not very expensive. They serve a specific function that a hearing aid often cannot. People need to know that "you get what you pay for." High quality narrow band FM and directional boom microphones are worth the price.

If financial constraints are an issue, have the client prioritize his communication needs and select the most versatile system. Prioritization is an effective way of involving the client as an active participant in the solution to his or her communication problems.

X. *Rechargeable or throwaway batteries or both?:*

Many clients prefer the convenience of rechargeable batteries. Some companies have better and more "user friendly" recharging systems than others. Depending upon the type of NICAD battery used, some systems maintain a charge longer than others. Some battery compartments are more difficult to open and close than others—important consideration for users with reduced vision and/or manual dexterity.

XI. *Human factors engineering/complexity of the system:*

Is the system too complicated for the client to manage? Will additional training/counseling be needed? If so, this service and the time it commands must be built into the audiologist's fee structure.

Physical design of the device is also important. Are the batteries easy to remove/replace? Is a raised volume control wheel needed? Can the device be re-charged without removing the batteries?

Demonstration/Evaluation of Equipment When demonstrating assistive technology, it is important to provide the client with "ears on" and "hands on" experience so he or she can gain an appreciation and a comfort level for it. The demonstration should be made as relevant as possible to the client's real life communication needs. Some examples:

1. If a client is experiencing difficulty on the telephone, then the hearing aid telecoil, telephone amplifier, or other device should be demonstrated on the telephone using telephone recordings or actual conversations.

2. A client desiring to once again enjoy music can be shown how to connect his or her hearing aid to a portable stereo tape player via a binaural, stereo DAI cord or a neckloop connected to a stereo-to-mono adapter.

3. Demonstration of television as played through an ALD or closed captioned decoder can be made using recordings of interesting programs. (A library of relevant audio and video tapes can be developed. [e.g., music: classical to jazz; television: Sesame Street for kids, music videos for teens, Wheel of Fortune for elders, Wall Street Week for bankers.])

4. If desired, a hardwired or wireless remote microphone system can be demonstrated in a test booth in background noise or in a room set aside for assistive device demonstrations. This room might be equipped with a loudspeaker system through which various types of background noise could be played.

5. A small display of selected alerting devices is helpful in explaining their set up and use.

Objective Measurement Choosing an assistive *listening* device for a client involves an analysis of that client's hearing impairment and listening needs in a variety of relevant everyday situations. Once the type of device needed is determined, then a brand must be selected. A serious impediment to the objective selection of assistive listening devices is the lack of standardized protocols for electroacoustic and probe-tube measurement.

Although electroacoustic measurement procedures have been suggested (Sinclair, Freeman, and Rigg 1981; Lewis et al. 1989; Thibodeau 1990a), until there is a national standard, we will not see unity of measurement across the various brands of products, and this makes it difficult to judge the quality of the various types of systems. Clinical test equipment and protocols are also needed for electroacoustic evaluation of telephone amplifiers, adapters, and specialty telephones.

If probe-tube measurement is considered de rigueur in the hearing aid fitting process, then a comparable protocol must be developed for evaluation of assistive listening devices. ALDs can be used alone or in conjunction with personal hearing aids. Either way, objective measurement of the system must be made if one is to ascertain that an appropriate frequency response, without the risk of excessive harmonic distortion, uncomfortable and/or over-amplification, is being provided.

Research has shown that when hearing aids are coupled to FM systems, the hearing aid characteristics are not necessarily maintained (Hawkins 1985; Thibodeau, McCaffrey, and Abrahamson 1988; Thibodeau 1990b). Currently, there are very limited assessment techniques being developed to look at the real ear performance of ALDs (Hawkins 1987; Lewis, Feigin, and Stelmachowicz 1991; Thibodeau 1990a). Before an accepted probe-tube measurement protocol is developed, several logistical questions need to be answered:

1. How should the test equipment be set up to duplicate a real world situation? If the remote microphone is placed in front of the loudspeaker at the same distance as it would be worn on a person, near-field effects are created. If the remote microphone is placed next to the ear does that really simulate how the FM or ALD is being worn in real life—even if a signal of 80 dB HL (Hawkins 1987; Lewis, Feigin, and Stelmachowicz 1991) is used?

2. Where should the volume control of the ALD be set? Hawkins (1987) matched the output of the FM system to that of the hearing aid at 1000 Hz. Lewis, Feigin, and Stelmachowicz (1991) found that matching it at either 1,000 Hz or 500

Hz did not result in the same frequency for the FM system and the hearing aid. They concluded that "due to current technological limitations[12] it often is not possible to achieve the same frequency response for the FM system and the hearing aid" (p. 18).

Even if it were possible to match the outputs, frequency by frequency, of the ALD and the hearing aid, would that be necessary? Research is needed to determine if, in fact, matched frequency responses are necessary. After all, it might be possible that a slightly different frequency response is acceptable or even more appropriate when using an ALD (and remote microphone) than when using a hearing aid only.

The establishment of a measurement protocol is essential if clients are to be fitted in a scientific and safe manner. This is particularly important for young children or others who cannot provide subjective feedback regarding potentially inappropriate fittings.

Speech Perception Testing Once appropriate coupling method and settings have been chosen, speech recognition or discrimination testing may be carried out to determine the performance of the ALD or to compare performance between the personal hearing aid and the ALD. Lewis et al. (1989) provide a step-by-step method for documenting the advantage of an FM system. This protocol could also be adapted for other assistive listening devices as well. Documentation of the ALD performance may be needed for educational purposes, for third party and/or employer financial support for ALDs or simply to prove to a client that he or she can be assisted by the technology.

Follow Up/Aural Rehabilitation

Just as with personal hearing aid fittings, follow-up counseling and evaluation is essential following the recommendation of assistive technology. Additional orientation and training also may be necessary. For example, some clients may require repeated instruction on how to use their hearing aid telecoil circuit with the telephone and ALDs. Others may need intensive practice in setting up and using ALDs.

---

[12]Technology is available that could eventually make it possible to fit a "smart" FM system which, when coupled to a hearing aid, would re-adjust itself to mimic the response of the hearing aid, thus providing a transparent fitting.

Some clients may require several weeks of practice in the use and care of the hearing aid and ALD as well as speech reading, auditory, and telephone training, training in the use of communication/ environmental strategies, and counseling (coping strategies). Furthermore, assertiveness training may be required, as the use of ALDs often requires the cooperation of others. It can be especially anxiety-producing to have to ask a lecturer to wear an FM transmitter or to request that colleagues at a staff meeting take turns talking into a microphone. For these reasons, it is important to assist the client, via instruction and role playing, in developing the skills and psychological strength necessary to assure successful assistive device usage.

Cultural Issues

Although hearing impairment is often treated from a medical model point of view, many hearing-impaired people also view it from a cultural perspective. Cultural orientation can have an important impact on a person's acceptance or rejection of technology. Clients who have lost their hearing gradually usually consider themselves "hard of hearing" and from an auditory world. Consequently, they may be reticent, and even fearful, to use nonauditory technologies representative of deaf culture (TDDs, decoders, and visual and vibrotactile alerting devices). Similarly, clients who, despite their significant auditory skills, identify themselves with the deaf culture, are often fearful of using auditory technologies. This may be due to negative past experiences as well as current conceptions that the use of auditory technology will cause them to be labeled by their peers as "hearing minded."

It is critical to provide clients with a comfortable, supportive, and nonjudgmental atmosphere in which a client can examine his or her technology options. It is important to communicate to the client that assistive devices are simply tools for communication access and that the use of these tools does not suggest that one must abandon his or her cultural identity.

The support of the client's family, friends, and colleagues is often instrumental in the successful use of assistive devices. It is important to involve them in counseling sessions. Introduction of clients to support groups such as Self Help for Hard of Hearing People (SHHH) is helpful.

It is advisable also to remember that some clients, despite counseling, may choose not to use assistive technology for communication access. Some,

for example, may elect to employ a sign language interpreter on the job. This viewpoint should be respected. Technology never should be forced upon a client.

Summary

A broad assortment of auditory and nonauditory technology is available to assist in removing the communication barriers that can prevent hearing impaired people from leading independent and productive lives. Unfortunately, the lack of standardized electroacoustic and real ear measurement protocols makes it difficult (if not frustrating) to incorporate assistive technology routinely into audiologic practice. Nonetheless, assistive devices can often solve communication problems that personal hearing aids cannot.

By evaluating our clients' telephone, interpersonal, media, and alerting communication needs carefully and by being familiar with today's hearing aids and assistive devices, we can select appropriate technology to meet these needs and can incorporate it into appropriate and comprehensive rehabilitative programs that will improve our clients' communication skills, not only in sound attenuated booths, but in the everyday world—which is why they come to us in the first place.

References

Anderson, J. 1990. Audio Enhancement, Inc. Personal communication.

Beck, L.B., and Nance, G.C. 1989. Hearing aids, assistive listening devices, and telephones: Issues to consider. Assistive Devices, *Seminars In Hearing* 10(1): 78–89.

Binnie, C. and Hession, C. 1990. A four week communication skillbuilding program. *ADA Feedback* Winter 1990: 37–41.

Brunved, P. 1989. Oticon Corporation. Personal communication.

Compton, C.L. 1989. Assistive devices. *Seminars in Hearing* 10(1).

Compton, C.L. 1990. Assistive devices: An overview. *ADA Feedback* Winter 1990: 19–29.

Compton, C.L. 1991. *Assistive Devices: Doorways to Independence*. Washington, DC: Gallaudet Publications and Production. Videotape and book distributed by The Academy of Dispensing Audiologists, 1-800-445-8629.

Harkins, J.E. In Press. Visual devices for deaf and hard of hearing people: State-of-the-art. *GRI Monograph Series*, Series A, No 2. Washington, DC: Gallaudet Research Institute.

Hawkins, D. 1985. Methods of improving speech recognition in the presence of noise and reverberation. *Audiological Acoustics* 9/10.

Hawkins, D.B. 1987. Assessment of FM systems with an ear canal probe tube microphone system. *Ear and Hearing* 8:301–303.

Hawkins, D.B., and Schum, D.J. 1985. Some effects of FM coupling on hearing aid characteristics. *Journal of Speech and Hearing Disorders* 50:132–41.

Lewis, D., Feigin, J., Karasek, A., and Stelmachowicz, P. 1989. Evaluation and assessment of FM systems. Paper read at American Speech-Language Hearing Association Convention, November, 1989, St. Louis.

Lewis, D., Feigin, J., and Stelmachowicz, P. 1991. Evaluation and assessment of FM systems. *Ear and Hearing*.

Mahon, W. 1990. BTE hearing instruments: At one of every five hearing aids sold, still a force in the market. *The Hearing Journal* 43(5):11–16.

Matkin, N., and Olsen, W. 1970. Induction loop amplification systems: Classroom performance. *ASHA* 12:239–44.

Mendosa, R. 1990. Phonic Ear, Inc. Personal communication.

Nybakki, K. 1989. Starkey Labs, Inc. Personal communication.

Preves, D. 1989. Argosy Electronics. Personal communication.

Sievers, D. E. 1990. D.E. Sievers & Associates, LTD. Personal communication.

Sinclair, J.S., Freeman, B.A. and Riggs, D.E. 1981. The use of the hearing aid test box to assess the performance of FM auditory training units. In *Amplification In Education* eds. F.H. Bess, B.A. Freeman, and J.S. Sinclair. Washington, DC: A.G. Bell Association, Inc.

Thibodeau, L. 1990a. Clinical considerations in using classroom amplfication systems. Paper read at the Second Annual Meeting of the American Academy of Audiology, April 26, 1990, New Orleans.

Thibodeau, L., McCaffrey, H., and Abrahamson, J. 1988. Effects of coupling hearing aids to FM systems via neckloops. *Journal of the Academy of Rehabilitative Audiology* 21:49–56.

Thibodeau L. 1990b. Electroacoustic performance of direct-input hearing aids with FM amplification systems. *Language, Speech and Hearing Services in the Schools* 21:49–56.

Weiss, M. 1990. Graduate Center of the City University of New York. Personal communication.

APPENDIX I

Vanderbilt/VA Hearing Aid Conference 1990 Consensus Statement
Research Needs in Amplification for the Hearing Impaired

Following the conference, Dr. Allen E. Boysen, Director of the Central Office Audiology and Speech Pathology Service, Department of Veterans Affairs (VA), charged a small working group from the conference faculty with the development of a consensus statement on research needs in hearing aids. The committee did not prioritize research needs, but rather identified areas in need of further exploration. The members of the committee who prepared the following statement are: Gerald A. Studebaker, Chair, Memphis State University; Robyn M. Cox, Memphis State University; Harry Levitt, City University, University of New York Graduate School; Stephen Fausti, VA Medical Center, Portland, Oregon.

I. Psychoacoustics of Hearing Impairment
    A. Psychoacoustic profile (intensity, temporal, spectral, binaural)
    B. Aging effects
    C. Links to speech perception
    D. Implications for amplification

II. Prescriptive Procedures
    A. New prescriptive procedures
        1. Multimemory aids
        2. Adaptive aids
        3. Maximum power output
        4. Compression aids
        5. Binaural aids
    B. Procedures for specific subgroups (e.g., elderly, precipitous and severe losses)
    C. Validation
        1. Laboratory
        2. Field
    D. Candidacy (aid type-person match)
    E. Efficient techniques to implement (or realize) a prescription

III. Evaluation Procedures
    A. Validation measures
        1. What measures to use? (long and short term measures, e.g., self-assessment, real ear, speech recognition)
        2. Develop improved measures
    B. Models for predicting performance, benefit, user satisfaction, etc.
    C. Factors affecting success (e.g., combined deficits)
    D. Measuring effect on life quality
    E. Negative effects of rehabilitation measures (e.g., excessive amplification, infection)

IV. Rehabilitation
    A. Efficacy
        1. Pre- and postfitting techniques
        2. Counseling (communication strategies)
    B. Improved procedures
        1. Speech reading
        2. Auditory training
        3. Role of others (family members, etc.)
        4. Augmentative devices
    C. Special groups
        1. Elderly
        2. Combined deficits (e.g., visual, cognitive, manual dexterity)
    D. Application of new technology (e.g., interactive videodisk)

V. Electroacoustic Measures
    A. Improved methods for conventional devices
        1. Nonlinear distortion

2. Broad and test signals (noise, speech)
3. Assistive listening devices

B. New Methods for Developing Technology
   1. Multiband compression
   2. Adaptive signal processing
   3. Noise reduction

VI. New Technologies
   A. Device Development and Evaluation
      1. Personal hearing instruments
      2. Assistive listening devices (e.g., telephone)
      3. Implantable devices
   B. Component Development
      1. Transducers
      2. Earmolds
      3. Controls (easier to use and more effective for user and clinician)
      4. Electronic components (e.g., circuits, batteries)
   C. Advanced signal processing
      1. Speech enhancement (e.g., compression, temporal and spectral manipulation)
      2. Noise reduction
      3. Dereverberation
      4. Feedback suppression

Vanderbilt/VA Hearing Aid Conference
1990 Consensus Statement
Recommended Components of a
Hearing Aid Selection Procedure for Adults

Following the conference, Dr. Allen E. Boysen, Director of Central Office, Audiology and Speech Pathology Service, Department of Veterans Affairs (VA), charged a small working group from the conference faculty with the development of a consensus statement on hearing aid selection procedures for adults. The members of the committee who prepared the following statement are: David B. Hawkins, Chair, University of South Carolina, Columbia, South Carolina; Lucille B. Beck, Department of Veterans Affairs, Washington, D.C.; Gene W. Bratt, Veterans Administration Medical Center, Nashville, Tennessee; David A. Fabry, Mayo Clinic, Rochester, Minnesota; H. Gustav Mueller, Letterman Army Medical Center, San Francisco, California; Patricia G. Stelmachowicz, Boys Town National Research Hospital, Omaha, Nebraska.

I. Introduction

Significant changes have occurred in hearing aid circuitry, the measurement of hearing aid performance, and hearing aid selection procedures in the ten years since the first Vanderbilt/VA Hearing Aid Report. Although much of this new technology has been integrated into the clinical setting, there still is no universally accepted protocol for selecting an appropriate hearing aid for a given individual. Certain aspects of the selection procedure, however, can be agreed upon by most individuals familar with both the research literature and the constraints of clinical practice. The purpose of this consensus statement is to outline the recommended components of a hearing aid selection procedure which meets the following

five criteria: (1) it is defensible based upon current research literature, (2) the responsibility for decision making rests with the audiologist, (3) the goals for hearing aid performance are clearly stated, (4) these amplification goals are measured and verified, and (5) counseling and follow-up procedures are viewed as essential.[1]

II. Hearing Aid Candidacy

The first decision that must be addressed is whether a person is a candidate for hearing aids. It is inappropriate to determine hearing aid candidacy by referring only to hearing sensitivity as represented by thresholds for pure-tone signals or scores on word recognition tests. Anyone who describes hearing difficulties in communicative situations should be considered a potential candidate for hearing aids or other assistive devices. Unless clear contraindications exist, binaural hearing aids should be considered the preferred fitting for the prospective hearing aid user.

III. Determination of Initial Electroacoustic Characteristics
A. Selection of SSPL90

Some accepted type of suprathreshold judgment (e.g. loudness discomfort levels, uncomfortable loudness levels, or highest comfortable levels) should be used to determine an appropriate maximum output of the hearing aid. If the person is unable to perform such judgments, a data-based predic-

---

[1]This procedure is not intended to address issues related to selection of hearing aids for young children.

tion method should be used to determine the SSPL90 setting. For instance, Cox (1985) has suggested that SSPL90 could be determined by the equation 100 + ¼ HL. Other recommendations for selecting SSPL90 based upon pure-tone thresholds can be found in Cox (1988), Seewald and Ross (1988), and Skinner (1988).

B. Selection of Gain/Frequency Response

Two-cm³ coupler gain should be determined which will yield desired real-ear performance as specified by a published gain/frequency response selection procedure (e.g. Berger, Hagberg, and Rane 1988; Byrne and Dillon 1986; Cox 1988; Libby 1986; McCandless and Lyregaard 1983; Schwartz, Lyregaard, and Lundh 1988; Seewald, Ross, and Stelmachowicz 1987; Skinner 1988). Many procedures provide corrections from desired real-ear gain to 2-cm³ coupler gain for the average person. The best approach would be to obtain corrections on an individual basis rather than relying upon average values incorporated into the prescription procedure. An example of such a correction procedure can be found in Punch, Chi, and Patterson (1990). The particular corrections will depend upon the style of hearing aid used. (Use of certain programmable or newer hearing aid circuitry may obviate the need for some 2-cm³ coupler real-ear conversions.)

C. Selection of Special Circuit Options

Decisions concerning output limitation options, special circuitry needs, etc. should be made at this point.

IV. Determination of Important Hearing Aid Features

Considerations of a variety of important hearing aid features must be incorporated into the decision making process. A needs assessment should be determined for a number of options or features, such as style of hearing aid, telecoil, direct audio input, raised volume control wheels, and directional microphone.

V. Selection of Hearing Aid(s) that Meet Desired Electroacoustic Characteristics

For behind-the-ear (BTE) hearing aids, the audiologist must select a hearing aid with the appropriate electroacoustic characteristics and options from available specification sheets. For in-the-ear (ITE) hearing aids, the audiologist should order the instrument by either (a) specifying the desired SSPL90 and full-on 2-cm³ coupler gain (assuming a reserve gain of 10-15 dB), or (b) selecting an appropriate specific circuit designation described by the manufacturer.

VI. Verification of Selected or Ordered Electroacoustic Characteristics

Upon receipt of the hearing aid and prior to delivery to the hearing aid user, electroacoustic measurements performed according to ANSI standards (S3.22 1987) should be completed to verify that the hearing aid functions according to the manufacturer's specifications. Additionally, in the case of an ITE hearing aid, the 2-cm³ coupler gain and SSPL90 should be examined to determine if an appropriate circuit was delivered from the manufacturer.

VII. Performance Assessment of Hearing Aid Characteristics on the User

A. Setting and Verification of SSPL90

The SSPL90 should be set to an appropriate level based upon earlier measurements. Verification of the chosen SSPL90 setting for prevention of loudness discomfort and overamplification should be performed for each ear. This determination can be accomplished through a variety of methods, such as Real Ear Saturation Response (RESR), or presentation of controlled signals or intense environmental sounds to saturate the hearing aid.

B. Verification of Desired Real-Ear Gain/Frequency Response

The hearing aid should be adjusted to approximate as closely as possible the previously determined target values for each ear. Verification methods may include functional gain, aided sound-field thresholds, Real Ear Aided Response (REAR), or Real Ear Insertion Response (REIR). A determination that adequate reserve gain is available at the chosen use volume control position should be made as well.

C. Other Assessments

Some type of assessment, formal or informal, should be made of special features of the hearing aid, such as a determination of whether adequate telecoil strength is available for the use of the telephone. The person's subjective reactions to amplified sound should be included in the evaluation. An assessment of the person's ability to understand amplified speech should be made. A number of different approaches, such as speech recognition scores, speech intelligibility ratings, or informal subjective responses, can be used for this purpose.

VIII. Counseling and Follow-up Procedures

Regardless of the selection strategy employed, proper counseling during the fitting and orientation and careful follow-up procedures are necessary if hearing aids are to be used successfully. During the initial stages of adjustment to amplification, electroacoustic characteristics may need to be altered based upon reactions and experiences of the hearing aid user. In addition, questions may arise that were not considered at earlier sessions, and misunderstandings about information provided earlier and expectations may need to be clarified. Finally, other concerns about communicative strategies, remaining difficulties, and use of other devices may need to be explored. Without adequate counseling and follow-up, a well-selected hearing aid can be used improperly, inadequately, or not at all.

References

Berger, K., Hagberg, E., and Rane, R. 1988. *Prescription of Hearing Aids: Rationale, Procedures, and Results*. Kent, OH: Herald Publishing Co.

Byrne, D., and Dillon, H. 1986. The National Acoustic Laboratories' (NAL) new procedure for selecting the gain and frequency response of a hearing aid. *Ear and Hearing* 7:257–65.

Cox, R. 1985. A structured approach to hearing aid selection. *Ear and Hearing* 6:226–39.

Cox, R. 1988. The MSU hearing instrument prescription procedure. *Hearing Instruments* 39:6–10.

Libby, E. 1986. The 1/3–2/3 insertion gain hearing aid selection guide. *Hearing Instruments* 37:27–28.

Martin, M., Grover, B., Worrall, J., and Williams, V. The effectiveness of hearing aids in a school population. *British Journal of Audiology* 10:33–40.

McCandless, G., and Lyregaard, P. 1983. Prescription of gain/output (POGO) for hearing aids. *Hearing Instruments* 34:16–21.

Punch, J., Chi, C., and Patterson, J. 1990. A recommended protocol for prescriptive use of target gain rules. *Hearing Instruments* 41(4):12–19.

Schwartz, D., Lyregaard, P., and Lundh, P. 1988. Hearing aid selection for severe-to-profound hearing loss. *Hearing Journal* 41:13–17.

Seewald, R., and Ross, M. 1988. Amplification for young hearing-impaired children. In *Amplification for the Hearing Impaired*, ed. M. Pollack. NY: Grune & Stratton.

Seewald, R., Ross, M., and Stelmachowicz, P. 1987. Selecting and verifying hearing aid performance characteristics for children. *Journal of the Academy of Rehabilitative Audiology* 20:25–37.

Skinner, M. 1988. *Hearing Aid Evaluation*. Englewood Cliffs, NJ: Prentice Hall.

Author Index

(Page numbers in italics indicate legends or captions on pages.)

Subject Index

(Page numbers in italics indicate material in figures or tables.)

329